MW00715266

Compliments of

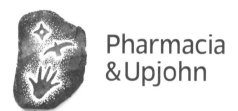
Pharmacia
&Upjohn

Critical Decisions in

THROMBOSIS
AND HEMOSTASIS

Jeffrey Ginsberg, MD, FRCP(C)
McMaster University
Hamilton, Ontario

Clive Kearon, MD, PHD, FRCP(C)
McMaster University
Hamilton, Ontario

Jack Hirsh, MD, PHD, FRCP(C), FRACP
McMaster University
Hamilton, Ontario

1998
B.C. Decker Inc.
Hamilton • London

B.C. Decker Inc.
4 Hughson Street South
P.O. Box 620, L.C.D. 1
Hamilton, Ontario L8N 3K7
Tel: 905-522-7017
Fax: 905-522-7839
e-mail: info@bcdecker.com
website: http://www.bcdecker.com

©1998 Jeffrey Ginsberg, Clive Kearon, Jack Hirsh

All rights reserved. No part of this publication may be reproduced, stored in a retrieval system, or transmitted, in any form or by any means, electronic, mechanical, photocopying, recording, or otherwise, without prior written permission from the publisher.

98 99 00 01 02 / PC / 6 5 4 3 2 1
ISBN 1-55009-043-7
Printed in Canada

Sales and Distribution

United States
Blackwell Science Inc.
Commerce Place
350 Main Street
Malden, MA 02148
U.S.A.
Tel: 1-800-215-1000

Canada
B.C. Decker Inc.
4 Hughson Street South
P.O. Box 620, L.C.D. 1
Hamilton, Ontario L8N 3K7
Tel: 905-522-7017
Fax: 905-522-7839

Japan
Igaku-Shoin Ltd.
Foreign Publications Department
3-24-17 Hongo, Bunkyo-ku
Tokyo 113-8719, Japan
Tel: 3 3817 5680
Fax: 3 3815 7805
e-mail: tmbook@ba2.so-net.or.jp

U.K., Europe, Scandinavia, Middle East
Blackwell Science Ltd.
c/o Marston Book Services Ltd.
P.O. Box 87
Oxford OX2 0DT
England
Tel: 44-1865-79115

Australia
Blackwell Science Pty, Ltd.
54 University Street
Carlton, Victoria 3053
Australia
Tel: 03 9347 0300
Fax: 03 9349 3016

Notice: The authors and publisher have made every effort to ensure that the patient care recommended herein, including choice of drugs and drug dosages, is in accord with the accepted standard and practice at the time of publication. However, since research and regulation constantly change clinical standards, the reader is urged to check the product information sheet included in the package of each drug, which includes recommended doses, warnings, and contraindications. This is particularly important with new or infrequently used drugs.

Contributors

Sonia S. Anand, MSc, MD, FRCPC
Hamilton Health Sciences Corporation
Hamilton General Hospital Division
Hamilton, Ontario, Canada

David R. Anderson, MD
Assistant Professor, Department of Medicine
Dalhousie University
Queen Elizabeth II Health Sciences Centre
Halifax, Nova Scotia, Canada

Shannon M. Bates, MDCM, FRCP(C)
Clinical Scholar, Department of Medicine
McMaster University
Hamilton Civic Hospitals Research Centre
Hamilton, Ontario, Canada

Rebecca J. Beyth, MD
Assistant Professor, Department of Medicine
Case Western Reserve University
University Hospitals of Cleveland
Cleveland, Ohio

Patrick Brill-Edwards, MD
Associate Professor, Department of Medicine
McMaster University
Hamilton, Ontario, Canada

Anthony Chan, MD, FRCP(A), FRACP
Hamilton Civic Hospitals Research Centre
Hamilton, Ontario, Canada

Paul L. Cisek, MD
Clinical Fellow in Vascular Surgery
Temple University Hospital
Philadelphia, Pennsylvania

G. Patrick Clagett, MD
Professor of Medical Sciences
University of Texas
Southwestern Medical Center at Dallas
Dallas, Texas

Alberto Cogo, MD, PhD
Department of Medicine
Casa di Cura "Villa Berica"
Vicenza, Italy

Eric A. Cohen, MD, FRCPC
Assistant Professor, Department of Medicine
Sunnybrook Health Science Centre
Toronto, Ontario, Canada

Anthony J. Comerota, MD, FACS
Department of Surgery
Temple University
Philadelphia, Pennsylvania

Marc A. Crowther, MD, FRCP(C)
Clinical Scholar, Department of Medicine
McMaster University
Hamilton Civic Hospitals Research Center
Hamilton, Ontario, Canada

Robert J. Duke, MD
Associate Clinical Professor, Department
    of Medicine
McMaster University
Hamilton, Ontario, Canada

Michael D. Ezekowitz, MD, PhD
Professor, Department of Medicine
Section of Cardiovascular Medicine
Yale University School of Medicine
New Haven, Connecticut

Stephen E. Fremes, MD
Associate Professor of Surgery
University of Toronto
Sunnybrook Health Science Centre
Toronto, Ontario, Canada

Jeffrey S. Ginsberg, MD, FRCP(C)
Associate Professor, Department of Medicine
McMaster University
Hamilton, Ontario, Canada

Eric Grubman, MD
Cardiovascular Division
University of Pennsylvania
Hospital of the University of Pennsylvania
Philadelphia, Pennsylvania

Ryan T. Hagino, MD
Assistant Professor of Surgery
University of Texas
Health Science Center at San Antonio
San Antonio, Texas

Jack Hirsh, MD, PhD, FRCP(C), FRACP
Director, Hamilton Civic Hospitals Research
    Centre
Professor Emeritus, Faculty of Health Sciences,
    McMaster University
Hamilton, Ontario, Canada

Douglas A. Holder, MD, FRCP(C)
Associate Professor, Department of Medicine
McMaster University
Hamilton Health Sciences Corporation
Hamilton General Hospital Division
Hamilton, Ontario, Canada

Said A. Ibrahim, MD
Assistant Professor, Department of Medicine
Case Western Reserve University
Cleveland, Ohio

Clive Kearon, MD, PhD, FRCP(C)
Assistant Professor, Department of Medicine
McMaster University
Henderson General Hospital Campus
Hamilton, Ontario, Canada

John G. Kelton, MD, FRCP(C)
Professor and Chair, Department of Medicine
McMaster University
Hamilton, Ontario, Canada

C. Seth Landefeld, MD
Professor, Department of Medicine
Case Western Reserve University
University Hospitals of Cleveland
Cleveland, Ohio

Agnes Y.Y. Lee, MD, FRCP(C)
Clinical Scholar, Department of Medicine
McMaster University
Hamilton Civic Hospitals Research Centre
Hamilton, Ontario, Canada

Negin Liaghati-Nasseri, BSc
Master of Science Student, University of Toronto
Sunnybrook Health Science Centre
Toronto, Ontario, Canada

Evan Loh, MD
Medical Director, Heart Failure and Cardiac
    Transplantation Program
University of Pennsylvania School of Medicine
Hospital of the University of Pennsylvania
Philadelphia, Pennsylvania

Michael D. Malone, MD
Department of Vascular Surgery
Cooper Health Systems
Camden, New Jersey

Paul Monagle, MBBS, FRACP, FRCPA
Hamilton Civic Hospitals Research Centre
Hamilton, Ontario, Canada

Marc A. Rodger, MD, FRCP(C)
Hematology Fellow, University of Ottawa
Ottawa Civic Hospital
Ottawa, Ontario, Canada

Stephen J. Skehan, MB, FFRRCSI
Department of Gastroenterology
Hamilton Health Sciences Corporation
McMaster University Medical Centre
Hamilton, Ontario, Canada

Pierre Théroux, MD, FACC
Professor, Department of Medicine
University of Montreal
Montréal, Québec, Canada

Gervais Tougas, MD, FRCPC
Associate Professor, Department of Medicine
McMaster University
Hamilton, Ontario, Canada

Alexander G.G. Turpie, MB, FRCP(UK), FACP,
    FACC, FRCP(C)
Professor of Medicine, McMaster University
Hamilton Health Sciences Corporation
Hamilton General Hospital Division
Hamilton, Ontario, Canada

Irwin Walker, MBBS, FRCP(C), FRACP
Professor, Department of Medicine
Head, Hematology Service
McMaster University Medical Centre
Hamilton, Ontario, Canada

Theodore E. Warkentin, MD, FRCP(C)
Associate Professor, Department of Medicine
McMaster University
Hamilton Health Sciences Corporation
Hamilton General Hospital Campus
Hamilton, Ontario, Canada

Margaret Warner, MD, FRCP(C)
Assistant Professor, Department of Medicine
McGill University, Royal Victorial Hospital
Montreal, Quebec, Canada

Jeffrey I. Weitz, MD, FRCP(C), FACP
Professor, Department of Medicine
McMaster University
Hamilton Civic Hospitals Research Centre
Hamilton, Ontario, Canada

Philip S. Wells, MD, FRCP(C), MSc (Clin Epi)
Assistant Professor, Department of Medicine
University of Ottawa, Ottawa Civic Hospital
Ottawa, Ontario, Canada

Salim Yusuf, MBBS, DPhil, FRCP(UK),
    FRCP(C), FACC
Professor, Department of Medicine
McMaster University
Hamilton Health Sciences Corporation
Hamilton General Hospital Division
Hamilton, Ontario, Canada

Preface

Over the last two decades, there has been an exponential growth in understanding the diagnosis, treatment, and prevention of thrombotic and hemostatic disorders. Virtually all healthcare workers interact with patients who have had such disorders. Consequently, we believe that a text which presents a clear and logical approach to the management of these disorders will be useful to a wide variety of physicians and other healthcare workers.

In *Critical Decisions in Thrombosis and Hemostasis*, the algorithm or decision tree is the focus of each chapter, and the text is intended to be "telegraphic" in nature. In general, the algorithms begin with a common clinical presentation and depict the process of diagnosis or treatment or both, taking into consideration possible alternatives and complications that could modify the management. In general, references are restricted to a minimum and are intended to point the interested reader in the right direction, rather than be comprehensive. Management choices often have to be made in the absence of definitive evidence from the medical literature to guide these decisions. Where evidence has not been available, the authors have been encouraged to describe their personal approach to management.

This book should be of interest to internists, hematologists, cardiologists, cardiac and vascular surgeons, intensivists, as well as medical students, residents, and interns.

We wish to acknowledge all of the authors who took valuable time out of their busy schedules to contribute to this book.

Jeffrey S Ginsberg, MD, FRCP(C)
Clive Kearon, MD, FRCP(C)
Jack Hirsh, MD, FRCP(C)

Dedication

Dedicated to the memory of Marion McEwen, Abraham Ginsberg, and Basil Kearon.

Contents

Section 2   Arterial Thrombosis

Section 3   Hemostasis

Section I

VENOUS THROMBOSIS

Chapter 1

RISK STRATIFICATION FOR VENOUS THROMBOEMBOLISM

Clive Kearon

The risk of developing venous thromboembolism (VTE) depends on the presence of intrinsic (patient) and extrinsic (environmental) risk factors. Surgery and acute illness are the most important extrinsic risk factors; the magnitude of risk differs between procedures and medical conditions. There are many risk factors, and the greater their prevalence, the higher the risk of VTE.[1] Risk factor evaluation allows patients to be stratified according to high, moderate, or low risk of developing VTE (Table 1.1).[2–6] The purpose of risk stratification is to identify which patients should receive VTE prophylaxis and how intensive prophylaxis should be. (See Chapter 16.)

A Nonhospitalized Patients

Risk stratification is used primarily in hospitalized patients with a high prevalence of risk factors[1] and in whom prophylaxis is cost effective;[7,8] however, some outpatients have a sufficiently high risk of VTE that primary prophylaxis may be worthwhile. Patients with metastatic breast cancer have a risk of about 3.5% of developing symptomatic VTE during a 6-month course of combination chemotherapy.[9] Outpatient prophylaxis may also be justified in patients with lower limb injuries that require plaster-cast immobilization. Patients with previous episodes of VTE, or hereditary hypercoagulable states, who do not normally take warfarin may benefit from prophylaxis as outpatients during situations which exacerbate their risk (e.g., prolonged travel, leg injuries, bed bound). Long-term anticoagulation after an acute episode of VTE is considered in Chapter 16.

B Hospitalized Surgical Patients

Surgery itself is an important risk factor for VTE because of venous stasis, venous trauma, and an induced hypercoagulable state and its association with other risk factors (e.g., advanced age, malignancy[1]). The individual risk of VTE can be determined by considering intrinsic and extrinsic risk factors.

Table 1.1   Rates of VTE by Risk Category (%)

| | Venographic DVT* | | Pulmonary Embolism | |
	Calf	Proximal	Clinical	Fatal
Low risk	2	0.4	0.2	<.01
Moderate risk	20	5	2	0.5
High risk	50	15	5	2

*detected by screening venography 7 to 14 days after surgery

C High-Risk Patients

Independent of the type of surgery or acute medical condition, some patients have a high intrinsic risk for VTE (Table 1.2). In combination with a minor acute risk factor, these patients are prone to developing VTE. Conditions such as activated protein C resistance, hyperhomocystinemia, and the presence of an antiphospholipid antibody are also associated with VTE; however, their importance as risk factors for postoperative VTE is unknown.

D Extent of Surgery

Venous stasis (intraoperatively, postoperatively) and venous trauma (i.e., during orthopedic and pelvic surgery) are the most important pathophysiological factors that predispose surgical patients to VTE.

E Anesthesia of More Than 30 Minutes in High-Risk Patients

The intraoperative and postoperative immobility associated with surgery requiring more than 30 minutes of anesthesia (general or regional) places patients at high risk of VTE.

F Anesthesia of Less Than 30 Minutes in High-Risk Patients

The intraoperative and postoperative immobility associated with surgery requiring up to 30 minutes of anesthesia places patients at moderate risk of developing VTE. This risk also occurs with surgery not requiring overnight hospitalization.

G Very High-Risk Surgery

Some surgical procedures are associated with a high risk of developing VTE regardless of patient factors. Hip and knee replacement and surgery for a hip fracture are associated with a very high risk of developing VTE owing to associated venous trauma (e.g., intraoperative venous torsion, tourniquet application) and immobilization. Radical pelvic surgery for malignancy is associated with a very high risk of developing VTE due to a combination of venous trauma and a malignancy-induced hypercoagulable state, in addition to immobility. Major trauma or spinal cord injury is also associated with a very high risk of VTE.[10]

H *Anesthesia for More Than 30 Minutes in Non-High-Risk Patients*
Without additional major risk factors, general surgery that lasts longer than 30 minutes is associated with a moderate risk of VTE.

I *Anesthesia for Less Than 30 Minutes in Non-High-Risk Patients*
After age 40, the risk of VTE increases markedly with age.[11] Patients who are less than 40 years old and do not have additional risk factors (e.g., immobilization) have a low risk of VTE after minor surgery involving less than 30 minutes of anesthesia.

J *Non-Surgical Patients*
Medical patients generally have a lower risk of VTE than surgical patients but the period of risk is less defined and often prolonged.

K *Immobilized High-Risk, Nonsurgical Patients*
"Immobilized" refers to patients who are bed bound or confined to a chair with minimal capacity for weight bearing. These patients have a high risk of developing VTE; however, patients with the highest intrinsic risk of VTE may receive long-term anticoagulants, which can usually be continued, assuming no surgery is scheduled.

L *High-Risk, Ambulatory Nonsurgical Patients*
Hospitalized patients who are ambulatory still have an increased risk of VTE owing to reduced mobility and activation of coagulation due to their acute condition.

Table 1.2   High Intrinsic Risk for VTE

Biochemical Hypercoagulable State
Protein C deficiency
Protein S deficiency
Antithrombin deficiency
Previous Symptomatic VTE

Risk Stratification for Venous Thromboembolism

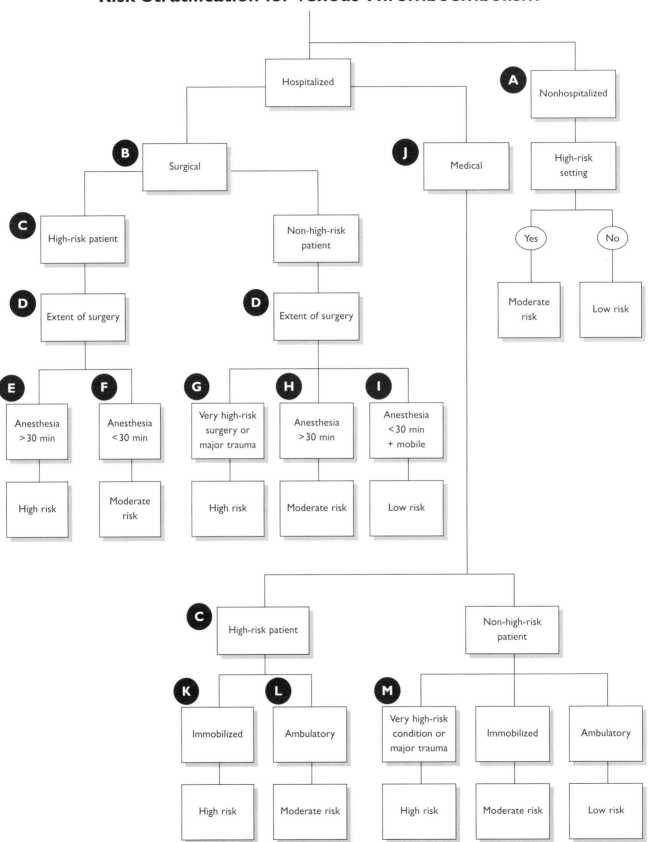

◼ *Very High-Risk, Nonsurgical Conditions*

Some medical conditions are associated with a high risk of VTE regardless of other patient factors. These conditions include stroke or brain tumors (primary or secondary) with hemiparalysis. Major trauma patients also have a high risk of VTE, even if they do not require surgery,[10] as do patients who develop heparin-induced thrombocytopenia[12] (see Chapter 18).

Bibliography

1. Anderson FA, Wheeler HB, Goldberg RJ, Hosmer DW, Forcier A. The prevalence of risk factors for venous thromboembolism among hospital patients. Arch Intern Med 1992;152:1660–4.

2. THRIFT Consensus Group . Risk of and prophylaxis for venous thromboembolism in hospital patients. Br Med J 1992;305:567–74.

3. Gallus AS, Salzman EW, Hirsh J. Prevention of venous thromboembolism. In: Colman RW, Hirsh J, Marder VJ, Salzman EW, eds. Hemostasis and Thrombosis: Basic Principles and Clinical Practice. 3rd edn. Philadelphia: J.B. Lippincott Co., 1993.

4. Salzman EW, Hirsh J. Clinical aspects of thrombotic disorders: the epidemiology, pathogenesis, and natural history of venous thrombosis. In: Colman RW, Hirsh J, Marder VJ, Salzman EW, eds. Hemostasis and Thrombosis; Basic Principles and Clinical Practice. 3rd edn. Philadelphia: J.B. Lippincott Co., 1994:1275–96.

5. European Consensus Statement. Prevention of venous thromboembolism. Int Angiol 1992; 11:151–9.

6. Clagett GP, Anderson FA, Heit J, Levine MN, Wheeler HB. Prevention of venous thromboembolism. Chest 1995;108(Suppl.):312S–34S.

7. Salzman EW, Davies GC. Prophylaxis of venous thromboembollism: analysis of cost effectiveness. Ann Surg 1980;191:207–18.

8. Hull R, Hirsh J, Sackett DL, Stoddart GL. Cost-effectiveness of primary and secondary prevention of fatal pulmonary embolism in high-risk surgical patients. Can Med Assoc J 1982;127:990–5.

9. Levine M, Hirsh J, Gent M, et al. Double-blind randomised trial of very-low-dose warfarin for prevention of thromboembolism in stage IV breast cancer. Lancet 1994;343:886–9.

10. Geerts WH, Code KI, Jay RM, Chen E, Szalai JP. A prospective study of venous thromboembolism after major trauma. N Engl J Med 1994;331:1601–6.

11. Anderson FA, Wheeler HB, Goldberg RJ, et al. A population-based perspective of the hospital incidence and case-fatality rates of deep vein thrombosis and pulmonary embolism. Arch Intern Med 1991;151:933–8.

12. Warkentin TE, Levine MN, Hirsh J, et al. Heparin-induced thrombocytopenia in patients treated with low-molecular-weight heparin or unfractionated heparin. N Engl J Med 1995;332:1330–5.

Additional Reading

Cogo A, Bernardi E, Prandoni P, et al. Acquired risk factors for deep-vein thrombosis in symptomatic outpatients. Arch Intern Med 1994;154:164–7.

Chapter 2

PREVENTION OF VENOUS THROMBOEMBOLISM IN SURGICAL PATIENTS

Clive Kearon

Surgical patients are at risk of developing venous thromboembolism (VTE) that can cause fatal pulmonary embolism (PE). Thrombosis usually starts in the calf, and extends to the proximal veins before it can cause PE; however, screening patients for leg symptoms and signs is unreliable for detecting VTE. Most patients with PE have no symptoms or signs of deep vein thrombosis (DVT) although venography reveals DVT in 70% of PE patients.[1] Consequently, primary prophylaxis is the best way of preventing fatal postoperative PE.

A *Risk Stratification for VTE*

The first step in deciding if and what method of prophylaxis should be used is an assessment to determine if a patient has a high, moderate, or low risk of developing VTE (see Chapter 1).

B *Moderate or High Risk of VTE*

Patients with a moderate or high risk of VTE should receive prophylaxis.[2–4] Unless contraindicated, this will involve the use of an antithrombotic agent alone or in combination with a mechanical method of prophylaxis.

C *Low Risk of VTE*

Prophylaxis is not required for patients with a low risk of VTE. Low-risk patients are generally less than 40 years of age, have had minor surgery performed (general anesthesia less than 30 minutes), and do not have additional risk factors for VTE. They should be mobilized as quickly as possible.

D *Moderate or High Risk of VTE When Antithrombotic Agents Are Not Contraindicated*

Antithrombotic agents, usually heparin or warfarin, are the mainstay of VTE prophylaxis. More aggressive antithrombotic regimens are required for high-risk patients.

E *High Risk of VTE When Antithrombotic Agents Are Not Contraindicated*

Low-dose, subcutaneous, unfractionated heparin (UFH) (5000 U bid or tid) is inadequate prophylaxis for high-risk patients.[2] The antithrombotic regimens shown in Table 2.1 are suitable for high-risk patients. Studies that have used screening venography (asymptomatic DVT) as a surrogate outcome for symptomatic VTE suggest that low-molecular-weight heparin (LMWH) regimens are the most effective; however, it is not known if LMWHs are associated with a lower incidence of symptomatic VTE. Compared to oral anticoagulants, LMWH does not require laboratory monitoring. The combination of an antithrombotic agent and a mechanical method may be more effective than either type of prophylaxis alone.[5–7]

F *High-Risk Patients with High Risk of VTE after Discharge*

Prophylaxis during hospitalization is adequate for most high-risk surgical patients; however, some patients remain at high risk following discharge and may benefit from extended prophylaxis. Early discharge following hip or knee replacement (i.e., within 7 days of surgery) reduces the duration of therapy and may also reduce the efficacy of

Table 2.1   Antithrombotic Regimens

High-Risk Patients
Low-molecular-weight heparin
Postoperative start (North America)
Preoperative start (Europe)
Adjusted dose of unfractionated heparin
Preoperative start with adjusted tid dose to raise activated partial thromboplastin time to upper limit of normal range (average daily dose: 10,000 U to 19,000 U)
Warfarin
Start 5 mg the day before or the same day as surgery. Adjust dose to achieve International Normalization Ratio of 2.0 to 3.0.
Moderate-Risk Patients
Unfractionated heparin
5000 U SQ 2 hours preoperatively, and bid or tid postoperatively.
Low molecular weight heparin
Preoperative start, and 2500 to 3500 U daily postoperatively

inpatient prophylaxis. If feasible (i.e., geographic accessibility, compliance), we continue prophylaxis following discharge in patients who have had major orthopedic surgery if they are non-weight bearing or if they have additional risk factors for VTE (e.g., pathological fracture with metastatic cancer). If continuing prophylaxis is anticipated, we generally use warfarin for both inpatient and outpatient care.

G *Moderate-Risk Patients for Whom Antithrombotic Agents Are Not Contraindicated*

These patients have not had orthopedic surgery with anesthesia for longer than 30 minutes. Low-dose subcutaneous UFH (5000 U bid or tid) with the first dose given 2 hours preoperatively is the most widely used method of prophylaxis; LMWH (2500 to 3500 U once daily) is also suitable. Recommended doses differ for different LMWHs. Graduated compression stockings may be combined with an antithrombotic agent to increase efficacy.[5,6] Intermittent pneumatic compression can also be used but the associated inconvenience is not justified in moderate-risk patients.

H *Antithrombotic Agents Contraindicated*

All antithrombotic agents are associated with a small increase in the risk of postoperative bleeding which is acceptable following most types of surgery; however, if patients are actively bleeding postoperatively or have a high risk of intracranial or spinal cord bleeding, antithrombotic medication is contraindicated. The most important groups in the latter categories are neurosurgical patients, and patients with major trauma who have had intracerebral bleeding at presentation (patients with cerebral contusion, localized petechial hemorrhages, or diffuse axonal damage can be treated).[8] If feasible, mechanical methods of prophylaxis (e.g., graduated compression stockings and/or intermittent pneumatic compression devices) should be used in such patients.

I *High Risk of VTE When Antithrombotic Agents Are Contraindicated*

Major trauma and intracerebral bleeding or neurosurgery account for most of these patients. Intermittent pneumatic compression, usually with graduated compression stockings, should be used, if feasible; however, patients with major trauma often have associated leg injuries that prevent the use of mechanical methods of prophylaxis.

J *High Risk of VTE, Antithrombotic Agents Contraindicated, Mechanical Methods of Prophylaxis Cannot be Used*

If no effective means of prophylaxis is feasible, secondary prevention can be performed whereby asymptomatic DVT is detected and treated before VTE becomes clinically apparent. Fibrinogen leg scanning was once used for this purpose but is no longer widely available. Duplex venous ultrasonography is currently the best available method although there is little published evidence validating its use for this purpose. Venous ultrasound assesses the popliteal and common femoral veins and can be performed twice weekly for the first 2 weeks and weekly thereafter. However, because the positive predictive value of venous ultrasound is low in asymptomatic patients (about 70% overall), an abnormal ultrasound should be confirmed by venography, unless DVT is extensive, since anticoagulation is problematic in this population (see Chapter 5). Although antithrombotic agents may be contraindicated shortly after surgery or major trauma, it may become safe to use these agents subsequently. Efficacy of antithrombotic agents is likely to be reduced if there is a marked delay between surgery and their initiation.

K *High Risk of VTE, Antithrombotic Agents Contraindicated, Mechanical Methods of Prophylaxis Feasible*

Graduated compression stockings and/or intermittent pneumatic compression devices can be used, provided that legs are not injured below the knees. In high-risk patients, however, intermittent pneumatic compression in combination with graduated compression stockings may be superior to graduated compression stockings alone. A mechanical device may serve as an interim method of prophylaxis until it is safe to use an antithrombotic agent.

L *Moderate Risk of VTE, Antithrombotic Agents Contraindicated*

Neurosurgical patients constitute the most important group in this category. Graduated compression stockings applied prior to surgery should be used. Thigh-level stockings have generally been used[9] but below-knee stockings may be just as effective. It is uncertain if intermittent pneumatic compression provides additional benefit for these patients.

Prevention of Venous Thromboembolism in Surgical Patients

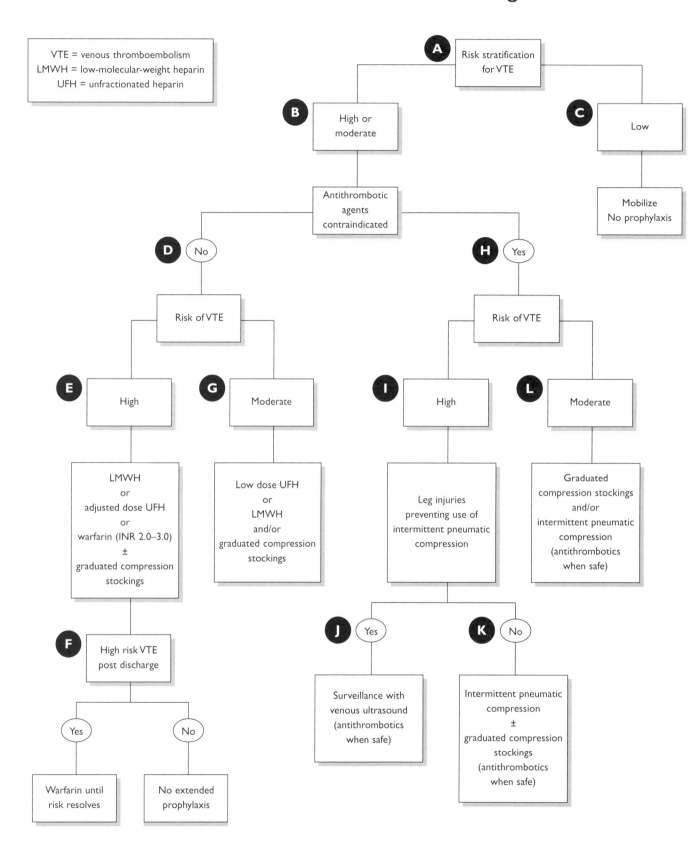

Bibliography

1. Hull RD, Hirsh J, Carter CJ, et al. Pulmonary angiography, ventilation lung scanning, and venography for clinically suspected pulmonary embolism with abnormal perfusion lung scan. Ann Intern Med 1983;98:891–9.

2. Clagett GP, Anderson FA, Heit J, Levine MN, Wheeler HB. Prevention of venous thromboembolism. Chest 1995;108(Suppl.):312S–34S.

3. THRIFT Concensus Group. Risk of and prophylaxis for venous thromboembolism in hospital patients. Br Med J 1992;305:567–74.

4. European Consensus Statement. Prevention of venous thromboembolism. Int Angiol 1992;11:151–9.

5. Torngren S. Low dose heparin and compression stockings in the prevention of postoperative deep venous thrombosis. Br J Surg 1980;67:482–4.

6. Wille-Jorgensen P, Thorup J, Fischer A, Holst-Christensen J, Flamsholt R. Heparin with and without graded compression stockings in the prevention of thromboembolic complications of major abdominal surgery: a randomized trial. Br J Surg 1985;72:579–81.

7. Ramos R, Salem BI, De Pawlikowski MP, Coordes C, Eisenberg S, Leidenfrost R. The efficacy of pneumatic compression stockings in the prevention of pulmonary embolism after cardiac surgery. Chest 1996;109:82–5.

8. Geerts WH, Jay RM, Code KI, et al. A comparison of low-dose heparin with low-molecular-weight heparin as prophylaxis against venous thromboembolism after major trauma. N Engl J Med 1996;335:701–7.

9. Wells PS, Lensing AWA, Hirsh J. Graduated compression stockings in the prevention of postoperative venous thromboembolism: a meta-analysis. Arch Intern Med 1994;154:67–72.

Chapter 3

PREVENTION OF VENOUS THROMBOEMBOLISM IN MEDICAL PATIENTS

Clive Kearon

Compared to experience with surgical patients, few clinical trials have been performed evaluating venous thromboembolism (VTE) prophylaxis in medical patients.[1] As the control arms of randomized trials provide valuable natural history data, less is known about the rates of, and contributing factors to, VTE in medical patients. Generally, the risk of VTE is lower in medical patients as the acute immobilization and venous trauma that often accompanies surgery is less common. Although the risk of VTE is less acute in medical patients, it is often prolonged because of irreversible risk factors. This may reduce the efficacy of prophylactic measures,[2] which are usually undertaken during the highest risk period, namely, while the patient is hospitalized. Recommendations for VTE prophylaxis in medical patients are not as firm as for surgical patients because there is less evidence available. Approaches to VTE prophylaxis in medical patients are often extrapolations from experience with surgical patients.

A *Hospitalized Patients*

Patients who are hospitalized with acute medical conditions are often temporarily or permanently immobilized. They are also elderly and have conditions (i.e., malignancy, paralysis, heart failure) that further predispose them to VTE. The first step in deciding if, and what method of, prophylaxis should be used in such patients is an assessment of risk factors to determine if the patient has a high, moderate, or low risk of developing VTE (see Chapter 1).

B *High or Moderate Risk of VTE*

Hospitalized patients who are immobilized (bed bound, or largely confined to a chair) have a moderate or high risk of developing VTE. If the patient has a high-risk profile (e.g., biochemical hypercoagulable state, previous VTE) or a very high-risk condition (e.g., hemiparalysis), the risk of VTE is highest; however, the distinction between moderate and high risk status is less important in medical patients because it does not determine the approach to VTE prophylaxis to the same degree as it does in surgical patients.

C Low Risk of VTE

Medical patients who remain mobile, particularly if they are younger, have a low risk of VTE and do not require specific VTE prophylaxis. Mobility should be encouraged throughout hospitalization.

D Antithrombotic Agents Contraindicated

The hemorrhagic potential of antithrombotic agents is usually less of a concern in medical patients than it is following surgery; however, if patients have been hospitalized because of bleeding, particularly in the form of a hemorrhagic stroke, antithrombotic agents are contraindicated.

E Antithrombotic Agents Not Contraindicated

Low-dose, unfractionated heparin (5000 U SQ bid) is the mainstay of VTE prophylaxis in medical patients. Low-molecular-weight heparin (2500 to 3500 U per day) is also effective. Based on experience in surgical patients, graduated compression stockings can be combined with a heparin preparation to further reduce the risk of thrombosis in high-risk medical patients. Prophylaxis should be continued as long as patients have an increased risk of VTE. This presents problems in hemiparesis patients and others who will remain immobile indefinitely. It is not known if these patients should remain on long-term prophylaxis.

F Antithrombotic Agents Are Contraindicated

Based on experience with surgical patients, graduated compression stockings and/or intermittent pneumatic compression devices should be used to reduce the risk of VTE.

G Medical Outpatients

Prophylaxis for VTE is rarely undertaken in nonhospitalized medical patients because the risk of VTE is generally not high enough to warrant the cost and inconvenience, and there is little evidence available to support the use of primary VTE prophylaxis in outpatients.

Prevention of Venous Thromboembolism in Medical Patients

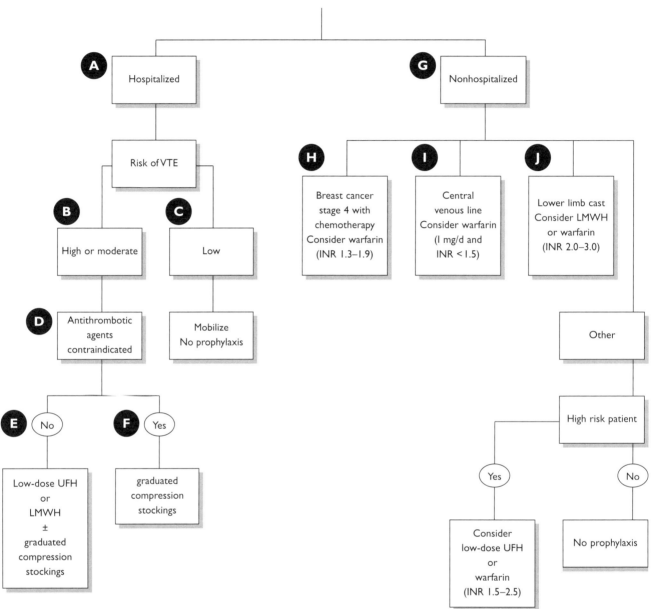

H *Stage IV Metastatic Breast Cancer Patients Receiving Chemotherapy*

These patients have a high risk of developing VTE, which can be markedly reduced with low intensity anticoagulation (i.e., international normalized ratio [INR] 1.3 to 1.9) (rates of symptomatic VTE of 0.4% versus 4.4% during 4 months of treatment).[3] Low-intensity warfarin also reduces costs in this setting[4] but because of concerns about safety, VTE prophylaxis has not been widely used for this indication.

I *Central Venous Catheters*

Indwelling central venous catheters (i.e., subclavian vein) are often complicated by thrombosis, which can be reduced with very low dose warfarin (1 mg per day, generally without prolongation of the INR)(rates of venographically confirmed VTE of 10% versus 38% during 3 months of treatment).[5] Safety, scepticism, inconvenience, and cost are some reasons why VTE prophylaxis has not been widely used for these patients.

J *Lower-Limb Plaster Cast Immobilization without Surgery*

These patients have an increased risk of developing VTE, which can be reduced with daily low-molecular-weight heparin (rates of ultrasound-detected VTE of 6% versus 17% after 2 to 3 weeks of immobilization).[6] Warfarin (INR 2.0 to 3.0) is also likely to be effective for these patients. It is unclear how often symptomatic DVT or PE occurs in this setting; consequently, VTE prophylaxis has not been widely used.

Bibliography

1. Clagett GP, Anderson FA, Heit J, Levine MN, Wheeler HB. Prevention of venous thromboembolism. Chest 1995;108(Suppl.):312S–34S.

2. Gårdlund B. Randomised, controlled trial of low-dose heparin for prevention of fatal pulmonary embolism in patients with infectious diseases. Lancet 1996;347:1357–61.

3. Levine M, Hirsh J, Gent M, et al. Double-blind randomised trial of very-low-dose warfarin for prevention of thromboembolism in stage IV breast cancer. Lancet 1994;343:886–9.

4. Rajan R, Gafni A, Levine M, Hirsh J, Gent M. Very low-dose warfarin prophylaxis to prevent thromboembolism in women with metastatic breast cancer receiving chemotherapy: an economic evaluation. J Clin Oncol 1995;13:42–6.

5. Bern MM, Lokich JJ, Wallach SR, et al. Very low doses of warfarin can prevent thrombosis in central venous catheters. Ann Intern Med 1990;112:423–8.

6. Kock HJ, Schmit-Neuerburg KP, Hanke J, Rudofsky G, Hirche H. Thromboprophylaxis with low-molecular-weight heparin in outpatients with plaster-cast immobilisation of the leg. Lancet 1995;346:459–61.

Chapter 4

CLINICAL ASSESSMENT
OF DEEP VEIN THROMBOSIS

Clive Kearon

The diagnosis of deep vein thrombosis (DVT) needs to be considered in two distinct clinical settings: when patients present with symptoms and/or signs that are suggestive of DVT (symptomatic DVT), and in asymptomatic patients who have a high risk of thrombosis, for example, following orthopedic surgery. This chapter only discusses patients suspected of having a first episode of symptomatic DVT.

A *Symptoms and Signs*

The clinical presentation of DVT varies from absence of leg symptoms and signs to extreme pain and swelling of the entire limb. Clinical features are caused by venous distention, which results in localized pain and/or tenderness; venous obstruction, which results in heaviness, swelling, edema, and/or dilated superficial veins; and tissue inflammation, which results in erythema, swelling, and/or tenderness. Although about one half of patients with proximal DVT have evidence of pulmonary embolism (PE) on lung scanning, clinical features suggestive of PE are present in a minority (~10%). This discussion will be confined to patients with suspected DVT who are not suspected of having PE.

   Symptoms: Leg pain and swelling are the most common presenting symptoms of DVT.[1-3] The average duration of symptoms before patients present for investigation is about 10 days but this varies markedly. The duration of symptoms does not discriminate between patients with or without DVT. Calf pain, either on its own or in association with thigh discomfort, is common. The location of symptoms is poorly predictive of the extent of DVT: patients with symptoms that are confined to the calf often have proximal DVT (i.e., involving the popliteal or the more proximal veins). The majority (~85%) of patients with symptomatic DVT have proximal thrombi that usually also involve the calf whereas the remainder have isolated calf DVT. This distinction is important because proximal DVT may cause PE and should be diagnosed rapidly. On the other hand, isolated calf DVT rarely causes PE unless it subsequently extends into the proximal veins, which occurs in about a quarter of untreated cases.

Signs: Leg swelling, and tenderness along the distribution of the deep veins, are the most common signs of DVT.[1-3] Tenderness is assessed by applying pressure along the course of the deep veins, which run from the midinguinal area, medial to the femur to the popliteal fossa, and into the calf posteriorly. Leg swelling that involves the whole leg, is associated with a 3-centimeter or greater increase in the circumference of the affected leg (measured 10 centimeters below the tibial tuberosity), and is associated with pitting edema increases the probability that a patient has DVT.[1] Dilated, nonvaricose, superficial veins are also suggestive of DVT. The probability of DVT increases with the severity of the physical findings. Patients with swelling and tenderness along the veins in both legs are considered to have a "typical" presentation of DVT whereas patients with only one or neither of these signs are considered to have an "atypical" presentation.

B *Alternative Diagnoses to Account for Presentation*

The probability of DVT is influenced by an alternative diagnosis that may explain the patient's symptoms and signs.[1] Many conditions can cause clinical findings that are often confused with DVT (Table 4.1); however, before a patient is considered to have an alternative diagnosis, this condition should be judged at least as likely DVT to account for the clinical findings. Although these conditions offer an alternative explanation for leg symptoms and signs, many of these conditions are also risk factors for DVT, and their presence may include concomitant DVT.

C *Risk Factors for DVT*

Most DVT occurs in high-risk situations[4,5]; consequently, independent of other clinical features, the probability that a patient has DVT increases as the prevalence of risk factors for thrombosis increases (see Chapter 1).[1] Risk factors for DVT can be severe or moderate (Table 4.2). Mild risk factors, such as obesity, advanced age, varicose veins, long journeys, and the use of oral contraceptives, are not included in this

Table 4.1   Conditions That May Be Confused with DVT

Leg trauma (e.g., hematoma, muscle rupture)
Cellulitis
Ruptured Baker's cyst
Superficial phlebitis
Pelvic venous obstruction
Recent hip or knee surgery
Venous insufficiency (e.g., varicose veins)

Suspected Deep Vein Thrombosis (DVT)

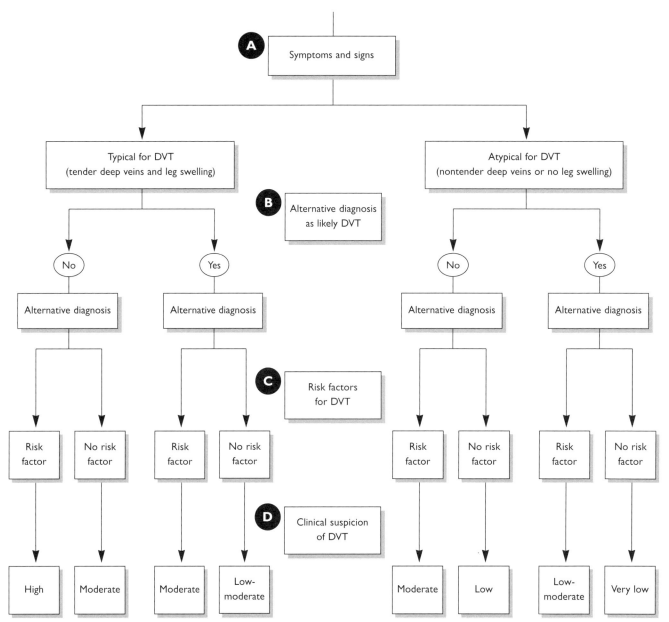

algorithm because they are common and do not help discriminate between patients with and without DVT.

D *Clinical Suspicion of DVT*

Based on typical symptoms or signs, an alternative diagnosis at least as likely DVT to account for presentation, and risk factors, patients can be stratified as having a low, moderate, or high clinical suspicion of DVT. In a prospective study performed

Table 4.2 Risk Factors for DVT

Severe	Moderate
Major orthopedic surgery	General surgery
Metastatic cancer	Hospitalization
Paralysis	Cancer chemotherapy
Major trauma	
Hypercoagulable states	
Heparin-induced thrombocytopenia	

by Wells et al.,[1] which is the basis for the algorithm, the prevalence of DVT in outpatients with different categories of clinical suspicion of DVT was as follows: high clinical suspicion, 85%; moderate clinical suspicion, 33%; and low clinical suspicion, 5%. Of outpatient referrals to thromboembolism clinics, approximately 20% of patients have high, 30% have moderate, and 50% have low clinical suspicion for DVT. It is unknown if clinical assessment of DVT in inpatients is as accurate as it is in outpatients because the prevalence of risk factors for DVT and comorbid illness is higher in inpatients.

The results of a structured clinical assessment that categorizes patients as having a low, moderate, or high probability of having DVT can be used in combination with other investigations to optimize the management of patients with suspected DVT[1] (see Chapter 5). However, it must be emphasized that clinical assessment is complementary to, rather than a substitute for, objective testing for DVT.

Bibliography

1. Wells P, Hirsh J, Anderson DR, et al. Accuracy of clinical assessment of deep-vein thrombosis. Lancet 1995;345:1326–30.
2. McLachlin J, Richards T, Paterson JC. An evaluation of clinical signs in the diagnosis of venous thrombosis. Arch Surg 1962;85:738–44.
3. Sandler DA, Duncan JS, Ward P, et al. Diagnosis of deep vein thrombosis: comparison of clinical evaluation, ultrasound, plethysmography, and venoscan with x-ray venogram. Lancet 1984;2:716–9.
4. Cogo A, Bernardi E, Prandoni P, et al. Acquired risk factors for deep-vein thrombosis in symptomatic outpatients. Arch Intern Med 1994;154:164–7.
5. Anderson FA, Wheeler HB, Goldberg RJ, Hosmer DW, Forcier A. The prevalence of risk factors for venous thromboembolism among hospital patients. Arch Intern Med 1992;152:1660–4.

Additional Reading

Sackett DL. A primer on the precision and accuracy of the clinical examination. JAMA 1992; 267:2638–44.

Chapter 5

Diagnosis of a First Episode of Deep Vein Thrombosis

Clive Kearon

Approximately 20% of patients who are investigated for deep vein thrombosis (DVT) have the diagnosis confirmed at presentation.[1,2] A majority (~85%) of symptomatic DVT are proximal thrombi involving the popliteal or more proximal veins whereas the remainder are confined to the calf (distal DVT).[1–3] Consequently, only about 4% of patients who are investigated for DVT have isolated distal thrombi at presentation, and of these 1 in 4 (~1% of evaluated patients) will develop thrombus extension into the proximal veins if they are not treated.[4,5] Venography is the only test which reliably diagnoses isolated distal DVT but it is not suitable for routine diagnostic testing because of its cost, side effects, and inconvenience. Venous ultrasound is an accurate test for diagnosing large proximal DVT (sensitivity and specificity of over 95%) but cannot reliably diagnose isolated distal DVT.[1,2,6] Consequently, follow-up venous ultrasound is required a week after an initial normal test to detect possible extension of calf DVT into the proximal veins. If isolated distal DVT does not extend within a week, subsequent extension is rare. Therefore, if serial venous ultrasound testing is normal on two occasions 1 week apart, anticoagulants can be safely withheld. The algorithm outlines an approach to the diagnosis of a first episode of symptomatic DVT using the combination of a structured clinical assessment (see Chapter 4) and venous ultrasound.

A Structured Clinical Assessment

A structured clinical evaluation assessing symptoms and signs, an alternative diagnosis to account for the patient's presentation, and risk factors for DVT, can stratify a patient's probability of having DVT into high, moderate, and low categories[2] (see Chapter 4). In our experience, approximately 20% of patients are classified as having a high clinical suspicion of DVT (prevalence of DVT ~ 85%), 30% are classified as having a moderate clinical suspicion of DVT (prevalence of DVT ~ 33%), and 50% of patients are classified as having a low clinical suspicion of DVT (prevalence of DVT ~ 5%). The results of venous ultrasound should be interpreted in combination with this clinical assessment.

B Venous Ultrasound

The most reliable ultrasound criterion for the diagnosis of DVT is lack of a fully compressible venous segment with the application of ultrasound probe pressure during real time, gray-scale (B-scan) ultrasonography.[1] Other ultrasound criteria such as Doppler changes (color or spectral analysis), intraluminal appearance, or changes in venous diameter during a Valsalva maneuver may compromise accuracy. Although venous ultrasound is very accurate for the assessment of the proximal veins, it is not reliable for the diagnosis of isolated distal DVT. Examination of the popliteal vein down to and including the calf vein trifurcation increases the sensitivity of the ultrasound examination; however, the finding of an isolated abnormal calf vein trifurcation has a positive predictive value of only 80%.[5,7] Similarly, the presence of short segments of noncompressibility confined to the common femoral vein, the superficial vein, or the popliteal vein without involvement of the calf trifurcation, also has positive predictive values for DVT of about 80%.[7]

C High Clinical Suspicion of DVT, Normal Venous Ultrasound

The negative predictive value of venous ultrasound (examination of the proximal veins and calf trifurcation) for all DVT in patients with a high clinical suspicion of thrombosis is about 70%.[2] In general, these patients can be managed by performing a follow-up venous ultrasound after a week to exclude the possibility of extension of a missed thrombus (see section H); however, if at presentation patients only have calf symptoms and signs or if they have severe symptoms, venography should be considered to exclude a false-negative venous ultrasound (missed proximal DVT in ~ 5%, or isolated distal DVT in ~ 25%).

D Low Clinical Suspicion of DVT, Normal Ultrasound

The negative predictive value of venous ultrasound for all DVT in patients with a low clinical suspicion of thrombosis is about 98%,[2,7] and of the remaining 2% of patients, only 1 in 4 are expected to have a subsequent clinically important extension of their thrombosis. Therefore, a normal venous ultrasound effectively excludes DVT in patients with a low clinical suspicion of thrombosis, and it is not necessary to perform a follow-up ultrasound a week later.

Suspected First Episode of Deep Vein Thrombosis

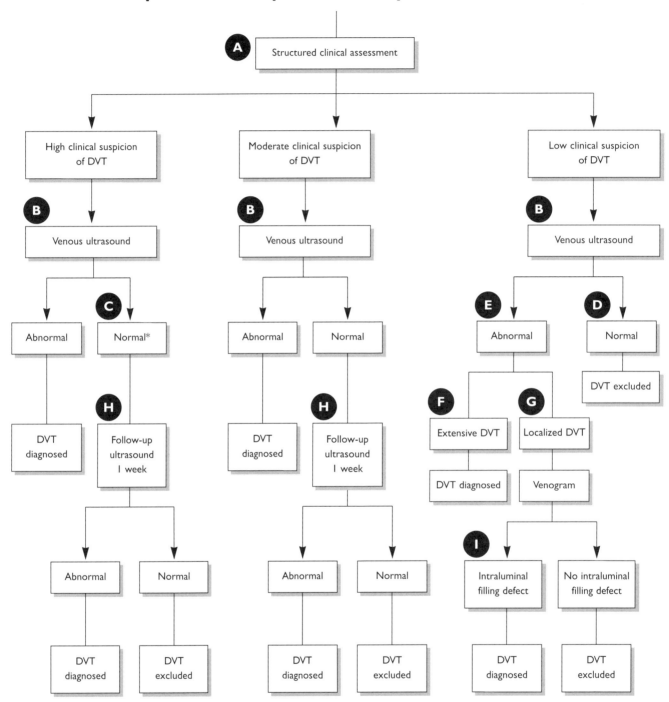

*Venography should be considered to rule out a false-negative venous ultrasound if symptoms are severe.

E *Low Clinical Suspicion of DVT, Abnormal Ultrasound*

The positive predictive value of venous ultrasound for DVT in patients with a low clinical suspicion of venous thrombosis is about 65%.[2] Consequently, venography should be considered to exclude the possibility of a false-positive result.

F If there is evidence of extensive DVT (e.g., unequivocal lack of compressibility of the common femoral vein and the popliteal vein or the popliteal vein and the calf trifurcation), confirmatory venography need not be performed unless there is a suspicion that the DVT may be old or inactive, or the risk of bleeding associated with anticoagulation is high.

G The risk of a false-positive venous ultrasound is high (40% or greater) if patients have a short segment of venous compressibility and a low clinical suspicion of DVT. Venography is recommended in these patients.

H *High or Moderate Clinical Suspicion of DVT, Normal Initial Venous Ultrasound*

An initial normal venous ultrasound effectively excludes proximal DVT but patients may still have distal DVT. If the initial venous ultrasound is normal in patients with a high or moderate clinical suspicion of DVT, follow-up venous ultrasound is performed a week later to detect proximal extension, which is expected in approximately 25% of cases of distal DVT. If the initial venous ultrasound does not include assessment of the calf trifurcation, two follow-up ultrasound examinations over a 7- to 10-day period are recommended.[1]

I *Venography*

An intraluminal filling defect that is constant in appearance on more than one view is diagnostic for acute DVT.

Bibliography

1. Lensing AWA, Prandoni P, Brandjes D, et al. Detection of deep-vein thrombosis by real-time B-mode ultrasonography. N Engl J Med 1989;320:342–5.
2. Wells P, Hirsh J, Anderson DR, et al. Accuracy of clinical assessment of deep-vein thrombosis. Lancet 1995;345:1326–30.
3. Cogo A, Lensing AWA, Prandoni P, Hirsh J. Distribution of thrombosis in patients with symptomatic deep-vein thrombosis: implications for simplifying the diagnostic process with compression ultrasound. Arch Intern Med 1993;153:2777–80.

4. Heijboer H, Buller HR, Lensing AWA, Turpie AGG, Colly LP, ten Cate WJ. A comparison of real-time compression ultrasonography with impedance plethysmography for the diagnosis of deep-vein thrombosis in symptomatic outpatients. N Engl J Med 1993;329:1365–9.

5. Cogo A, Lensing AWA, Koopman MMW, et al. Compression ultrasound for the diagnostic management of clinically suspected deep-vein thrombosis. Thromb Haemost 1995;73:1098 (758a).

6. White RH, McGahan JP, Daschbach MM, Hartling RP. Diagnosis of deep-vein thrombosis using duplex ultrasound. Ann Intern Med 1989;111:297–304.

7. Wells PS, Hirsh J, Anderson DR, et al. Comparison of the accuracy of impedance plethysmography and compression ultrasonography in outpatients with clinically suspected deep vein thrombosis. Thromb Haemost 1995;74:1423–7.

Additional Reading

Lensing AWA, Hirsh J, Buller H. Diagnosis of venous thrombosis. In: Coleman RW, Hirsh J, Marder VJ, Salzman EW, eds. Hemostasis and thrombosis: basic principles and clinical practice. 3rd edn. Philadelphia: J.B. Lippincott Co., 1993.

Heijboer H, Cogo A, Buller HR, Prandoni P, ten Cate JW. Detection of deep vein thrombosis with impedance plethysmography and real-time compression ultrasonography in hospitalized patients. Arch Intern Med 1992;152:1901–3.

Wells PS, Lensing AWA, Davidson BL, Prins MH, Hirsh J. Accuracy of ultrasound for the diagnosis of deep venous thrombosis in asymptomatic patients after orthopedic surgery. Ann Intern Med 1995;122:47–53.

Becker DM, Philbrick JT, Bachhuber TL, Humphries JE. D-dimer testing and acute venous thromboembolism. A shortcut to accurate diagnosis? Arch Intern Med 1996;156:939–46.

Wells PS, Brill-Edwards P, Stevens P, et al. A novel and rapid whole-blood assay for d-dimer in patients with clinically suspected deep vein thrombosis. Circulation 1995;91:2184–7.

Chapter 6

Diagnosis of Recurrent Deep Vein Thrombosis

Clive Kearon

Recurrent deep vein thrombosis (DVT) is more difficult to diagnose than a first episode of DVT for the following reasons. First, previous thrombosis can cause symptoms and signs that are indistinguishable from recurrent DVT (e.g., "postphlebitic syndrome"). Second, DVT commonly causes persistent abnormalities in the deep veins, which can obscure recurrent thrombosis or, alternatively, can be misinterpreted as representing new thrombosis.[1,2] Therefore, it is necessary to have objective evidence of new thrombus formation before diagnosing recurrent DVT. Third, few well-designed studies have been performed evaluating diagnostic strategies for recurrent DVT.[1,3,4] Fourth, a number of tests that have been validated for the diagnosis of recurrent DVT are not widely available (e.g., impedance plethysmography [IPG], fibrinogen leg scanning).[3,4] The algorithm outlines an approach to the diagnosis of recurrent DVT using venous ultrasound and venography, supplemented by IPG, if available. As clinical assessment has not been adequately evaluated in patients with suspected recurrent DVT, it is not included in this approach although it is likely to be helpful.

A *Venous Ultrasonography*

Assessment of full compressibility of the common femoral and the popliteal veins is performed initially (see Chapter 5). The accuracy of other ultrasound criteria for the diagnosis of recurrent DVT has not been adequately assessed, and the use of such criteria is not recommended.

B *Noncompressibility of the Common Femoral Vein and/or the Popliteal Vein*

Patients with noncompressible common femoral or popliteal veins cannot be assumed to have recurrent DVT as persistent abnormalities in the deep veins are common in patients with previous DVT (abnormal in about half the patients 1 year after diagnosis and treatment).[1,2] Comparison of the venous ultrasound with a previous venous ultrasound may reveal if new thrombosis has occurred (sections E, F, and G).

C *Fully Compressible Common Femoral and Popliteal Veins*

This finding excludes proximal DVT;[1] however, the possibility of isolated calf vein thrombosis remains. Consequently, venous ultrasound should be repeated twice over the next 7 to 10 days to detect extension of DVT into the common femoral vein and/or popliteal vein segments. If the clinical suspicion of DVT is high, venography can be performed (section J).

D *Abnormal Venous Ultrasound, No Previous Ultrasound Available for Comparison*

In this situation, impedance plethysmography may distinguish between new and old DVT (section H). If impedance plethysmography is not available, venography should be performed (section J).

E *A New Noncompressible Common Femoral or Popliteal Vein*

This finding is diagnostic for recurrent DVT.[1,2]

F *Abnormal Venous Ultrasound with Previous Ultrasound Comparison, No New Noncompressible Common Femoral or Popliteal Vein*

In this situation, impedance plethysmography may distinguish between new and old DVT (section H). If impedance plethysmography is not available, a comparison of the current venous ultrasound with a previous venous ultrasound may be able to distinguish between new and old DVT (section G).

G *Comparison of Thrombus Diameter at Common Femoral and Popliteal Veins, Measured on a Current, and a Previous Venous Ultrasound*

Although complete resolution of thrombosis occurs slowly following diagnosis and treatment of DVT, the diameter of residual clot as assessed by ultrasound decreases substantially over the first 3 months.[1] One small study suggests that an increase in diameter of the common femoral or popliteal veins of 2 mm on a current ultrasound, compared to a previous baseline, is diagnostic for recurrent DVT and that failure to find an increase in diameter of either venous segment of 2 mm excludes recurrent DVT.[1] More conservative criteria are to exclude recurrent DVT if venous diameter has not increased by 1 mm, diagnose recurrence if venous diameter has increased by 4 mm, and consider the ultrasound comparison as nondiagnostic if there has been an increase in diameter of 1.1 to 3.9 mm. Venography should be performed in the latter group of patients (section J).

H *Diagnosis of Recurrent DVT Using Impedance Plethysmography*

Impedance plethysmography returns to normal more rapidly than venous ultrasound, with about 90% of tests being normal a year after diagnosis and treatment of proximal DVT.[3,4] A normal impedance plethysmograph, which remains normal during serial testing performed over a 7- to 10-day period, can be used to exclude recurrent proximal DVT. An abnormal impedance plethysmography can be used to diagnose DVT if a previous test was normal, or if the last episode of DVT was over a year previously, and a diagnosis of recurrent DVT is consistent with the overall clinical picture (i.e., clinical presentation, other investigations). If the last IPG was abnormal and the current IPG is abnormal, or the results of IPG testing are not consistent with the clinical suspicion of recurrent DVT, venography should be performed (section J).

I *Venography for the Diagnosis of Recurrent DVT*

The presence of an intraluminal filling defect is diagnostic for recurrent DVT. Venography which outlines all the deep veins and does not show an intraluminal filling defect excludes recurrent DVT. Venography which fails to outline all the deep veins and does not show an intraluminal filling defect is nondiagnostic (section K).

J *Nondiagnostic Venography*

An intraluminal filling defect is considered a sensitive criterion for diagnosing recurrent DVT. Consequently, most patients without an intraluminal filling defect and with segments of the deep venous system that are not outlined by venography, are unlikely to have recurrent DVT. The decision whether or not to anticoagulate these patients is influenced by clinical presentation (i.e., clinical suspicion of recurrent DVT, cardiopulmonary reserve, risk of bleeding on anticoagulants) and the results of previously noted investigations (i.e., extent of thrombosis on venous ultrasound, extent of nonfilling on venography) and additional investigations that

Diagnosis of Recurrent DVT

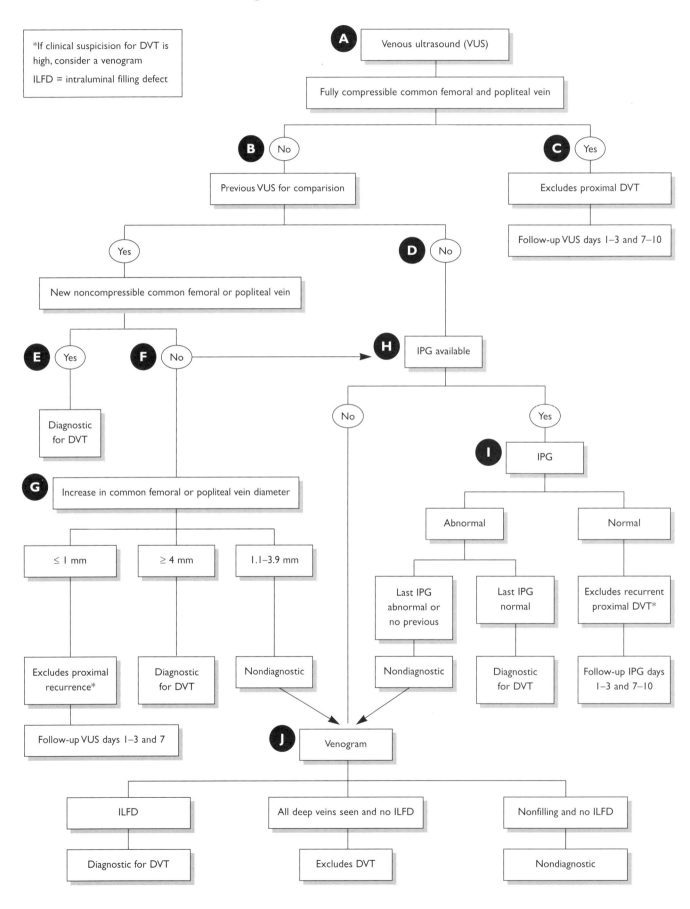

*If clinical suspicision for DVT is high, consider a venogram

ILFD = intraluminal filling defect

A Venous ultrasound (VUS)

Fully compressible common femoral and popliteal vein

B No

C Yes

Previous VUS for comparision

Excludes proximal DVT

Follow-up VUS days 1–3 and 7–10

Yes

D No

New noncompressible common femoral or popliteal vein

E Yes

F No

H IPG available

Diagnostic for DVT

No

Yes

I IPG

G Increase in common femoral or popliteal vein diameter

Abnormal

Normal

≤ 1 mm

≥ 4 mm

1.1–3.9 mm

Last IPG abnormal or no previous

Last IPG normal

Excludes recurrent proximal DVT*

Excludes proximal recurrence*

Diagnostic for DVT

Nondiagnostic

Nondiagnostic

Diagnostic for DVT

Follow-up IPG days 1–3 and 7–10

Follow-up VUS days 1–3 and 7

J Venogram

ILFD

All deep veins seen and no ILFD

Nonfilling and no ILFD

Diagnostic for DVT

Excludes DVT

Nondiagnostic

may have been performed (i.e., D-dimer assays, fibrinogen leg scanning, magnetic resonance imaging). On the basis of all evidence, unless recurrent DVT is thought to be highly likely, we usually withhold anticoagulation in this setting and perform serial venous ultrasound over the next 7 to 10 days to detect evidence of thrombus extension (i.e., increase in venous diameter, extension of thrombus length).

Bibliography

1. Prandoni P, Cogo A, Bernardi E, et al. A simple ultrasound approach for detection of recurrent proximal vein thrombosis. Circulation 1993;88:1730–5.
2. Heijboer H, Jongbloets LMM, Buller HR, Lensing AWA, ten Cate JW. Clinical utility of real-time compression ultrasonography for diagnostic management of patients with recurrent venous thrombosis. Acta Radiol 1992;33:297–300.
3. Hull RD, Carter CJ, Jay RM, et al. The diagnosis of acute recurrent deep vein thrombosis: a diagnostic challenge. Circulation 1983;67:901–6.
4. Huisman MV, Buller HR, ten Cate JW. Utility of impedance plethysmography in the diagnosis of recurrent deep-vein thrombosis. Arch Intern Med 1988;148:681–3.

Additional Reading

Lensing AWA, Hirsh J, Buller H. Diagnosis of venous thrombosis. In: Coleman RW, Hirsh J, Marder VJ, Salzman EW, eds. Hemostasis and thrombosis: basic principles and clinical practice. 3rd edn. Philadelphia: J.B. Lippincott Co., 1993.

Becker DM, Philbrick JT, Bachhuber TL, Humphries JE. D-dimer testing and acute venous thromboembolism. A shortcut to accurate diagnosis? Arch Intern Med 1996;156:939–46.

Chapter 7

Diagnosis of
Deep Vein Thrombosis
during Pregnancy

Shannon M Bates

Jeffrey S Ginsberg

Venous thromboembolic disease is an important cause of obstetric morbidity and mortality. The true incidence of deep vein thrombosis (DVT) during pregnancy and the postpartum period is unknown. While some studies have made estimates of the incidence of DVT based on clinical diagnosis, these are likely to be inaccurate. Few studies have used objective diagnostic techniques but in those that have, the estimated incidences of symptomatic venous thrombosis during pregnancy in patients without prior events have ranged from 0.018 to 0.27 per 100 deliveries.[1] Symptomatic pulmonary embolism will occur in 15 to 24% of patients with untreated DVT, resulting in a 12 to 15% mortality. With appropriate therapy, the incidence of pulmonary embolism declines to 4.5%, with an overall mortality rate of 0.7%.[2–4]

Traditionally, the risk of thrombosis has been considered greatest during the third trimester and the postpartum period.[5] Recent studies using objective diagnosis have suggested that antepartum venous thrombosis is at least as common as postpartum DVT.[6,7] However, prospective studies using objective diagnostic tests have not found the incidence of DVT to be higher during the third trimester than during the first two trimesters.[8]

During pregnancy, DVT appears to have a predilection for the left leg.[6,8] The reason for this preponderance is unknown. It has been suggested that the usual compression of the left iliac vein where it is crossed by the right iliac artery is exaggerated,[9] leading to increased venous stasis.

Several factors may be important in the development of DVT during pregnancy. Venous stasis, which may be caused by several factors, probably increases the likelihood of DVT. Increased venous distensibility and capacity, with a resultant reduction in lower extremity blood flow velocity, are demonstrable from the first trimester of pregnancy.[10] Also, obstruction of the inferior vena cava and the left iliac vein by the gravid uterus may result in decreased venous flow.[11] Vascular damage may occur during cesarean section or with placental separation during vaginal delivery. Altered levels of coagulation factors and natural inhibitors of coagulation in association with a reduction in fibrinolytic activity during pregnancy may produce a relative hypercoagulable state.[1]

A *Clinical Assessment of Deep Vein Thrombosis*

While the common clinical findings of DVT are lower extremity pain, tenderness, and swelling, many patients with DVT are asymptomatic. In pregnant women, non-thrombotic causes of leg pain and swelling are common. The clinical diagnosis of DVT is unreliable and the presence of venous thrombosis is confirmed by objective investigations in less than 50% of suspected cases.[12] Accurate objective diagnosis of DVT is essential because while treatment of venous thromboembolic disease is effective, it is not without significant risks (see Chapter 15); moreover, failure to treat patients with DVT can have devastating results.

B *Differential Diagnosis*

The differential diagnosis of DVT is extensive (see Chapter 4). Venous stasis due to compression of the common iliac veins, venous insufficiency, superficial phlebitis, cellulitis, hematoma, congestive heart failure, ruptured Baker's cyst, and tumor can all mimic deep vein thrombosis.

C *Laboratory Diagnosis of Deep Vein Thrombosis*

The objective diagnosis of DVT during pregnancy presents special problems because the enlarged uterus may cause false-positive tests for DVT, and many diagnostic tests expose the fetus to ionizing radiation. With low-dose in-utero radiation exposures of <5 rads, there is probably a slight increase in the incidence of subsequent childhood cancers but no increase in congenital malformations.[13] While the dose of radiation delivered to the fetus varies with radiographic technique, maternal anatomy, and fetal gestational age, in general, it is possible to establish a diagnosis of DVT with a fetal radiation exposure of <0.50 rads.[13] This level of radiation is likely to be associated with trivial rates of adverse events.[13]

Validated objective tests for the diagnosis of DVT include impedance plethysmography (IPG), compression ultrasound (CUS), and contrast venography.

D *Impedance Plethysmography*

Impedance plethysmography is a safe, inexpensive, and relatively sensitive and specific test for the diagnosis of occlusive proximal DVT.[11] It measures alterations in electrical impedance that result from changes in blood volume within a limb. Because it is insensitive to calf vein and some nonocclusive proximal DVT, serial testing should be performed over 7 to 14 days in patients with a normal initial IPG to exclude extending or nonocclusive proximal DVT. The safety of withholding anticoagulant therapy in pregnant patients with negative serial IPGs has been validated.[14] If the repeat IPG becomes positive, this is sufficient to diagnose DVT. An abnormal IPG during the first two trimesters of pregnancy can be used to make the diagnosis of DVT. As compression of the pelvic vessels by the gravid uterus can cause a false-positive IPG during the last trimester of pregnancy, a positive test should be repeated after the patient has been in the lateral recumbent position for 20 to 30 minutes. If the test remains abnormal, a limited venogram should be performed to differentiate between a proximal DVT and compression of the pelvic vessels by an enlarged uterus. If the limited venogram is negative, a complete venogram should be performed to detect iliofemoral vein thrombosis.

E *Compression Ultrasound*

Compression ultrasound can directly visualize the deep veins and distinguish venous thrombosis from extrinsic venous obstruction. The finding of a noncompressible venous segment has a very high positive predictive value for the diagnosis of DVT.[1] While CUS is sensitive and specific for the diagnosis of proximal DVT in symptomatic nonpregnant patients,[1] it does not reliably detect isolated iliac vein thrombi,[13] which are thought to occur more commonly in pregnancy, or calf vein thrombi.[15] If CUS reveals a noncompressible venous segment, proximal DVT can be diagnosed. If the CUS reveals no thrombus, and isolated iliac vein thrombosis is not suspected, it is reasonable to monitor the patient with serial CUS to rule out proximal extension of a calf vein thrombus. While no large prospective series have evaluated the safety of this approach in pregnancy, the safety of withholding treatment in nonpregnant patients with normal serial CUS has been demonstrated.[16] Isolated iliac vein thrombosis should be suspected when a pregnant patient develops unilateral leg pain and swelling that involves the entire lower extremity with or without associated lower abdominal, hip, or buttock pain. If this diagnosis is considered, duplex ultrasonography assessing common iliac vein patency, pulsed Doppler examination of the common iliac vein, or IPG can be used to detect isolated iliac vein thrombosis.[1]

Diagnosis of Deep Vein Thrombosis during Pregnancy

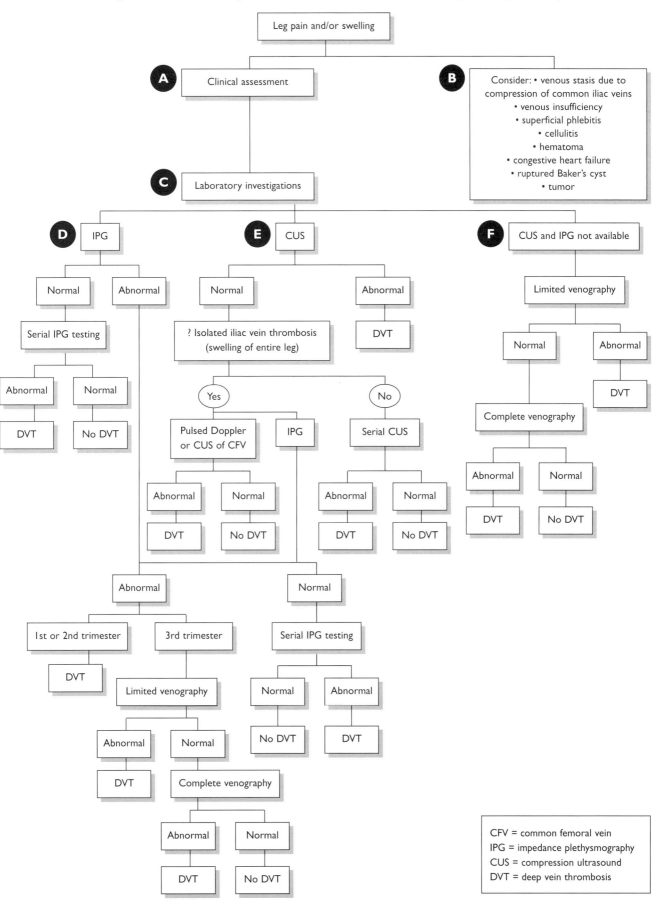

F *Venography*

Ascending contrast venography is the reference standard for the diagnosis of DVT.[1] Venography should be performed if noninvasive tests are equivocal or if serial non-invasive tests cannot be performed. When adequately performed, a normal test excludes DVT.[1] A persistent intraluminal filling defect present in two or more views is diagnostic of DVT.[1]

A limited venogram with pelvic and abdominal shielding reduces the amount of radiation absorbed by the fetus but does not allow visualization of the iliac veins. Therefore, if limited venography is normal, iliac vein thrombosis cannot be excluded unless a complete venogram is performed.

Bibliography

1. Douketis JD, Ginsberg JS. Diagnostic problems with venous thromboembolic disease in pregnancy. Haemostasis 1995;25:58–71.

2. Villasanta U. Thromboembolic disease in pregnancy. Am J Obstet Gynecol 1965;93:142–60.

3. Ullery J. Thromboembolic disease complicating pregnancy and puerperium. Am J Obstet Gynecol 1965;68:1243–8.

4. Hirsh J, Cade JF, Gallus AS. Anticoagulants in pregnancy: a review of the indications and complications. Am Heart J 1972;83:301–5.

5. Aaro LA, Juergens JL. Thrombophlebitis associated with pregnancy. Am J Obstet Gynecol 1971;109:1128–33.

6. Rutherford S, Montoro M, McGehee W, Strong T. Thromboembolic disease associated with pregnancy: an 11-year review (abstract). Am J Obstet Gynecol 1991;164(Suppl):286.

7. Tengborn L, Bergqvist D, Matzsch T, Bergqvist A, Hedner U. Recurrent thromboembolism in pregnancy and puerperium. Am J Obstet Gynecol 1985;28:107–18.

8. Ginsberg JS, Brill-Edwards P, Burrows RF, et al. Venous thrombosis during pregnancy: leg and trimester of presentation. Thromb Haemost 1992;67:519–20.

9. Cockett FB, Thomas ML. The iliac compression syndrome. Br J Surg 1965;52:816–21.

10. Irkard RW, Ueland K, Folse R. Lower limb venous dynamics in pregnant women. Surg Gynecol Obstet 1971;132:483–8.

11. Kerr MG, Scott DB, Samuel E. Studies of the inferior vena cava in late pregnancy. Br Med J 1964;1:532–3.

12. Barnes RW, Wu KK, Hoak JC. Fallibility of clinical diagnosis of venous thrombosis. JAMA 1975;234:605–7.

13. Ginsberg JS, Hirsh J, Rainbow AJ, Coates G. Risks to the fetus of radiologic procedures used in the diagnosis of maternal venous thromboembolic disease. Thromb Haemost 1989;61:189–96.

14. Hull RD, Raskob GE, Leclerc JR, Jay RM, Hirsh J. The diagnosis of clinically suspected venous thrombosis. Clin Chest Med 1984;5:439–55.

15. Hull RD, Raskob GE, Carter CJ. Serial impedance plethysmography in pregnant patients with clinically suspected deep vein thrombosis. Ann Intern Med 1990;112:663–7.

16. Cronan JJ, Dorfman GS, Scola FM, Schepps B, Alexander J. Deep vein thrombosis: ultrasound assessment using vein compression. Radiology 1987;162:191–4.

Additional Reading

Heijboer H, Brandjes DPM, Lensing AWA, Buller HR, ten Cate JW. Efficacy of real time B-mode ultrasonography versus impedance plethysmography in the diagnosis of deep vein thrombosis in symptomatic outpatients. Thromb Haemost 1991;65:804a.

Chapter 8

Diagnosis of Pulmonary Embolism during Pregnancy

Shannon M Bates

Jeffrey S Ginsberg

Pulmonary embolism (PE) has been estimated to occur in 1 in 2000 pregnancies.[1] After toxemia of pregnancy, PE is the most common cause of maternal mortality.[2,3] Moreover, PE during pregnancy can cause long-term morbidity in the form of chronic thromboembolic pulmonary hypertension.[4] In the pregnant patient with suspected PE, accurate diagnosis is important because while adequate anticoagulant therapy reduces mortality and may prevent long-term sequelae, it is not without risk.

A Clinical Assessment

The clinical presentation of PE in pregnant patients is, like that in nonpregnant patients, deceptively nonspecific (see Chapter 10). While small emboli may go unrecognized by the patient, dyspnea, tachypnea, and pleuritic chest pain are present in some 70% of patients with documented PE.[5] Other symptoms suggestive of PE include apprehension, cough, palpitations, and hemoptysis. While tachypnea is the most common sign of PE, tachycardia, diaphoresis, wheezing, pleural friction rub, evidence of a pleural effusion, pulmonary rales, an accentuated pulmonic valve second heart sound, and gallop rhythm may be seen. Patients with massive PE may present with cyanosis, syncope, hypotension, and signs of right heart failure. Symptoms or signs of lower extremity venous thrombosis occur in less than 25% of patients with proven PE.[6]

History, physical examination, electrocardiography, and chest X-ray are useful in the initial assessment of patients with possible PE, not because they are specific for the diagnosis but because they can establish an alternative diagnosis and, therefore, exclude PE.

B *Alternative Diagnoses*

Pneumonia, "pleurisy," pleurodynia, congestive heart failure, pneumothorax, musculoskeletal injury, and myocardial infarction can all mimic PE.

C *Objective Tests for the Diagnosis of PE*

Fear of exposing the fetus to radiation makes the use of necessary radiologic procedures worrisome during pregnancy. A literature review of outcomes following low-dose in-utero radiation exposures of < 5 rads suggests that there is probably a slight increase in subsequent childhood cancer but no increase in congenital malformations.[7] The same study suggested that the amount of radiation absorbed by the fetus during lung scanning could be reduced to < 0.05 rads by halving the amount of ^{99m}Tc-MAA used in perfusion scanning.[7] Using a brachial route rather than a femoral route for pulmonary angiography decreases the estimated fetal radiation exposure from approximately 0.30 rads to < 0.05 rads.[7] The dose of radiation delivered to the fetus varies with the radiographic technique, maternal anatomy, and gestational age; however, with the judicious use of available techniques, the diagnosis of PE is possible, with a fetal radiation exposure of < 0.05 rads if lung scanning alone is performed and < 0.50 rads if angiography is required after lung scanning.[7] This level of radiation exposure is likely associated with minimal rates of adverse events.

D *Perfusion Lung Scan*

The ventilation-perfusion lung scan (V/Q lung scan) is the most useful noninvasive test in patients with suspected PE[8] and, consequently, is the accepted initial diagnostic test.[9] A perfusion scan should be performed first, as a normal scan excludes PE.[9,10] Fetal radiation exposure can be limited by using a dose of 1 mCi of radiolabelled ^{99m}Tc-MAA.[7]

E *Ventilation Lung Scan*

An abnormal perfusion scan necessitates a ventilation scan. In nonpregnant patients, a "high-probability scan" in which there is a segmental or large subsegmental perfusion defect with normal ventilation is diagnostic of PE in most cases.[9,10] However, some 40 to 50% of nonpregnant patients with suspected PE have neither a high-probability nor a normal lung scan.[9,10] In this group of patients with non-diagnostic scans, the prevalence of PE is approximately 25%.[9,10] Therefore, further investigations are required to find the source of embolism or to definitively diagnose or exclude PE.[4]

Diagnosis of Pulmonary Embolism during Pregnancy

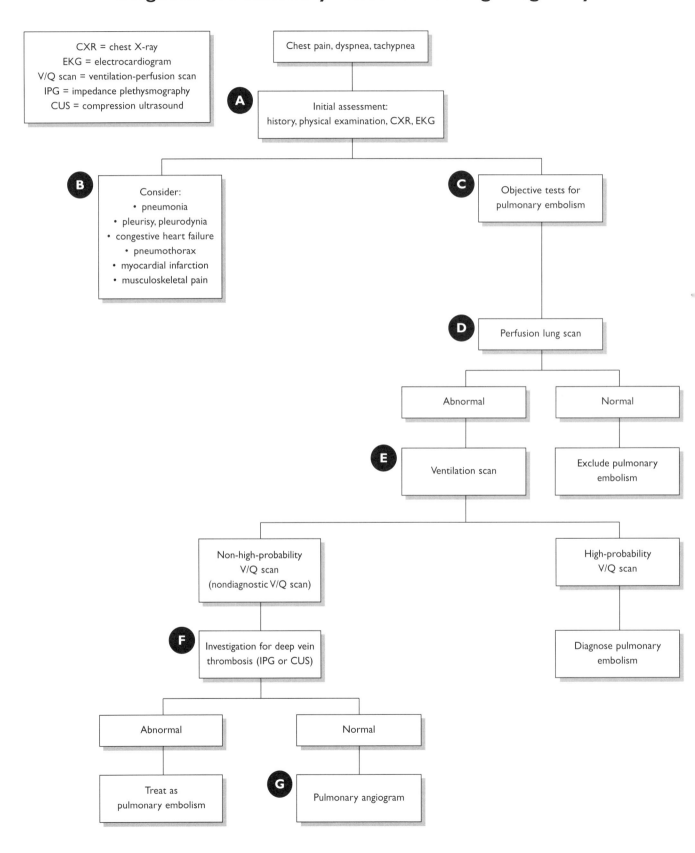

F *Investigations for Deep Vein Thrombosis*

As the majority of PEs originate in the proximal veins of the legs,[8,9,11] impedance plethysmography or compression ultrasound testing should be performed to detect deep vein thrombosis in patients with nondiagnostic V/Q scans. The presence of thrombosis in patients with clinically suspected PE provides reasonable grounds for initiating anticoagulant therapy.

G *Pulmonary Angiogram*

Pulmonary angiography is the diagnostic reference standard for PE.[12] The radiation absorbed by the fetus can be minimized by using the brachial route and by shielding the abdomen with a lead-lined apron.[7]

Bibliography

1. Sipes S, Weiner CP. Venous thromboembolic disease in pregnancy. Semin Perinatol 1990; 14:103–18.

2. Kaunitz AM, Hughes JM, Grimes DA, Smith JC, Rochat RW, Katrisen ME. Causes of maternal mortality in the U.S. Obstet Gynecol 1985;65:605–12.

3. Sachs BP, Brown DA, Driscoll SG, Schulman E, Acker D, Ransil BJ, Jewett JF. Maternal mortality in Massachusetts. Trends and prevention. N Engl J Med 1987;316:667–72.

4. Douketis JD, Ginsberg JS. Diagnostic problems with venous thromboembolic disease in pregnancy. Haemostasis 1995;25:58–71.

5. UPET Investigators. The Urokinase Pulmonary Embolism Trial: a national cooperative study. Circulation 1973;47(Suppl 2):1–108.

6. Hull RD, Raskob GE, Coates G, Panju AA, Gill GJ. A new noninvasive management strategy for patients with suspected pulmonary embolism. Arch Intern Med 1989;149:2549–55.

7. Ginsberg JS, Hirsh J, Rainbow AJ, Coates J. Risks to the fetus of radiologic procedures used in the diagnosis of maternal venous thromboembolic disease. Thromb Haemost 1989;61:189–96.

8. Hull RD, Hirsh J, Carter CJ, et al. Pulmonary angiography, ventilation lung scanning and venography for clinically suspected pulmonary embolism with abnormal perfusion lung scan. Ann Intern Med 1983;98:891–9.

9. Hull RD, Hirsh J, Carter CJ, et al. Diagnostic value of ventilation-perfusion lung scanning in patients with suspected pulmonary embolism. Chest 1985;88:819–28.

10. PIOPED Investigators. Value of the ventilation-perfusion lung scan in acute pulmonary embolism. Results of the Prospective Investigation Of Pulmonary Embolism Diagnosis (PIOPED). JAMA 1990;262:2753–9.

11. Moser KM. Venous thromboembolism. Am Rev Respir Dis 1990;141:235–49.

12. Stein PD, Athanasoulis C, Alavi A, Greenspan RH, Hales CA, Saltzman HA. Complications and validity of pulmonary angiography in acute pulmonary embolism. Circulation 1992;85:462–8.

Chapter 9

Clinical Assessment of Pulmonary Embolism

Marc A Rodger

Philip S Wells

The clinical diagnosis of pulmonary embolism is problematic. Although the frequency of pulmonary embolism is probably referral-centre-specific, in general, less than 35% of patients suspected of pulmonary embolism (PE) will have the diagnosis confirmed.[1] Thus, the majority of patients suspected of having PE do not actually have this condition. However, less than half of all cases of fatal PE will be suspected prior to death and hence a low threshold for investigating suspected pulmonary embolism may be justified. Many patients with fatal PE do not have antecedent signs and symptoms, making antemortem diagnosis difficult.[2]

Two well-designed studies have established that clinical assessment can categorize patients as having a high, moderate, or low probability of PE. Clinical assessment has been shown to be complementary to the findings of ventilation-perfusion lung scanning; positive and negative predictive values are higher when both clinical assessment and the lung scan are concordant (i.e., both clinical assessment and lung scan are low or high probability for PE) compared to when they are discordant.

As outlined below, the individual components of the clinical assessment (e.g., a particular physical examination finding or a specific ECG change) are often of limited value but the synthesis by clinicians of all the individual components of the clinical assessment provides a reliable means to assess the probability of PE in a patient. In this chapter, we provide a structured approach to the clinical determination of pretest probability of PE. The algorithm provides a suggested approach to the clinical determination of pretest probability. It is based on an assessment of symptoms and signs (typical/atypical), presence or absence of an alternative diagnosis likely as PE, and the presence of risk factors for venous thromboembolism (VTE).

Subsequently (Chapter 10), we describe how the results of this assessment can be combined with the results of objective tests for VTE to manage patients with suspected PE.

A Signs and Symptoms

A careful history and physical examination are essential to the diagnostic process in patients with suspected PE. While individual presenting symptoms do not reliably differentiate between patients with and without PE, even in those patients without previous cardiopulmonary disease (Table 9.1), the synthesis of the presenting symptoms with other clinical factors allows the clinician to determine whether the presentation is typical or atypical of PE, develop a differential diagnosis, and subsequently

Table 9.1   Summary of Reported Prevalence for a Number of Signs, Symptoms, Risk Factors, and Test Results in Patients with Suspected Pulmonary Embolism Comparing Patients with and without a Final Diagnosis of Pulmonary Embolism

Predictive Factor	Number with Predictive Factor/Outcome	
	Pulmonary Embolism	No Pulmonary Embolism
Pleuritic pain or hemoptysis[†]	76/117 (65%)	147/248 (59%)
Isolated dyspnea[†]	26/117 (22%)	52/248 (21%)
Circulatory collapse[†]	9/117 (8%)	22/248 (9%)
One or more DVT risk factors[†]	96/117 (82%)	162/248 (65%)*
Immobilization[†]	66/117 (56%)	81/248 (33%)*
Surgery[†]	63/117 (54%)	78/248 (31%)*
Malignancy[†]	27/117 (23%)	38/248 (15%)
Previous DVT or PE[†]	16/117 (14%)	19/248 (8%)
Crackles[†]	60/117 (51%)	98/248 (40%)*
Fourth heart sound[†]	28/117 (24%)	34/248 (14%)*
Increased pulmonic sound[†]	27/117 (23%)	33/248 (13%)*
Any ECG abnormality[†]	62/89 (70%)	not reported
S-T or T wave changes[†]	44/89 (49%)	not reported
ECG evidence of RV overload[§]	37/49 (76%)	not reported
CXR: atelectasis or pulmonary parenchymal abnormality[†]	79/117 (68%)	119/247 (48%)*
Pleural effusion on CXR[†]	56/117 (48%)	77/247 (31%)*
Pleural-based opacity[†]	41/117 (35%)	53/247 (21%)*
Normal A-a gradient[‡]	31/277 (11%)	78/491 (16%)*
Normal A-a; no prior DVT or PE[‡]	2/132 (1.5%)	130/807 (16%)*

* p = < .05; [†] from[3]; [§] from[6]; [‡] from[7]

determine pretest probability. Similarly, individual physical findings often do not reliably distinguish between patients who have PE and those who do not have PE. While the presence of a fourth heart sound (S4), loud second pulmonary heart sound (P2), and inspiratory crackles on chest auscultation are more common in patients with pulmonary embolism than in those without pulmonary embolism, in isolation, none of these signs is sensitive or specific for pulmonary embolism (see Table 9.1). Other findings such as tachypnea and pleural rubs are equally likely in patients suspected to have pulmonary embolism regardless of whether this diagnosis is ultimately confirmed or excluded (see Table 9.1).[3] Of note, the presence of chest wall tenderness in patients with pleuritic chest pain does not exclude pulmonary embolism.

The synthesis of presenting signs and symptoms by clinicians to 1) determine whether the presentation is typical or atypical for pulmonary embolism and 2) ascertain whether an alternative diagnosis is or more likely to be PE is a key feature of our suggested algorithm.

B *Typical or Atypical Clinical Constellation*

In the Prospective Investigation of Pulmonary Embolism Diagnosis (PIOPED) study, which investigated the diagnostic accuracy of ventilation-perfusion lung scans, almost all patients without antecedent cardiopulmonary disease and with confirmed pulmonary embolism presented with one of three clinical syndromes:

1) Pleuritic chest pain or hemoptysis suggesting pulmonary infarction and inflammation—65% of patients;
2) Unexplained dyspnea, suggesting increased dead space ventilation or intrapulmonary shunting—22% of patients;
3) Shock or loss of consciousness, suggesting circulatory collapse secondary to obstruction of right ventricular outflow—8% of patients.[4]

Approximately 10% of patients did not present with any one of these syndromes. These patients presented with unexplained radiographic abnormalities such as atelectasis, pleural effusion, or pleural-based opacities. Atrial fibrillation, other tachyarrhythmias, confusion without hypotension, new onset wheezing, or paradoxical arterial embolism may, on rare occasions, be the presenting symptoms or signs of PE. These presentations should be considered atypical.

C *Alternative Diagnosis*

After signs and symptoms have been assessed and the presentation has been determined to be typical or atypical of PE, other investigations should be considered to decide if an alternative diagnosis is, or more likely to be, PE. These investigations should include a chest x-ray and may include an ECG or arterial blood gases.

Chest x-rays are of limited diagnostic value for pulmonary embolism; radiologists agree on the presence of pulmonary embolism in only one-third of patients, and in only one-third of these is the diagnosis correct.[5] In PIOPED, atelectasis or a parenchymal abnormality was more commonly seen in those with (68%), than those without (48%), PE. Pleural effusions and pleural-based densities are also more common with PE (see Table 9.1). None of these chest x-ray findings was specific or sensitive enough to use in isolation. However, the chest x-ray is important because it may reveal an alternative diagnosis (e.g., pneumothorax).

An abnormal ECG is present in 70% of those patients with PE but the frequency of ECG abnormalities in patients with suspected PE, in whom the diagnosis is excluded, has not been reported. Hence, an abnormal ECG cannot be used to rule in or rule out PE. The most common ECG abnormalities in those with PE are S-T or T-wave changes (49%).[3] A combination of ECG changes associated with right ventricular overload have been reported to have a sensitivity of 76% for PE.[6] Also, ECGs may reveal findings consistent with an alternative diagnosis (e.g., pericarditis, myocardial infarction).

It is a common misconception that a normal A-a gradient excludes pulmonary embolism. In fact, up to 28% of patients with suspected PE and a normal A-a gradient have pulmonary embolism.[7] However, as with the other individual signs and symptoms discussed above, a normal A-a gradient may be a useful component in a synthesis of the global clinical assessment.

In summary, individual features of an ECG, chest x-ray, and blood gas are neither sensitive nor specific for PE. However, these investigations form important components of the clinical assessment and may provide an alternative diagnosis which is, or more likely to be, PE.

D Risk Factors

The presence of significant risk factors for VTE increases the probability of PE. However, the predictive value of individual factors is low. For example, in one study, the presence of one or more risk factors for VTE was more commonly seen in patients with, than without, PE. However, the only individual risk factors that were significantly associated with pulmonary embolism in the same study were immobilization (the longer the immobilization, the greater the risk) and surgery (within 12 weeks)[3] (see Table 9.1). Other important risk factors to consider include malignancy (treatment ongoing or within the last 6 months or in the palliative stages), previous DVT, lower extremity fracture, family history of VTE (two or more family members with objectively proven events or a first-degree relative with thrombophilia), lower extremity paralysis, and the postpartum period.

E *Pretest Probability*

After combining B,C, and D a clinical pretest probability can be determined. The assessment of clinical probability is then used in combination with the V/Q scan findings in the management strategy discussed in the next chapter.

Determining the Pretest Probability of Pulmonary Embolism

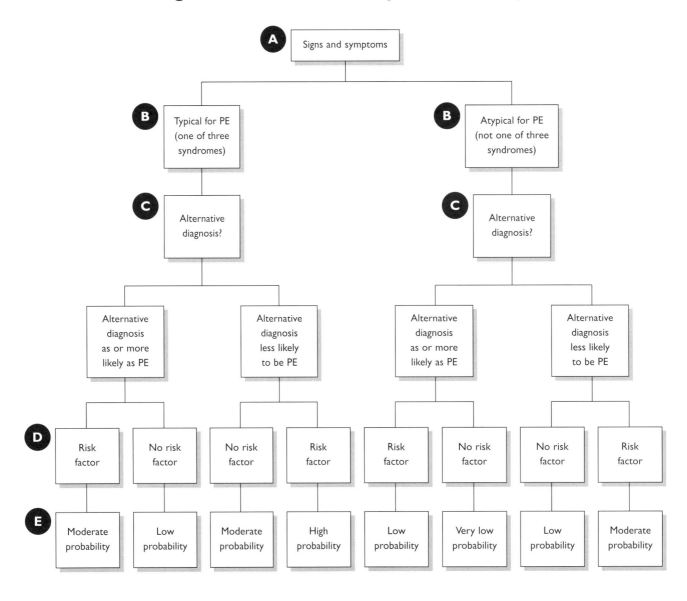

Bibliography

1. The PIOPED Investigators. Value of the ventilation/perfusion scan in acute pulmonary embolism: results of the Prospective Investigation of Pulmonary Embolism Diagnosis (PIOPED). JAMA 1990;263:2753–9.

2. Stein PD, Henry JW. Prevalence of acute pulmonary embolism among patients in a general hospital and at autopsy. Chest 1995;108:978–81.

3. Stein PD, Terrin ML, Hales CA, et al. Clinical, laboratory, roentgenographic, and electrocardiographic findings in patients with acute pulmonary embolism and no pre-existing cardiac or pulmonary disease. Chest 1991;100:598–603.

4. Stein PD, Gottschalk A, Saltzman HA, Terrin ML. Diagnosis of acute pulmonary embolism in the elderly. J Am Coll Cardiol 1991;18:1452–7.

5. Greenspan RH, Ravin CE, Polansky M, McLoud TC. Accuracy of the chest radiograph in diagnosis of pulmonary embolism. Invest Radiol 1982;17:539–43.

6. Sreeram N, Cheriex EC, Smeets JLRM, Gorgels AP, Wellens HJJ. Value of the 12-lead electrocardiogram at hospital admission in the diagnosis of pulmonary embolism. Am J Cardiol 1994;73:298–303.

7. Stein PD, Goldhaber SZ, Henry JW, Miller AC. Arterial blood gas analysis in the assessment of suspected acute pulmonary embolism. Chest 1996;109:78–81.

Chapter 10

Diagnosis of Pulmonary Embolism

Marc A Rodger

Philip S Wells

The mortality rate for untreated pulmonary embolism in hospitalized patients is 30% but falls to 8% with anticoagulant therapy.[1] However, anticoagulant therapy is not without its own risk of morbidity and mortality.[2] Therefore, once pulmonary embolism is suspected, the diagnosis must be excluded or confirmed with objective testing. The gold standard diagnostic test is pulmonary angiography but this test is not widely applied because of limited availability, cost, and perceived risk. In this chapter, we describe an approach to the diagnosis of pulmonary embolism that limits the use of pulmonary angiography.

A Clinical Assessment

The assignment of a pretest probability of pulmonary embolism has the potential to improve the diagnostic accuracy of noninvasive tests (that is, post-test probability).[3] Prior to diagnostic testing, clinicians should determine if patients have a low, moderate, or high pretest probability for pulmonary embolism. Pretest probability is assigned by an assessment of signs, symptoms, risk factors, and the presence of an alternative diagnosis, as described in Chapter 9.

B Ventilation-Perfusion (V/Q) Lung Scan

A normal or near-normal perfusion scan is associated with a probability of pulmonary embolism of about 1% and thus essentially excludes this diagnosis.[3]

C Combination of Clinical Assessment and V/Q Scan Findings

The V/Q scan can reliably diagnose pulmonary embolism if the scan is interpreted as being high probability (e.g., one or more mismatched segments or segment equivalents) and the clinical pretest suspicion is moderate or high. In these situations, the post-test probabilities for pulmonary embolism are 88% and 96%, respectively. Most physicians accept these probabilities as being high enough to obviate the need for further testing.[3] However, patients with low pretest probability and high probability V/Q scans have a post-test probability for pulmonary embolism of about 56%; so we recommend further testing in this situation (see Section G).

The greatest difficulty in the diagnosis of pulmonary embolism occurs in those 45 to 60% of patients who have nondiagnostic V/Q scan results (i.e., low or intermediate probability V/Q scans). Only 20 to 40% of such cases will ultimately have pulmonary embolism proven if angiography is performed. In most of these cases, further testing is required.[3]

D *Further Testing*

If the combination of the clinical assessment and the V/Q scan does not provide a definitive diagnosis, further testing is warranted. The combinations in which further testing are warranted are 1) low probability lung scan with low pretest suspicion (see Section E), 2) low probability scan and moderate or high pretest suspicion (see Section F), or 3) intermediate probability scan regardless of pretest probability (see Section F), and 4) high probability scan with low pretest suspicion (see Section G).

E *Low Probability Scan and Low Pretest Suspicion*

In most patients with pulmonary embolism, the source is the deep veins of the lower extremities; thus, evaluation for deep vein thrombosis is potentially useful. We recommend a single ultrasound test in patients with low pretest probability and a low probability V/Q scan; if the ultrasound is normal, pulmonary embolism is unlikely (prevalence of PE ~2%). If ultrasonography is abnormal, treatment with anticoagulants is indicated.

It should be noted that the presence of a thrombus in the leg in patients with suspected pulmonary emboli does not necessarily confirm the latter. The subgroup of patients with suspected PE who do not have PE may have risk factors for VTE and hence may have incidental DVT. In one study performing pulmonary angiography and venography in all patients with suspected PE, the positive predictive value of venography was only 72%.[4] Thus, other etiologies for the index chest symptoms should always be considered in patients with nondiagnostic lung scans even when DVT is diagnosed.

F *Low Probability Scan and Moderate or High Pretest Suspicion or Intermediate Probability V/Q Scan with Any Pretest Suspicion*

Patients with a low probability scan and moderate or high pretest suspicion or an intermediate probability V/Q scan with any pretest suspicion should undergo bilateral lower extremity venous ultrasonography. If ultrasonography is abnormal, treatment with anticoagulants is indicated but other etiologies for the index chest symptoms should also be excluded. A normal ultrasound result should be followed with serial ultrasound testing or pulmonary angiography depending on the patient's cardiopulmonary reserve.

It has been demonstrated that patients with nondiagnostic V/Q scans and reasonable cardiopulmonary reserve can be safely managed using serial impedance plethysmography to detect evolving proximal DVT.[5] The rationale for this management approach is that the greatest risk to patients with recent PE is from a further embolism but that recurrent embolism is highly unlikely without preceding proximal DVT. The highest risk period for recurrent PE is within 2 weeks of the initial event. If proximal DVT is not detected during this period, the subsequent risk of recurrence is very low. As venous ultrasonography is at least as accurate for the diagnosis of proximal DVT as impedance plethysmography, it is reasonable to assume that serial venous ultrasound is also a valid management approach in this situation.[6] The safety of the serial impedance plethysmography approach is comparable to that of pulmonary angiography. Angiography is warranted if patients have poor cardiopulmonary reserve (either new or old) as a recurrent pulmonary embolism in these patients could be catastrophic.

G *High Probability V/Q Scan and Low Pretest Suspicion*
We would recommend a single ultrasound test in patients with low pretest probability and a high probability V/Q scan. If the ultrasound is normal, the patient should have angiography. If the ultrasound is abnormal, anticoagulant therapy is warranted.

FUTURE DIRECTIONS

D-dimers are cross-linked fibrin degradation products that become elevated in deep vein thrombosis and pulmonary embolism but also in many other conditions associated with fibrin formation (trauma, DIC, sepsis, etc.). Low D-dimer levels may help to exclude pulmonary embolism but high levels are nonspecific.[7,8] Continuous volume computed tomography (CVCT) and magnetic resonance angiography (MRA) enable much of the pulmonary arteries to be visualized noninvasively and may be helpful for the diagnosis of pulmonary embolism. However, at this point, the results of large prospective management trials using D-dimer, MRA, or CVCT have not been published.

Diagnostic Approach in Patients with Suspected Pulmonary Embolism

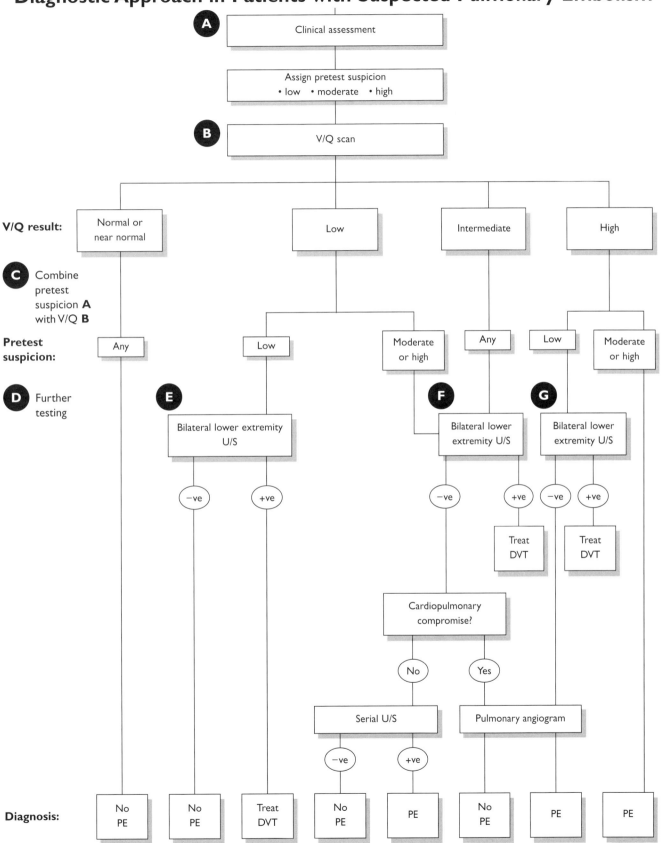

Bibliography

1. Carson JL, Kelley MA, Duff A, et al. Clinical course of pulmonary embolism. N Engl J Med 1992;326:1240–5.

2. Landefeld CS, Beyth RJ. Anticoagulant-related bleeding: clinical epidemiology, prediction and prevention. Am J Med 1993;95:315–28.

3. The PIOPED Investigators. Value of the ventilation/perfusion scan in acute pulmonary embolism: results of the Prospective Investigation of Pulmonary Embolism Diagnosis (PIOPED). JAMA 1990;263:2753–9.

4. Hull RD, Hirsh J, Carter CJ, et al. Pulmonary angiography, ventilation lung scanning, and venography for clinically suspected pulmonary embolism with abnormal perfusion lung scan. Ann Intern Med 1983;98:891–9.

5. Hull RD, Raskob G, Ginsberg JS, et al. A non-invasive strategy for the treatment of patients with suspected pulmonary embolism. Arch Intern Med 1994;154:289–97.

6. Wells PS, Hirsh J, Anderson DR, et al. Comparison of the accuracy of impedance plethysmography and compression ultrasonography in outpatients with clinically supected deep vein thrombosis. Thromb Haemost 1995;74:1423–7.

7. Ginsberg JS, Wells PS, Brill-Edwards P, et al. Application of a novel and rapid whole blood assay for D-Dimer in patients with clinically suspected pulmonary embolism. Thromb Haemost 1995;73:35–8.

8. Bounameaux H, de Moerloose P, Perrier A, Reber G. Plasma measurement of D-Dimer as diagnostic aid in suspected venous thromboembolism: an overview. Thromb Haemost 1994;71:1–6.

Chapter 11

INITIAL THERAPY OF DEEP VEIN THROMBOSIS AND PULMONARY EMBOLISM

Agnes YY Lee

Jeffrey S Ginsberg

Anticoagulation is the main therapy for the treatment of acute venous thromboembolism (VTE). Initial therapy requires an adequate dose of unfractionated heparin (UFH) or low-molecular-weight heparin (LMWH) and loading doses of warfarin. Recently, two randomized controlled studies showed that outpatient therapy with low-molecular-weight heparin (LMWH) is as safe and efficacious as traditional inpatient management with UFH for the initial treatment of deep vein thrombosis (DVT). For acute PE, two large randomized studies have also demonstrated the safety and efficacy of initial therapy with LMWH. For those presenting with hemodynamic instability, thrombolytic therapy or surgical intervention should be considered. In patients with acute VTE and contraindications for anticoagulation, insertion of an inferior vena cava filter is the standard alternative.

A Contraindications for Anticoagulation

The relative and absolute contraindications for anticoagulation are listed in Table 11.1. Prior to starting any patient on anticoagulants, the risk of thrombus extension and/or embolization must be weighed against the risk of hemorrhage. Patients with active hemorrhage, except those with mild bleeding from superficial and compressible sites, should not receive anticoagulants. If the bleeding and the underlying cause are likely to be transient and reversible, then anticoagulants can be started when hemostasis is achieved. If the patient has a permanent or prolonged risk of bleeding, such as an acquired or inherited coagulopathy, or severe thrombocytopenia (platelet count $< 20 \times 10^9$/l), then an inferior vena cava filter should be inserted (see Chapter 13).

Table 11.1   Contraindications for Anticoagulation

Absolute Contraindications
Active hemorrhage
Recent neurosurgery or intracranial bleed (< 7 days)
Severe thrombocytopenia (platelet count < 20 x 10^9/l)

Relative Contraindications
Recent gastrointestinal hemorrhage (< 14 days)
Recent major abdominal surgery (< 1 to 2 days)
Brain metastases
Uncontrolled hypertension
Moderate thrombocytopenia (platelet count 20 to 50 x 10^9/l)
Inherited coagulopathy

B *Heparin-Induced Thrombocytopenia*

An uncommon but absolute contraindication for, and a complication of, heparin therapy is heparin-induced thrombocytopenia (HIT). Patients with HIT can develop extensive venous or arterial thrombosis with exposure to heparin. When these patients require anticoagulation, either for prophylaxis or treatment, the options include danaparoid sodium (Orgaran, a heparinoid with less than 5% cross-reactivity with heparin), ancrod (Arvin, a defibrinogenating snake venom), argipidine (Argatroban, a synthetic antithrombin agent), or hirudin (a direct thrombin inhibitor from the medicinal leech). The diagnosis and management of these patients are discussed in Chapter 18.

C *Inferior Vena Cava Filter Insertion*

For patients with contraindications for anticoagulation (see Table 11.1), insertion of an inferior vena cava filter should be considered. Caval interruption is also indicated when patients develop recurrent PE despite adequate anticoagulation (failure of therapeutic anticoagulation), are noncompliant, or are inaccessible for monitoring. Many types of filters are available, including the Greenfield, Venatech, and Bird's Nest filters. (Despite their common use, there are no controlled studies examining the exact indications for filter insertion or their efficacy in preventing PE.[1]) The use and complications of vena cava filters are discussed in Chapter 13.

D *Hemodynamic Stability*

When a patient presents with acute pulmonary embolism, hemodynamic status must be quickly and routinely assessed. Important parameters to review are vital signs including the pulse and rhythm, blood pressure, and respiratory rate, jugular venous pressure, oxygen saturation, and mental status. The majority of patients present with shortness of breath and/or pleuritic chest pain but are hemodynamically stable and respond well to anticoagulation alone. However, if the clinical assessment indicates critical hemodynamic compromise or impending cardiovascular collapse, urgent intervention with thrombolysis or surgical thrombectomy should be considered. Table 11.2 lists the abnormal parameters that indicate the necessity for prompt intervention. While waiting for diagnostic tests or checking also the need for additional therapy, patients should be started on intravenous heparin.

E   *Thrombolysis and Surgical Thrombectomy*

When patients with acute massive pulmonary embolism are hemodynamically unstable, acute thrombolysis or surgical thrombectomy can rapidly reverse cardiovascular compromise.[1] The choice of pharmacological or surgical intervention will depend on local experience and the availability of a cardiovascular surgeon. There are no prospective studies comparing these options, and given the infrequency and urgency of the situation, it is unlikely that a randomized trial will be conducted. The indications and complications of these interventions are discussed in Chapters 14 and 28.

F   *Unfractionated Heparin*

Unfractionated heparin is the standard initial treatment for acute venous thrombosis. Studies have shown that adequate doses are required initially to prevent recurrence.[2,3] Provided that the activated partial thromboplastin time (aPTT) is monitored and maintained at therapeutic levels, unfractionated heparin can be given either via an

Table 11.2   Parameters Indicating Critical Hemodynamic Instability in Patients with Acute Pulmonary Embolism

Clinical Parameters	
Pulse and rhythm	Sinus tachycardia or arrhythmia
Blood pressure	Hypotensive (systolic pressure < 90 mm Hg)
Jugular venous pressure	Marked elevated or presence of v waves indicating tricuspid regurgitation
Respiratory rate	Markedly elevated (> 24)
Colour	Central cyanosis
Mental status	Altered or depressed mental status
Laboratory Parameters	
Oxygen saturation	< 90% on supplemental oxygen (40% concentration)
Electrocardiogram	S-T depression, T wave inversion, or other signs of myocardial ischemia

intravenous (IV) continuous infusion or subcutaneous (SQ) injection. Intermittent IV infusions are associated with a higher risk of bleeding and are not recommended.[4] The standard IV loading dose for UFH of 5000 units should be followed by a continuous infusion of at least 30,000 units per 24 hours. Subsequent doses should be adjusted based on a standard or weight-based nomogram to reach and maintain a therapeutic aPTT, corresponding to a heparin level of 0.2 to 0.4 units/ml by protamine sulfate titration, or 0.4 to 0.7 units/ml by antifactor Xa assay, as quickly as possible.[5–8] The therapeutic aPTT range differs for different reagents and the automated coagulation machines used, and a fixed ratio of 1.5 times control is not therapeutic for most aPTT reagents.[9] In patients requiring large doses of heparin (greater than 40,000 units per 24 hours), the heparin level should be monitored because of a dissociation between the aPTT and heparin concentration in heparin-resistant patients[2] (see Chapter 20). For patients without IV access, SQ heparin can be initiated at 17,500 units every 12 hours. When patients are receiving SQ heparin, the aPTT should be drawn at 6 hours after the last injection.

Initial treatment in uncomplicated acute venous thrombosis with heparin should be continued for at least 5 days. It can be discontinued when warfarin has reached therapeutic levels for 2 consecutive days, as indicated by the International Normalized Ratio (INR). For patients presenting with extensive disease, e.g., phlegmasia cerulea dolens or life-threatening PE, a longer course of heparin is indicated.

Because of the variable pharmacokinetics of UFH, it has a narrow therapeutic window, and monitoring is essential to ensure adequate dosing and avoid complications. The major complication of unfractionated heparin, like all other anticoagulants, is bleeding. The bleeding risk depends on the total dose of heparin, the age of the patient, underlying bleeding tendencies (e.g., peptic ulcer disease), and whether the patient is receiving concomitant antiplatelet therapy[4,5] (see Chapter 26). Heparin activity in patients with active bleeding can be rapidly reversed with protamine sulfate and by stopping the heparin infusion. Long-term heparin use is also associated with osteoporosis and, rarely, hirsutism. Heparin-induced thrombocytopenia can occur after any heparin exposure but it usually presents after 5 to 10 days of therapy and is more likely with larger doses and in patients who have undergone surgery (see Chapter 18).

G *Low-Molecular-Weight Heparins*

Low-molecular-weight heparins have both theoretical and clinical advantages over UFH.[10] Because of their predictable pharmacokinetics and high bioavailability, weight-adjusted doses of LMWH can be given as once or twice daily SQ injections without monitoring. In experimental animal models, LMWHs cause less microvascular bleeding but in clinical practice, this advantage has only been shown in large meta-analyses.[11–13] Recently, two randomized trials showed that for symptomatic proximal DVT, outpatient treatment with LMWH (enoxaparin 100 U/kg SQ twice daily or nadroparin-calcium weight-adjusted dose SQ twice daily) is as safe and efficacious as inpatient therapy with UFH.[14,15] The bleeding rates for both groups in both studies were similar. Although these studies strongly support that replacing UFH with LMWH in the treatment of acute DVT is safe and cost effective, it is uncertain whether these results can be translated to all types of LMWH because of the heterogeneity of the different preparations. Also, both randomized studies excluded patients with PE and previous VTE, and only 33 to 69% of all patients with acute DVT were eligible to be treated as outpatients. The Columbus Investigators[16] recently reported that patients with symptomatic DVT and/or PE can be safely and effectively treated initially with LMWH (reviparin sodium). This finding is supported by another large randomized study in which 612 patients with acute PE were randomized to SQ tinzaparin versus standard intravenous UFH.[17]

Low-molecular-weight heparins have side effects similar to heparin but they may be associated with a lower risk of bleeding, osteoporosis, and heparin-induced thrombocytopenia. When patients bleed while receiving LMWH, protamine sulfate will neutralize the larger heparin molecules present in circulation that are likely responsible for the bleeding.[5]

H *Warfarin Therapy*

Warfarin therapy is necessary to provide anticoagulation once the patient is discharged from hospital. It should be started within 24 hours of initial treatment with UFH or LMWH. There is no consensus on the starting dose of warfarin. A recent publication suggests that a loading dose of 5 mg, compared to 10 mg, is associated with less excessive anticoagulation and is less likely to produce a transient hypercoagulable state due to a faster drop in the protein C than the prothrombin level.[17] Subsequent doses of warfarin are adjusted according to the prothrombin time, expressed as the INR. For VTE, the therapeutic target range is an INR of 2.0 to 3.0. Once the patient reaches this target for 2 consecutive days, which usually takes 4 to 5 days, heparin can be stopped. This overlap ensures that the antithrombotic effect of warfarin (through lowering the prothrombin concentration) has occurred. The total duration of warfarin therapy will depend on the type of initial event (calf vein thrombosis or extensive, life-threatening presentation), presence of risk factors (transient or persistent), and the risk of bleeding. This is discussed in detail in Chapter 16.

Like heparin, there is a wide patient-to-patient variation in the warfarin requirement.[18] The INR should be monitored regularly and the dose adjusted appropriately. More frequent monitoring is indicated when the patient's drug regimen is changed because many medications, especially antibiotics, will interact with warfarin and alter the INR response. If the INR is excessive (over 5.0) but the patient is asymptomatic and not bleeding, warfarin can be held and vitamin K administered. Too large a dose of vitamin K can lower the INR to subtherapeutic levels and delay the recovery of a therapeutic value. If a patient is bleeding with an elevated INR, rapid correction can be achieved with fresh frozen plasma. A thorough search should be conducted to identify the cause and site of bleeding. Unless there is a localized lesion, spontaneous bleeding is unusual when the INR is within the therapeutic range (see Chapter 27).

Initial Therapy of VTE

A rare complication of warfarin therapy is warfarin-induced skin necrosis. This occurs primarily in patients with protein C or protein S deficiency who are started on anticoagulation with warfarin alone. This causes a further drop in the already low protein C or S level, without a parallel decrease in prothrombin and other coagulation factors, resulting in a hypercoagulable state and thrombotic occlusion of small vessels. These patients require initial therapy with heparin to provide antithrombotic protection prior to starting therapy with warfarin.

Bibliography

1. ten Cate JW, Koopman MMW, Prins MH, Büller HR. Treatment of venous thromboembolism. Thromb Haemost 1995;74:197–203.

2. Ginsberg JS. Management of venous thromboembolism. N Engl J Med 1996;335:1816–28.

3. Anand S, Ginsberg JS, Kearon C, Gent M, Hirsh J. The relation between the APTT response and recurrence in patients with venous thrombosis treated with continuous intravenous heparin. Arch Intern Med 1996;156:1677–81.

4. Levine MN, Raskob GE, Landefeld S, Hirsh J. Hemorrhagic complications of anticoagulant treatment. Chest 1995;108:(Suppl):276s–90s.

5. Hirsh J, Fuster V. Guide to anticoagulant therapy. Part 1: heparin. Part 2: oral anticoagulants. Circulation 1994;89:1449–80.

6. Hull RD, Raskob GE, Rosenbloom D, et al. Optimal therapeutic level of heparin therapy in patients with venous thrombosis. Arch Intern Med 1992;152:1589–95.

7. Raschke RA, Reilly BM, Guidry JR, Fontana JR, Srinivas S. The weight-based heparin dosing nomogram compared with a "standard care" nomogram: a randomized controlled trial. Ann Intern Med 1993;119:874–81.

8. Cruickshank MK, Levine MN, Hirsh J, Roberts R, Siguenza M. A standard heparin nomogram for the management of heparin therapy. Arch Intern Med 1991;151:333–7.

9. Brill-Edwards P, Ginsberg JS, Johnston M, Hirsh J. Establishing a therapeutic range for heparin therapy. Ann Intern Med 1993;119:104–9.

10. Hirsh J, Levine MN. Low-molecular-weight heparin. Blood 1992;79:1–17.

11. Lensing AWA, Prins MH, Davidson BL, Hirsh J. Treatment of deep vein thrombosis with low-molecular-weight heparins. A meta-analysis. Arch Intern Med 1995;155:601–7.

12. Leizorovicz A, Simonneau G, Decousus H, Boissel JP. Comparison of efficacy and safety of low-molecular-weight heparins and unfractionated heparin in initial treatment of deep vein thrombosis: a meta-analysis. Br Med J 1994;309:299–304.

13. Siragusa S, Cosmi B, Piovella F, Hirsh J, Ginsberg JS. Low-molecular-weight heparins and unfractionated heparin in the treatment of patients with acute venous thromboembolism: results of a meta-analysis. Am J Med 1996;100:269–77.

14. Koopman MMW, Prandoni P, Piovella F, et al. Treatment of venous thrombosis with intravenous unfractionated heparin administered in the hospital as compared with subcutaneous low-molecular-weight heparin administered at home. N Engl J Med 1996; 334:682–7.

15. Levine M, Gent M, Hirsh J, et al. A comparison of low-molecular-weight heparin administered primarily at home with unfractionated heparin administered in the hospital for proximal deep vein thrombosis. N Engl J Med 1996;334:677–81.

16. The Columbus Investigators. Low-molecular-weight heparin in the treatment of patients with venous thromboembolism. N Engl J Med 1997;337:657–62.

17. Simmoneau G, Sors H, Charbonnier B, et al. A comparison of low molecular weight heparin with unfractionated heparin for acute pulmonary embolism. N Engl J Med 1997;337:663–9.

18. Harrison L, Johnston M, Massicotte MP, Crowther M, Moffat K, Hirsh J. Comparison of 5-mg and 10-mg loading doses in initiation of warfarin therapy. Ann Intern Med 1997;126:133–6.

Chapter 12

THROMBOLYTIC THERAPY FOR PULMONARY EMBOLISM AND DEEP VEIN THROMBOSIS

David R Anderson

Pulmonary embolism and deep vein thrombosis are caused by fibrin deposition and subsequent obstruction of portions of the pulmonary arterial and deep venous circulation, respectively. The use of thrombolytic agents to lyse these thrombi and relieve the vascular obstruction would seem to be a rational treatment approach for patients with pulmonary embolism or deep vein thrombosis, especially given the benefits of lytic agents for the treatment of patients with acute myocardial infarction. In this chapter, we review the clinical data evaluating thrombolytic therapy for the treatment of pulmonary embolism and deep vein thrombosis and provide guidelines for its use.

THROMBOLYTIC THERAPY FOR PULMONARY EMBOLISM

Parenteral unfractionated heparin therapy followed by warfarin is the standard treatment for patients with acute pulmonary embolism. Deaths are uncommon, occurring in less than 3% of patients treated for acute pulmonary embolism.[1]

Thrombolytic therapy has been compared with unfractionated heparin for the treatment of acute pulmonary embolism in randomized controlled clinical trials. Studies involving tissue plasminogen activator, streptokinase, or urokinase have consistently demonstrated that thrombolytic agents cause more rapid lysis of pulmonary emboli than unfractionated heparin treatment alone.[2,3] However, the early benefits of thrombolytic therapy appear to be short lived, since by 5 to 7 days after the initiation of treatment, as much pulmonary arterial clot lysis has occurred in patients who have received thrombolytic therapy as in those patients treated with unfractionated heparin alone.[4,5]

Although thrombolytic agents clearly cause more rapid improvements in the hemodynamic and radiographic parameters associated with acute pulmonary embolism, to date these have not translated into improved patient outcomes. Results from individual studies and a pooled analysis of clinical trials comparing thrombolytic therapy with unfractionated heparin therapy have not demonstrated that thrombolytic therapy results in a reduction of either the morbidity or the mortality of patients with acute pulmonary embolism.[3,6] Furthermore, thrombolytic therapy is associated with an increased risk of major bleeding, including intracerebral hemorrhage. Estimates from acute myocardial infarction trials using thrombolytic therapy have reported intracerebral bleeding rates of about 0.5%.[7] Major bleeding complications occur in about 20% of patients with acute pulmonary embolism who receive thrombolytic therapy and are usually related to the performance of invasive procedures, namely, pulmonary angiography.[7]

Is there a role then for thrombolytic therapy for the treatment of acute pulmonary embolism? This consideration must be tempered with the potential for serious bleeding side effects and the lack of proven clinically important benefits with its use. However, the clinical trials performed to date have been underpowered to detect a significant benefit from thrombolytic therapy. There may be a therapeutic benefit of thrombolytic therapy to patients who are hemodynamically compromised with acute pulmonary embolism, in whom rapid clot lysis could have important clinical consequences.[8] Such patients may include those who present with cardiovascular compromise manifest by hypotension, severe right ventricular strain, and/or the presence of thrombus within the right atrium or ventricle of the heart. Subgroup analyses of clinical trials have suggested that these patients are at much higher risk of mortality from acute pulmonary embolism and, thus, may be more likely to benefit from the addition of thrombolytic therapy.[6,9] Thrombolytic therapy should be strongly considered in patients who are hemodynamically compromised by acute pulmonary embolism, especially if a deterioration in their condition occurs despite heparin therapy.

THROMBOLYTIC THERAPY FOR THE TREATMENT OF DEEP VEIN THROMBOSIS

As with acute pulmonary embolism, a parenteral heparin preparation (either unfractionated or low-molecular-weight heparin) followed by warfarin has been proven to be very safe and effective therapy for patients with acute deep vein thrombosis. Mortality from pulmonary embolism is very rare once anticoagulant therapy has been instituted for the treatment of acute deep vein thrombosis. The major argument for the use of thrombolytic therapy for the treatment of deep vein thrombosis is for its potential to prevent the development of postphlebitic syndrome. The postphlebitic syndrome is characterized by pain and swelling of the extremity along with a stasis dermatitis that may result in ulcer formation in the skin overlying the medial malleolus. It is caused by venous valvular incompetence and/or vessel obstruction that is a consequence of the damage from the deep vein thrombosis.[2]

Thrombolytic therapy has proven to be more efficacious than unfractionated heparin at inducing clot lysis and in maintaining venous valvular patency in patients with an acute deep vein thrombosis.[10] However, clinical trial results have been conflicting, and it remains controversial whether thrombolytic therapy significantly reduces the development of the postphlebitic syndrome.[11,12] The risk of major bleeding from thrombolytic therapy remains for patients with deep vein thrombosis tilting the benefit/risk ratio against using thrombolysis for the treatment of this condition.

Who, if anyone, should receive thrombolytic therapy for the treatment of acute deep vein thrombosis? The clear indication for use of thrombolytic therapy

Management of Acute Pulmonary Embolism

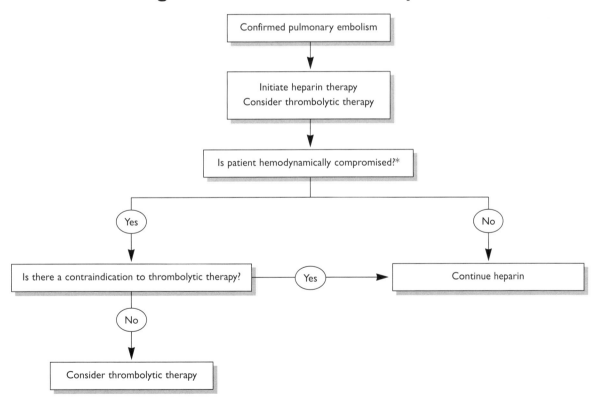

*Hemodynamic compromise may be defined as systolic blood pressure less than 90 mm Hg despite fluid support or as a decline of over 30 mm Hg in baseline systolic blood pressure with clinical evidence of end-organ hypoperfusion.

is a patient with massive deep vein thrombosis who, despite heparin, is developing limb gangrene secondary to the occlusion. Heparin-induced thrombocytopenia should be excluded in such patients. Patients presenting with their first episode of an acute massive proximal deep vein thrombosis without limb gangrene whose symptom onset is less than 72 hours duration may also possibly benefit from thrombolysis.[10] However, conclusive evidence to support use of thrombolytics for this latter indication await confirmation from controlled clinical trials.

THROMBOLYTIC AGENTS AND ROUTE OF ADMINISTRATION

Streptokinase, urokinase, and tissue plasminogen activator have all been used clinically for the treatment of pulmonary embolism and deep vein thrombosis. Streptokinase and urokinase regimens are administered by continuous infusion over a 12- to 24-hour period for the treatment of acute pulmonary embolism and over a 24- to 72-hour period for the treatment of acute deep vein thrombosis (Table 12.1). There is no clear correlation between in vitro tests of fibrinolysis and patient outcome. It is generally recommended that a thrombin time or an activated partial thromboplastin time (aPTT) be performed 2 to 4 hours after the initiation of streptokinase or urokinase. A prolongation of the thrombin time or aPTT by 10 seconds or more is sufficient to demonstrate the fibrinolytic effect of the drug, and no further monitoring of these thrombolytic agents is required. If a fibrinolytic effect has not been achieved, then the streptokinase or urokinase infusion dose could be increased by 25% and another thrombin time or aPTT repeated 4 hours later. A rapid bolus infusion of streptokinase is not recommended for the treatment of acute pulmonary embolism due to the hypotensive reaction that may occur in up to 10% of patients.

Table 12.1   Thrombolytic Regimens

Agent	Indication	Dose
Streptokinase	DVT/PE	250,000 U bolus over 30 minutes followed by infusion of 100,000 U/hr
Urokinase	DVT/PE	4400 IU/kg over 10 minutes followed by infusion of 4400 IU/kg/hr
Tissue plasminogen activator	PE	a) 100 mg infusion over 2 hours or b) 0.6 mg/kg over 15 minutes (maximum dose 50 mg)
	DVT	0.05 mg/kg/hr over 24 hours (maximum dose 150 mg)

DVT = deep vein thrombosis; PE = pulmonary embolism

Table 12.2   Contraindications to Use of Thrombolytic Therapy

Major bleeding within previous 6 months
Intracranial or intraspinal disease
Hypertension (>200 mm Hg systolic, >110 mm Hg diastolic)
Operation/biopsy, major trauma within 10 days
Endocarditis
Pericarditis
Aneurysm
Bleeding diathesis

For the treatment of pulmonary embolism, tissue plasminogen activator may be administered as a bolus or as an infusion over 2 hours as outlined in Table 12.1. A continuous infusion of tissue plasminogen activator over 24 hours has been used for the treatment of acute deep vein thrombosis. There is no need to measure the thrombin time or aPTT for patients receiving tissue plasminogen activator.

A continuous unfractionated heparin infusion should be instituted, without a bolus, following the completion of thrombolytic therapy, once the patient's aPTT is less than twice the midpoint of the normal aPTT range. For tissue plasminogen activator, heparin may be started immediately upon cessation of the thrombolytic infusion. An aPTT should be measured 4 hours after the initiation of heparin and subsequent dosing adjusted using a validated heparin nomogram.[11]

Clinical trials comparing different agents or routes of administration of thrombolytic therapy for the treatment of pulmonary embolism or deep vein thrombosis are limited and no one agent or regimen has been clearly demonstrated to be superior to another.[6,11]

SELECTION OF PATIENTS FOR THROMBOLYTIC THERAPY

Given the very narrow therapeutic index of thrombolytic therapy for the treatment of venous thrombosis, careful patient selection is mandatory. The diagnosis of venous thromboembolism should be confirmed by valid objective tests before consideration is given to using thrombolytic therapy. Thrombolytic therapy should be avoided in patients whose medical condition places them at considerable risk for clinically important bleeding complications. Such conditions are outlined in Table 12.2.

Bibliography

1. Carson JL, Kelley MA, Duff A, et al. The clinical course of pulmonary embolism. N Engl J Med 1992;326:1240–5.

2. Hirsh J, Hoak J. Management of deep vein thrombosis and pulmonary embolism. Circulation 1996;93:2212–45.

3. Ginsberg JS. Management of venous thromboembolism. N Engl J Med 1996;335:1816–28.

4. Levine M, Hirsh J, Weitz J, et al. A randomized trial of a single bolus dosage regimen of recombinant tissue plasminogen activator in patients with acute pulmonary embolism. Chest 1990;98:1473–9.

5. Urokinase pulmonary embolism trial. Phase 1 results. JAMA 1970;214:2163–72.

6. Anderson DR, Levine MN. Thrombolytic therapy for the treatment of acute pulmonary embolism. Can Med Assoc J 1992;146:1317–24.

7. Levine MN, Goldhaber SZ, Gore JM, Hirsh J, Califf RM. Hemorrhagic complications of thrombolytic therapy in the treatment of myocardial infarction and venous thrombo-embolism. Chest 1995;108:291S–301S.

8. Goldhaber SZ. Thrombolytic therapy in venous thromboembolism. Clin Chest Med 1995;16:307–20.

9. Tapson VF, Witty LA. Massive pulmonary embolism. Clin Chest Med 1995;16:329–40.

10. Rogers LQ, Lutcher CL. Streptokinase therapy for deep vein thrombosis: a comprehensive review of the English literature. Am J Med 1990;88:389–95.

11. Hyers TM, Hull RD, Weg JG. Antithrombotic therapy for venous thromboembolic disease. Chest 1995;108:335S–51S.

12. Kakkar VV, Lawrence D. Hemodynamic and clinical assessment after therapy of acute deep vein thrombosis. Am J Surg 1985;10:54–63.

Chapter 13

Inferior Vena Cava
Interruption

Paul L Cisek

Michael D Malone

Anthony J Comerota

The most feared complication of deep venous thrombosis (DVT) is fatal pulmonary embolism (PE), which continues to be a common cause of in-hospital mortality. In spite of the significant morbidity and mortality associated with DVT and PE, adequate prophylaxis is still underused.[1] Most patients suffering venous thromboembolic complications are managed successfully with anticoagulation. However, patients who cannot be anticoagulated require inferior vena caval (IVC) filtration for mechanical protection against recurrent embolism.

A *Patients with Significant Risk for Pulmonary Embolism*

Deep vein thrombosis represents a spectrum of disease patterns ranging from asymptomatic calf vein thrombosis to venous gangrene. Patients who have a significant risk for PE are those with proximal DVT or pre-existing PE.

A select group of high-risk trauma patients have been identified who have a high risk of DVT.[2] Placement of IVC filters in these patients may reduce the incidence of fatal and nonfatal PE and can be used as an adjunct to, or instead of, prophylactic anticoagulants.[3]

B *Contraindications to Anticoagulation*

Evaluation of patients includes their risk of bleeding from anticoagulation therapy. The well-documented benefits of anticoagulation include decreased clot propagation and embolization and reduced risk of recurrent DVT.[4,5] The benefits of anticoagulation must be weighed against the risk of bleeding.

The indications for vena caval filter placement have been liberalized due to a generally favorable experience and the relative ease of placement. However, vena caval filtration has potentially serious complications; so the decision to insert a filter should be carefully considered. Contraindication to anticoagulation remains the most common indication for IVC filtration (Table 13.1). Careful clinical judgment is necessary to determine whether the risk of anticoagulation outweighs the risk of filter placement in patients with relative contraindications.

C Complications with Anticoagulation

If no contraindication exists, the patient is treated with standard anticoagulation, usually initiated with intravenous unfractionated heparin and converted to oral anticoagulation. Low-molecular-weight heparin given subcutaneously is increasingly used in countries where it is available, and it will likely be approved for treatment in the United States in 1998. The incidence of major bleeding with heparin is approximately 4%. If bleeding occurs in the presence of supratherapeutic anticoagulation, the heparin infusion (oral anticoagulation dose) should be appropriately reduced. Significant bleeding that requires transfusion (> 2 units/24 hr) in the absence of excessive anticoagulation is an indication for an IVC filter.

Heparin-induced thrombocytopenia is an infrequent complication (approximately 3%) that typically occurs 5 to 15 days after the initiation of treatment. The important clinical implication of this syndrome is arterial and venous thrombosis (see Chapter 18).

D Recurrent Pulmonary Embolism, Pulmonary Hypertension, Marginal Cardiopulmonary Reserve

Patients with recurrent PE, pulmonary hypertension, and/or marginal cardiopulmonary reserve have a high risk of severe morbidity and mortality from small pulmonary emboli. Their limited cardiorespiratory reserve places them at increased risk for fatal PE, and, therefore, the physician should have a lower threshold for IVC

Table 13.1   Contraindications to Anticoagulation

Absolute	Relative
1. Active bleeding	1. Recent major surgery (< 5 days), organ biopsy
2. Recent hemorrhagic cerebrovascular accident	2. Active peptic ulcer disease/GI pathology
3. History of heparin sensitivity (urticaria, bronchospasm, anaphylaxis)	3. Recent major trauma
4. History of heparin-induced thrombocytopenia	
5. Underlying bleeding diathesis	
6. Intracranial pathology (subdural hematoma, etc.)	

interruption in such patients. Free-floating iliac or IVC thrombus is particularly susceptible to embolization[6] and patients with large-volume free-floating thrombi, are considered candidates for IVC filtration in some centers.

E IVC and Anticoagulation

Thrombolytic therapy accelerates the resolution of PE.[7,8] Therefore, in patients with hemodynamic instability from PE, thrombolytic therapy should be considered. Preventing recurrent thrombosis can be achieved in most cases with long-term anticoagulation.

F Re-evaluate Contraindication to Anticoagulation

Continued monitoring of the patient's clinical status is important to determining if long-term anticoagulation can be initiated in order to treat the deep venous thrombosis. If the original contraindication to anticoagulation has been eliminated or resolved, anticoagulation should be reinstituted to reduce the risk of recurrent thrombosis.

G Open Vena Caval Ligation

Operative vena caval plication or ligation is seldom performed. In light of the superior patency and reduced complications of percutaneously placed filters, operative vena caval plication is rarely indicated. In instances of poor percutaneous access to the vena cava, open exposure to facilitate placement may be required.

H Percutaneous Placement of Filter

The use of low profile percutaneously placed filters has essentially eliminated the use of an abdominal approach to inferior vena caval interruption. There are essen-

Table 13.2   Comparison of Inferior Vena Caval Filters

Type	Greenfield Stainless Steel	Greenfield Titanium	Vena Tech	Bird's Nest	Simon Nitinol
Number followed	469	123	77	440	102
Recurrent PE	4%	3%	2%	2.7%	4%
Caval patency	98%	100%	92%	97%	81%
Filter patency	98%	nr	63%	81%	nr

nr = not reported. (Data from Greenfield LJ. Caval interruption procedures. In: Rutherford RB, ed. Vascular surgery. 4th edn. W.B. Saunders, 1995.)

Selection for Vena Cava Interruption

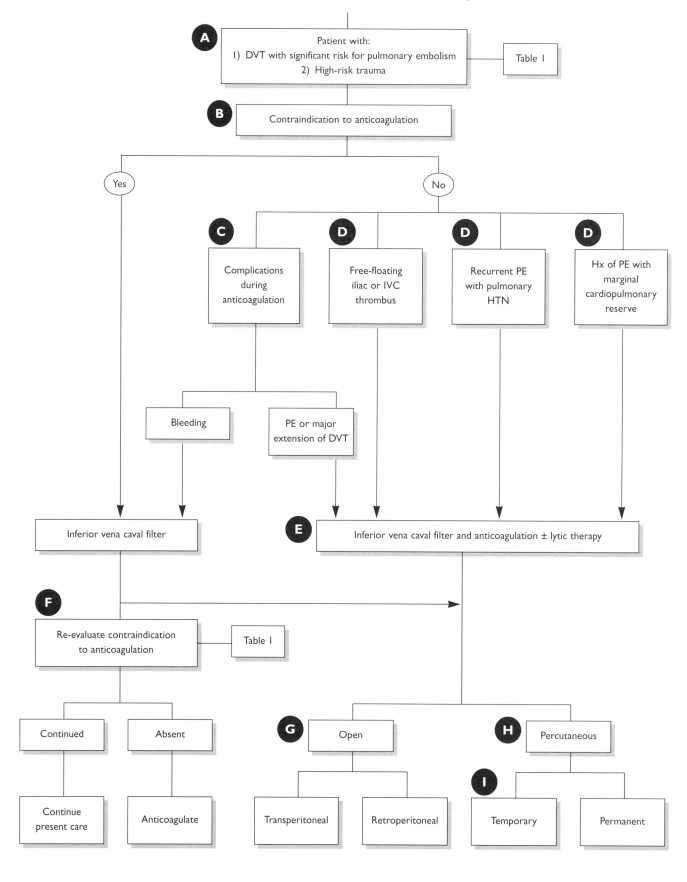

tially five filter types that have reasonably documented follow-up information to compare their effectiveness (Table 13.2)

▎ *Temporary IVC Filters*

Limited data exist on the use of temporary IVC filters.[9] This filter type does not appear to reduce the rate of insertion vein or IVC thrombosis compared with permanent filters; therefore, their advantage over permanent filters is presently unclear.

Bibliography

1. Anderson FA, Wheeler HB. Physician practices in the prevention of venous thromboembolism: a community wide survey. J Vasc Surg 1992;16:707–14.

2. Geerts WH, Code KI, Jay RM, et al. A prospective study of venous thromboembolism after major trauma. N Engl J Med 1994;331:1601–6.

3. Khansarinia S, Dennis JW, Veldenz HC, et al. Prophylactic Greenfield filter placement in selected high-risk trauma patients. J Vasc Surg 1995;22:231–6.

4. Barritt BW, Jordan SC. Anticoagulant drugs in the treatment of pulmonary embolism: a controlled clinical trial. Lancet 1960;1:1309–13.

5. Schulman S, Rhedin A, Lindmarker P, et al. A comparison of six weeks with six months of oral anticoagulant therapy after a first episode of venous thromboembolism. N Engl J Med 1995;332:1661–6.

6. Farber SP, O'Donnell TF, Deterling RA, et al. The clinical implications of acute thrombosis of the inferior vena cava. Surg Gynecol Obstet 1984;158:141–7.

7. Sharma GVRK, Burleson VA, Sasahara AA. Effect of thrombolytic therapy on pulmonary capillary blood volume in patients with pulmonary embolism. N Engl J Med 1980;303:842–7.

8. Sharma GVRK, Folland ED, McIntyre KM, Sasahara AA. Long term hemodynamic benefit of thrombolytic therapy in pulmonary embolic disease.[Abstract] J Am Coll Cardiol 1990;15:65A.

9. Millward SF, Bormanis J, Burbridge BE, Markman SJ, Peterson RA. Preliminary experience with the Gunther temporary inferior vena cava filter. J Vasc Interv Radiol 1994;6:863–8.

Chapter 14

VENOUS THROMBECTOMY

Anthony J Comerota

Iliofemoral venous thrombosis represents the most extreme form of deep venous thrombosis (DVT) and is associated with the most severe acute and long-term sequelae.[1,2] The most effective treatment options for prevention of long-term sequelae from postphlebitic syndrome are directed at eliminating the clot in the iliofemoral venous system thereby restoring unobstructed venous drainage from the leg to the vena cava. Therapeutic anticoagulation should be continued to avoid recurrent thrombosis.

Catheter-directed thrombolysis and surgical thrombectomy are currently popular treatment options that can be used to eliminate a clot from the iliofemoral venous system, and integration of these techniques is a reasonable treatment strategy.[3] Some patients have contraindications to thrombolysis, and there are others in whom thrombolysis fails. Contemporary surgical thrombectomy is a sensible alternative for these patients, provided that a capable and experienced surgeon is available.

Operative approaches in the management of acute DVT of the iliofemoral venous segment have been discouraged during the past two decades because of the results observed in the 1960s and early 1970s.[4,5] It is fair to say that most medical centers in North America do not have a surgeon who has experience with venous thrombectomy. This fact is disappointing since active individuals who develop symptomatic iliofemoral DVT and who are not candidates for, or who fail, catheter-directed thrombolysis can benefit from a properly planned and executed venous thrombectomy. During the past 9 years this author performed 18 venous thrombectomies from a wide referral base, which includes a university hospital. This fact suggests that the majority of patients continue to be treated with standard anticoagulation. It also reflects an increasing enthusiasm for catheter-directed thrombolysis, which is my initial approach if the patient does not have contraindication to thrombolytic therapy.

During the past two decades, the technique of venous thrombectomy has been refined and results have improved.[3,6–10] In a prospective, randomized trial, operative venous thrombectomy with arteriovenous fistula was found to be superior to anticoagulation alone in patients with iliofemoral venous thrombosis.[8] Table 14.1 summarizes technical differences between the contemporary procedure and that performed years earlier.

A *Patient Selection/Diagnostic Tests/Contralateral Iliocavagram*

Patients presenting with symptomatic iliofemoral venous thrombosis within 2 weeks of onset should be considered for a form of treatment that can eliminate their thrombus. Modest, nonpainful swelling in an elderly individual should be treated with anticoagulation. However, patients with pain and discoloration at rest, and previously active individuals with iliofemoral DVT should be considered candidates for catheter-directed lysis or venous thrombectomy. As the age of the thrombus increases, the likelihood of restoring complete patency diminishes. As previously mentioned, catheter-directed thrombolysis is the initial approach in these patients.

A complete evaluation of the full extent of venous thrombosis is required in all patients. Venous duplex imaging can define the limits of the infrainguinal venous thrombosis and that the thrombus extends above the inguinal ligament. A contralateral iliocavagram evaluates the opposite iliofemoral venous system, inferior vena cava, and the proximal extent of ipsilateral clot. If bilateral iliofemoral venous thrombosis is present, a bilateral operative procedure is recommended. If the thrombus extends into the vena cava, consideration must be given to a right retroperitoneal exposure of the vena cava for direct control and extraction. Alternatively, a double-balloon technique (via both femoral veins) with fluoroscopic guidance can be considered.

Table 14.1 Venous Thrombectomy: Comparison of Old and Contemporary Techniques

	Old	Contemporary
Pre Rx phlebography	Occasional	Yes
Venous thrombectomy catheter	No	Yes
Arteriovenous fistula	No	Yes
Operative fluoroscopy and phlebography	No	Yes
Identify and correct iliac vein stenosis	No	Yes
Continuous anticoagulation	Occasional	Yes
Intermittent pneumatic compression (post-operative)	No	Yes

B *Preparation of Operating Room*

The operating room is prepared for intraoperative fluoroscopy of the iliofemoral veins and vena cava and for the capability of completion phlebography.

C *General Anesthesia*

Patients are usually offered general anesthesia since spinal and epidural techniques are frequently contraindicated because of the need for anticoagulation. Local anesthesia is possible but usually unnecessary.

D *Inguinal Incision/Venotomy*

An inguinal incision is performed exposing the common femoral vein, sapheno-femoral junction and origin of the profunda femoral vein. The extent of the dissection and the location of the venotomy will depend upon the extent of the venous thrombosis. If the thrombus is limited to the suprainguinal iliofemoral system, a transverse venotomy is performed. If the patient has associated infrainguinal venous thrombosis, a longitudinal venotomy is made extending over the orifices of the profunda femoral and superficial femoral veins.

E *Iliofemoral ± Infrainguinal Thrombectomy*

An iliofemoral thrombectomy is performed with a #8 or #10 balloon venous thrombectomy catheter. The catheter is advanced part way into the iliac venous system, extracting portions of the thrombus prior to entry into the vena cava. Upon entry into the vena cava, positive airway pressure is applied that produces increased abdominal pressure and retrograde blood flow in the iliac veins, thereby reducing the potential for embolization.

The leg is elevated, and a snug-fitting rubber bandage is applied from the toes to the upper thigh to squeeze the loosely adherent thrombus from the infrainguinal venous segment. Retrograde passage of a balloon catheter through the infrainguinal veins is attempted but usually is unsuccessful due to the venous valves.

In patients with extensive infrainguinal venous thrombosis, in whom lower limb compression does not expel the thrombus, a cutdown to the posterior tibial vein is performed. A #3 Fogarty catheter is passed proximally, which exits through the common femoral venotomy. A balloon thrombectomy catheter (#4 Fogarty catheter) is attached to the #3 Fogarty catheter and is guided in retrograde fashion into the posterior tibial vein in order to perform an infrainguinal venous thrombectomy. This is repeated as indicated. The infrainguinal venous system is then flushed with copious amounts of heparinized saline via a large bore catheter placed in the posterior tibial vein. The irrigation solution and large amounts of thrombus are retrieved from the common femoral venotomy. A urokinase solution is then infused into the leg and a heparin infusion catheter placed in the posterior tibial vein for postoperative anticoagulation.

F *Completion Phlebography*

Completion phlebography is performed through the common femoral venotomy to evaluate for residual thrombus and the presence of an iliac vein stenosis.

G *Balloon Angioplasty/Stent*

A balloon angioplasty is performed if a focal iliac vein stenosis is present. If resolution is observed with balloon angioplasty, no further intervention is required. If recoil of the stenotic segment occurs, an appropriately sized stent is inserted.

H *Arteriovenous Fistula*

An arteriovenous fistula is constructed, frequently using the transected greater saphenous vein to the side of the superficial femoral artery. Often, a thrombectomy of the greater saphenous is required in order to restore patency. If a large proximal branch of the saphenous vein is available, it will be used in preference to the main saphenous vein. A small sleeve of polytetrafluoroethylene is placed around the proximal saphenous vein and looped with an "0" monofilament suture to be left in the subcutaneous space, in the event the arteriovenous fistula needs to be operatively closed in the future.

Common femoral venous pressures are recorded before and after the arteriovenous fistula is opened. If the venous pressure increases when the fistula is opened, one must suspect that there is a residual iliac vein stenosis or that the fistula is too large. After the iliac venous segment is re-evaluated to ensure unobstructed venous return, the fistula is narrowed to reduce venous pressure to normal. The purpose of the fistula is to increase venous velocity and thereby reduce recurrent thrombosis. It should not increase venous pressure. The arteriovenous fistula is generally considered to be permanent although some will close spontaneously due to neointimal fibroplasia.

I *Maintain Therapeutic Anticoagulation*

At the time of diagnosis, patients are fully anticoagulated with intravenous heparin and maintained at a therapeutic level throughout their operative and postoperative course. Patients are converted to oral anticoagulation with warfarin when oral intake begins postoperatively. However, a preoperative dose is frequently given if time allows. The duration of anticoagulant therapy is discussed elsewhere.

Iliofemoral Venous Thrombosis

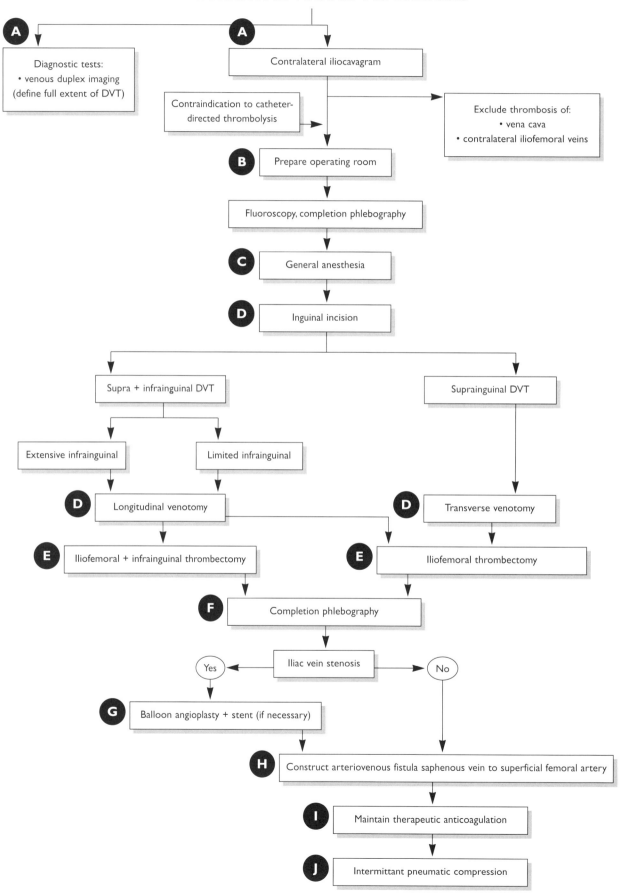

J *Intermittent Pneumatic Compression*

Intermittent pneumatic compression devices are applied to both lower extremities in the recovery room and continued until the patient is fully ambulatory.

Bibliography

1. O'Donnell TF, Browse NL, Burnard KG, et al. The socioeconomic effects of an iliofemoral thrombosis. J Surg Res 1977;22:483–8.
2. Cockett FB, Thomas L. The iliac compression syndrome. Br J Surg 1995;52:816–21.
3. Comerota AJ, Aldridge SC, Cohen G, et al. A strategy of aggressive regional therapy for acute iliofemoral venous thrombosis with contemporary venous thrombectomy or catheter-directed thrombolysis. J Vasc Surg 1994;20:244–54.
4. Karp RB, Wylie EJ. Recurrent thrombosis after iliofemoral venous thrombectomy. Surg Forum 1966;17:147.
5. Lansing AM, Davis WM. Five-year follow-up study of iliofemoral venous thrombectomy. Ann Surg 1968;168:620–8.
6. Juhan C, Cornillon B, Tobiana F, et al. Etude de la permeabilite des thrombectomies veineuse iliofemorales et ilio-caves. Ann Chir Vasc 1987;1:529–33.
7. Einarsson E, Albrechtsson V, Eklof B. Thrombectomy and temporary arteriovenous fistula in iliofemoral vein thrombosis: technical considerations and early results. Int Angiol 1986;5:65–70.
8. Plate G, Einarsson E, Ohlin P, et al. Thrombectomy with temporary arteriovenous fistula in acute iliofemoral venous thrombosis. J Vasc Surg 1984;1:867–76.
9. Eklof B, Juhan C. Revival of thrombectomy in management of acute iliofemoral venous thrombosis. Contemp Surg 1992;40:21–30.
10. Torngren S, Swedenborg J. Thrombectomy and temporary arteriovenous fistula for iliofemoral venous thrombosis. Int Angiol 1988;7:14–8.

Additional Reading

Comerota AJ. Venous thromboembolism. In: Rutherford RB, ed. Vascular surgery. Philadelphia: W.B. Saunders, 1995.

Chapter 15

ANTICOAGULATION
DURING PREGNANCY

Shannon M Bates

Jeffrey S Ginsberg

Indications for anticoagulant therapy during pregnancy include prevention of venous thromboembolism in patients with familial thrombophilia or previous venous thrombosis, treatment of acute venous thromboembolism, and prevention of systemic embolism in patients with prosthetic heart valves or native valvular heart disease. Heparin and/or acetylsalicylic acid are also used to prevent pregnancy loss in selected individuals with the antiphospholipid antibody syndrome.

A Unfractionated Heparin

Unfractionated heparin is a heterogeneous, sulfated, long-chain acidic glycosamino-glycan with a mean molecular weight of 12,000 to 15,000 daltons that is extracted from bovine or porcine lung or gut.[1] It functions as a catalytic cofactor for antithrombin, an endogenous inhibitor of serine proteases, increasing its ability to neutralize thrombin, factor Xa, factor IXa, factor XIa, and factor XIIa.[1] For most indications, heparin is the anticoagulant of choice during pregnancy since it does not cross the placenta.[2] While a review of published reports concluded that unfractionated heparin use during pregnancy was associated with adverse fetal outcomes in approximately one-third of cases,[3] both a critical review of the literature[4] and a retrospective cohort study of 100 consecutive pregnancies[5] concluded that maternal therapy with unfractionated heparin is safe for the fetus. The reported frequency of maternal bleeding in that cohort study was 2%.[5] Because unfractionated heparin does not cross the placenta, there is no increased bleeding risk for the fetus. Heparin-induced thrombocytopenia (see Chapter 18) is an immunologic phenomenon associated with a decrease in platelet count some 7 to 10 days after initiating heparin therapy.[6] In nonpregnant patients, it has been reported to occur in approximately 4% of those receiving therapeutic doses of unfractionated heparin.[6] Paradoxical thrombosis associated with heparin-induced thrombocytopenia can result in deep vein thrombosis, pulmonary embolism, major arterial thrombosis, gangrene, and limb loss.[6] Long-term heparin therapy has been reported to cause osteoporosis.[7] While the incidence of overt fracture is probably less than 5%,[7] subclinical bone density reduction has been reported in up to one-third of patients receiving greater than 1 month of therapeutic dose unfractionated heparin therapy.[7] There is some suggestion that heparin-induced osteoporosis is at least partly reversible.[7] Heparin appears to be safe for the infants of breastfeeding mothers.

B *Oral Anticoagulants*

The oral anticoagulants produce their anticoagulant effect by interfering with the hepatic synthesis of the vitamin K-dependent coagulation factors II, VII, IX, and X.[8] They cross the placenta readily and can produce a characteristic embryopathy, central nervous system abnormalities, and fetal bleeding.[7] Warfarin embryopathy is characterized by nasal hypoplasia and/or stippled epiphyses,[3] and it is associated with warfarin exposure between the 6th and 12th weeks of gestation.[9] While the true incidence of warfarin embryopathy is not known, up to 30% of all infants exposed to warfarin between 6 and 12 weeks of gestation have been reported to be affected.[9] The central nervous system abnormalities associated with maternal oral anticoagulant use include dorsal midline dysplasia with agenesis of the corpus callosum, Dandy-Walker malformations, midline cerebellar atrophy, ventral midline dysplasia with optic atrophy and blindness, and hemorrhage.[3] Unlike warfarin embropathy, which has only been reported with first trimester warfarin exposure, central nervous system abnormalities can occur after warfarin exposure at any point in gestation.[3] While the incidence of these anomalies appears low (i.e., <5%), their long-term sequelae have the potential to be more devastating than those associated with warfarin embryopathy.[3] When warfarin use is continued until term, the trauma of delivery can result in significant fetal hemorrhage.[7] Therefore, if warfarin is used during pregnancy, its use should be restricted to the second and third trimesters and avoided near term in order to prevent delivery of an anticoagulated fetus.[7] Warfarin appears safe for the breastfeeding infants of women receiving warfarin. Small studies have found no warfarin activity in the breast milk of warfarin-treated patients or in their infants' circulation.[7]

Two approaches can be taken to lessen the risk of thrombotic complications and warfarin embryopathy in women requiring long-term anticoagulation who wish to become pregnant. One approach is to continue warfarin therapy and perform frequent pregnancy tests. As soon as pregnancy is diagnosed and prior to the sixth week of gestation, heparin therapy is substituted. This assumes that warfarin is safe during the first 4 to 6 weeks of pregnancy.[7] The other approach is to discontinue warfarin and initiate heparin therapy once the decision is made to attempt pregnancy. This approach has the potential to expose the patient to many months of heparin therapy, increasing her risk of heparin-induced osteoporosis.[7]

C *Low-Molecular-Weight Heparin*

Low-molecular-weight heparins are heparin fragments produced by chemical or enzymatic depolymerization of unfractionated heparin, or heparin fractions that are separated by gel filtration on the basis of molecular weight.[10] Low-molecular-weight heparins may be advantageous during pregnancy because of their long half-life, which may allow once-daily dosing,[7] their more predictable anticoagulant response,[7] which may obviate the need for monitoring, and their decreased association with heparin-induced thrombocytopenia.[6] Their use is also likely associated with a decreased risk of heparin-induced osteoporosis.[7] In nonpregnant patients, low-molecular-weight heparins have been shown to be at least as effective and safe as unfractionated heparin in the treatment of acute proximal deep vein thrombosis[11,12] and in the prevention of deep vein thrombosis in patients who undergo both general and orthopedic surgery.[13] Numerous studies have demonstrated that these agents do not cross the placenta.[7] Although there is a growing experience with the use of low-molecular-weight heparins in pregnant patients, they are more expensive than unfractionated heparins, and there is a lack of published clinical trials comparing their efficacy and safety with unfractionated heparin in this patient population.

D *Aspirin*

Aspirin has the potential to cause both bleeding and birth defects in the fetus. While the safety of doses of more than 150 mg/day and/or aspirin ingestion in the first trimester of pregnancy is controversial, the use of low-dose aspirin (60 to 150 mg/day) during the second and third trimesters has not been associated with adverse fetal or neonatal effects.[14]

E *Valvular Heart Disease in Pregnancy*

Antithrombotic therapy of valvular heart disease in pregnancy is controversial and is reviewed in Chapter 45.

F *Treatment of Deep Vein Thrombosis and Pulmonary Embolism During Pregnancy*

Depending on the severity of the thrombosis and the response to therapy, patients should receive intravenous unfractionated heparin therapy for 5 to 10 days.[7] This is usually initiated with an intravenous bolus dose of 5000 units, followed by a main-tenance continuous infusion of at least 30,000 units per 24 hours titrated to prolong the activated partial thromboplastin time (aPTT) into the therapeutic range.[15] After the initial intravenous therapy, subcutaneous unfractionated heparin should be given for the duration of the pregnancy every 12 hours in doses adjusted to prolong the midinterval (6 hours postinjection) aPTT into the therapeutic range.[7] The aPTT should be monitored every 1 to 2 weeks, as heparin requirements may vary through-out pregnancy. To minimize the volume of injection, concentrated heparin solutions should be used. Although there is little data in pregnant patients, it is very likely that initial, followed by long-term, low-molecular-weight heparin is a reasonable substitute for unfractionated heparin in this patient population.

The anticoagulant response to subcutaneous unfractionated heparin can be prolonged, causing a persistent anticoagulant effect for up to 28 hours, when it is administered in high doses just before delivery.[7] Persistent anticoagulation at deliv-ery can make epidural analgesia hazardous and has the potential to cause excessive bleeding. The mechanism of this prolonged anticoagulant effect is unknown. This potential problem can be avoided by electively inducing labor close to term (e.g., at 37 weeks) and stopping heparin therapy 24 hours prior to induction.[7] The aPTT must be checked prior to delivery in order to ensure that it has normalized with the discontinuation of heparin. If the aPTT is greater than 1.5 times control, the heparin effect should be reversed with protamine sulfate.[7] An intravenous infusion of unfractionated heparin should be started after discontinuation of subcutaneous heparin in patients considered at high risk for thrombotic complications.[15] This infusion can then be discontinued 4 to 6 hours before the anticipated time of delivery, with the expectation that the aPTT will be within normal limits at delivery.[15] If a pregnant women receiving dose-adjusted subcutaneous heparin enters labor spontaneously, heparin injections should be discontinued immediately. Protamine sulfate may be necessary if the aPTT prior to delivery is excessively prolonged.

As the risk of postpartum venous thromboembolism is significant, therapeutic doses of subcutaneous or intravenous heparin should be restarted as soon as ade-quate hemostasis is achieved after delivery.[15] Warfarin should be started the same day. Heparin should be continued until the warfarin has reached a therapeutic level (international normalized ratio of 2.0 to 3.0) for 2 consecutive days.[15] Oral anti-coagulants should be continued for 4 to 6 weeks postpartum or for a minimum of 3 months when the venous thromboembolic event occurs late in pregnancy (i.e., third trimester).[15]

G *Thromboembolism Prophylaxis During Pregnancy*

Patients with previous venous thromboembolism have an increased risk for recurrent events.[7] There is a commonly held view that women with a previous history of deep vein thrombosis or pulmonary embolism have an increased risk of recurrence during pregnancy and the postpartum period. Reliable estimates of the rate of recurrent venous thromboembolism in these women are not available. Women who developed their initial thrombosis in the presence of a transient risk factor might be expected to have a lower risk of recurrence than those whose event was idiopathic, associated with a previous pregnancy, or who have an ongoing risk factor.[7]

The presence of inherited deficiencies of antithrombin (AT), protein C (PC), and protein S (PS) as well as activated protein C resistance (APC-R) is associated with an increased risk of venous thrombosis. While it is difficult to assess the increased risk of venous thromboembolism during pregnancy and the postpartum period in women with these inherited abnormalities, it appears to be greater for AT deficient than for PC or PS deficient patients.[15] Moreover, for each of these abnormalities, the risk appears to be greater in the postpartum than the antepartum period.[15]

H *Prophylaxis in Women with Previous Venous Thromboembolism*

The optimal management of pregnant women with previous venous thromboembolism is not known. The pattern of practice varies widely, from clinical surveillance to aggressive antepartum heparin therapy with postpartum warfarin therapy. There is no consensus on optimal prophylaxis among various consensus panels. The American College of Chest Physicians (1995) provides three options: (1) 5000 units of unfractionated heparin subcutaneously every 12 hours throughout pregnancy, (2) dose-adjusted unfractionated heparin to produce a heparin level of 0.1 to 0.2 U/ml by antifactor Xa activity throughout pregnancy, or (3) clinical surveillance combined with periodic impedance plethysmography or compression ultrasound for those women who cannot, or will not, use heparin or for those who developed their prior thrombosis in association with a transient risk factor. For each of these regimens, 4 to 6 weeks of postpartum warfarin is also recommended.[7] The British Society for Haematology Guidelines recommend prophylaxis with either 5000 units of unfractionated heparin every 12 hours during the first and second trimesters with an increase in dosage sufficient to prolong the midinterval aPTT to 1.5 times control in the third trimester or 10,000 units of unfractionated heparin every 12 hours throughout pregnancy (with a decrease in dose only if the heparin level is greater than 0.3 U/ml).[16] Meanwhile, the Maternal and Neonatal Haemostasis Working Party of the Haemostasis and Thrombosis Task[17] suggests delaying anticoagulation

Anticoagulants Required during Pregnancy

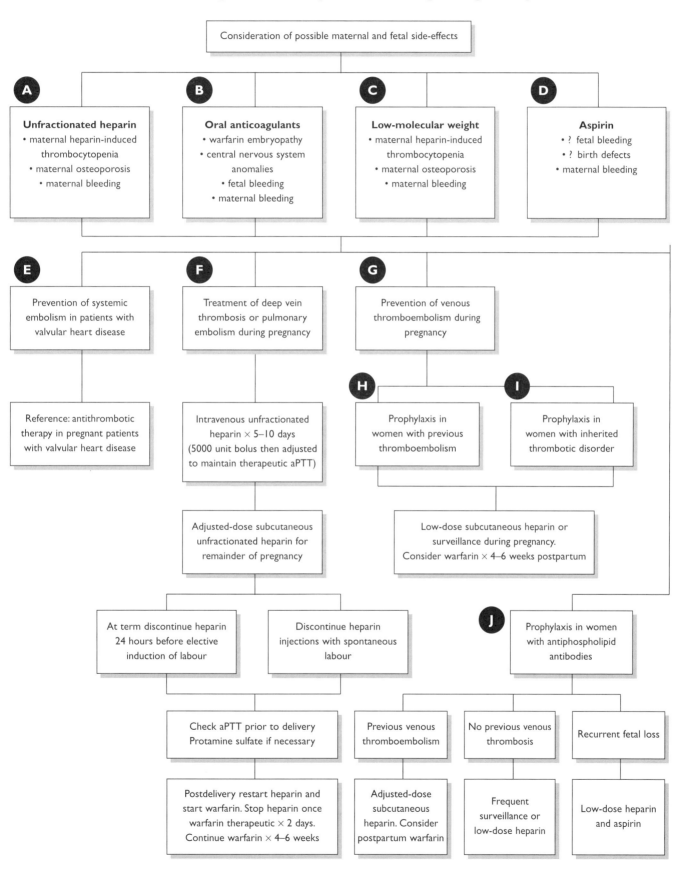

until the puerperium in those women in whom the episode occurred postnatally and introducing heparin 4 to 6 weeks before the stage at which thrombosis occurred in those patients with a history of thrombosis during pregnancy. Women whose thrombosis was not associated with pregnancy may be given prophylaxis through-out pregnancy if their previous episode was severe or during the third trimester and puerperium if the previous episode was less serious. Recommended doses include 7500 units of unfractionated heparin every 12 hours if used before 36 weeks gestation or postpartum and 10,000 units every 12 hours when used from 36 weeks to term. Again, prophylaxis with warfarin is recommended for at least 6 weeks postpartum.[17]

I *Prophylaxis in Women with Inherited Thrombotic Disorders*

The management of women with inherited deficiencies of AT, PC, or PS or APC-R is controversial. Patients with an inherited hypercoagulable state and previous deep vein thrombosis or pulmonary embolism are often receiving long-term anticoagu-lation. In these individuals, warfarin should be replaced by therapeutic doses of heparin (i.e., aPTT/heparin level) before 6 weeks gestation.[7] The optimal manage-ment of asymptomatic individuals not receiving long-term anticoagulation is unknown. Studies suggest that anticoagulant prophylaxis is worthwhile during the postpartum period.[7] It is not clear that prophylaxis is required during pregnancy, especially for PS deficient patients.[7] Clearly, each women must be considered indi-vidually. Those with a strong family history of thrombosis may merit prophylactic anticoagulation. Others could be managed with low-dose heparin throughout pregnancy or with regular surveillance consisting of clinical assessment combined with impedance plethysmography and/or compression ultrasonography.[7]

J *Prophylaxis in Women with Antiphospholipid Antibodies*

Antiphospholipid antibodies include anticardiolipin antibodies (detected by immunoassays) and lupus anticoagulant (detected using clotting-based assays). The presence of persistent antiphospholipid antibodies may be associated with recurrent venous thrombosis, arterial thrombosis, thrombocytopenia, and fetal loss.[7] It is not clear whether women with antiphospholipid antibodies but no prior history of thrombosis should receive anticoagulant prophylaxis. Clinical practice usually includes frequent surveillance or prophylactic low-dose heparin throughout preg-nancy.[7] Dose-adjusted subcutaneous unfractionated heparin is a reasonable approach to prophylaxis in pregnant women with antiphospholipid antibodies and previous venous thrombosis.[7] Patients receiving long-term oral anticoagulation should be switched to full-dose subcutaneous heparin before the sixth week of gestation. The optimal therapy for women with antiphospholipid antibodies and recurrent fetal loss is unknown. The best results to date have been obtained with the use of aspirin (75 to 80 mg of aspirin per day) throughout pregnancy and low-dose unfractionated heparin starting as soon as a viable pregnancy is confirmed.[18,19]

Bibliography

1. Salzman EW, Hirsh J, Marder VJ. Clinical use of heparin. In: Colman RW, Hirsh J, Marder VJ, Salzman EW, eds. Hemostasis and thrombosis: basic principles and clinical practice . 3rd edn. Philadelphia: J.B. Lippincott Co. 1994.

2. Flessa HC, Kapstrom AB, Glueck HI, Will J. Placental transport of heparin. Am J Obstet Gynecol 1965;93:570–3.

3. Hall JG, Pauli RM, Wilson KM. Maternal and fetal sequelae of anticoagulants during pregnancy. Am J Med 1980;68:122–40.

4. Ginsberg JS, Hirsh J, Turner DC, Levine MN, Burrows R. Risks to the fetus of anticoagulant therapy during pregnancy. Thromb Haemost 1989;61:197–203.

5. Ginsberg JS, Kowalchuk G, Hirsh J, Brill-Edwards P, Burrows R. Heparin therapy during pregnancy: risks to the fetus and mother. Arch Intern Med 1989;149:2233–6.

6. Warkentin TE, Levine MN, Hirsh J, et al. Heparin-induced thrombocytopenia in patients treated with low-molecular-weight heparin or unfractionated heparin. N Engl J Med 1995;332:1330–5.

7. Ginsberg JS, Hirsh J. Use of antithrombotic agents during pregnancy. Chest 1995;108(Suppl): 305S–11S.

8. Hirsh J, Ginsberg JS, Marder VJ. Anticoagulant therapy with coumarin agents. In: Colman RW, Hirsh J, Marder VJ, Salzman EW, eds. Hemostasis and thrombosis: basic principles and clinical practice. 3rd edn. Philadelphia: J.B. Lippincott Co. 1994.

9. Iturbe-Alessio I, Fonseca MC, Mutchnik O, Santos MA, Zajarias A, Salazar E. Risks of anticoagulant therapy in pregnant women with artificial heart valves. N Engl J Med 1986;315: 1390–3.

10. Hirsh J, Levine M. Low-molecular-weight heparin. Blood 1992;79:1–17.

11. Koopman MMW, Prandoni P, Piovella F, et al. Treatment of venous thrombosis with intravenous unfractionated heparin administered in the hospital as compared with subcutaneous low-molecular-weight heparin administered at home. N Engl J Med 1996;334:682–7.

12. Levine M, Gent M, Hirsh J, et al. A comparison of low-molecular-weight heparin administered primarily at home with unfractionated heparin administered in the hospital for proximal deep-vein thrombosis. N Engl J Med 1996;334:677–81.

13. Nurmohamed MT, Rosendaal FR, Buller HR, et al. Low-molecular-weight heparin in general and orthopaedic surgery: a meta-analysis. Lancet 1992;340:152–6.

14. CLASP Collaborative Group. CLASP: a randomized trial of low dose aspirin for the prevention and treatment of preeclampsia among 9,364 pregnant women. Lancet 1994;343:619–29.

15. Demers C, Ginsberg JS. Deep vein thrombosis and pulmonary embolism in pregnancy. Clin Chest Med 1992;13:645–56.

16. Colvin BT, Barrowcliff TW. The British Society for Haematology guidelines on the use and monitoring of heparin 1992: second revision. J Clin Pathol 1993;45:97–103.

17. Maternal and Neonatal Haemostasis Working Party of the Haemostasis and Thrombosis Task. Guidelines on the presentation, investigation, and management of thrombosis associated with pregnancy. J Clin Pathol 1993;47:489–96.

18. Cowchock FS, Reece EA, Balaban D, Branch DW, Plouffe L. Repeated fetal losses associated with antiphospholipid antibodies: a collaborative randomized trial comparing prednisone with low-dose heparin treatment. Am J Obstet Gynecol 1992;166:1318–23.

19. Rai RS, Regan L, Dave M, Colten H. Randomized trial of aspirin vs. aspirin and heparin in pregnant women with the antiphospholipid syndrome (Abstract). Lupus 1996;5:518.

Chapter 16

Duration of Anticoagulation in Venous Thromboembolism

Clive Kearon

Patients with acute venous thromboembolism (VTE) are treated with heparin for at least 5 days (see Chapter 11), followed by oral anticoagulation (warfarin). The optimal duration of anticoagulation after an acute episode of VTE is determined by assessment of the risk of recurrent VTE, the risk of bleeding, costs of continuing warfarin, and patient preference. The risk of recurrent VTE is highest immediately following an acute episode and falls rapidly with the duration of treatment. Anticoagulation is very effective (risk reduction of over 80%) at preventing recurrent VTE but unless the absolute risk of recurrence is high enough, the burden of anticoagulation is not justified. This chapter outlines an approach to selecting the duration of anticoagulation in individual patients with acute VTE based on a clinical assessment of risk factors for recurrent thrombosis. Additional factors that may influence this decision are shown in Table 16.1. The chapter focuses on patients with symptomatic VTE (DVT and PE) but asymptomatic deep vein thrombosis (DVT) (detected by screening of high-risk patients) is also considered.

A Asymptomatic VTE

Deep vein thrombosis detected by screening tests (i.e., bilateral venography or ultrasonography) following high-risk surgery is termed "asymptomatic." The natural history of these thrombi is uncertain but it is likely that without treatment a minority will cause symptomatic DVT or PE. The optimal treatment of these thrombi is also uncertain. We generally treat asymptomatic isolated distal (not involving the popliteal or more proximal veins) DVT with warfarin for 4 weeks, and until full mobility has been regained, often without initial heparin therapy. Patients with asymptomatic proximal DVT are treated with initial heparin therapy for 5 days and warfarin for

3 months. Ongoing studies will determine if 4 weeks of anticoagulation is adequate therapy for proximal DVT, which occurs following surgery.

B Risk Factors for VTE

Recent studies have identified factors that strongly influence the risk of recurrent VTE.[1-5] An assessment of these risk factors has important implications for the duration of therapy. Risk factor status is determined from clinical data, supplemented by laboratory testing in selected patients; however, the optimal duration of anticoagulation in patients with a first episode of VTE and different risk factor profiles has yet to be determined by prospective studies. Among these subgroups the risk of recurrent VTE differs, and ongoing studies may find that the optimum duration of anticoagulation also differs; they will be considered separately even though they are currently treated with anticoagulants for similar durations.

C First Episode of VTE with Continuing Risk Factors

Patients who develop VTE in association with ongoing risk factors (Table 16.2)

Table 16.1   Additional Factors That May Influence the Duration of Anticoagulation

Patient Factors
Patient preference
Fear of recurrent VTE or bleeding
Impact of anticoagulation on lifestyle
Compliance with medication
Cardiopulmonary reserve
Anticoagulation may be continued if ability to tolerate recurrent VTE is poor
Thromboembolism Factors
Pulmonary embolism may have a higher risk of recurrence than DVT
Distal (calf) DVT probably has a lower risk of recurrence than proximal DVT
Evidence of persistent DVT or PE (i.e., ultrasound, lung scan) may increase the risk of recurrence, and makes diagnosis of recurrence more difficult
Anticoagulant Factors
Geographic inaccessibility
Liver disease
Highly variable anticoagulant response
Additional indications for anticoagulants (i.e., atrial fibrillation)
Bleeding risk
Structural lesions associated with bleeding
A history of anticoagulant-related bleeding
Antiplatelet therapy requirements
Thrombocytopenia
Hereditary or acquired bleeding disorder

Table 16.2   Continuing Risk Factors for Recurrent VTE

Biochemical hypercoagulable states
    Antithrombin deficiency
    Protein C deficiency
    Protein S deficiency
Active malignancy
Lower limb paralysis

have a high risk of recurrent VTE (about 15% per year) if anticoagulants are stopped after 3 months. These patients should be treated for at least 6 months with anticoagulation, and if risk factors do not resolve during this period, treatment should be continued indefinitely. This decision will be strongly influenced by other factors (see Table 16.1).

D *First Episode of "Idiopathic" VTE*

Patients who develop VTE without a risk factor appear to have a high risk of recurrence (over 10% per year) when anticoagulants are stopped. The risk of recurrence is likely to be higher in patients with a first episode of VTE who have a biochemical abnormality known to be associated with thrombosis, compared to those without such abnormalities.[6–8] Screening for protein C, protein S, and antithrombin deficiency is appropriate in patients less than 40 years of age, those having a strong family history of thrombosis (more than one first-degree relative), previous episodes of thrombosis, and/or thrombosis involving unusual sites (see Chapter 21). If any of these biochemical conditions are found, patients are considered to have "continuing risk factors" for thrombosis (section C). The prognostic implications of having activated protein C resistance, a lupus anticoagulant, mild hyperhomocystinemia or an anticardiolipin antibody are less clear. Activated protein C resistance and a persistent lupus anticoagulant are likely associated with an increased risk of recurrence;[6,9–11] however, until the magnitude of the risk and the risk-benefit ratio of extended anticoagulation in patients with these conditions are clarified, we treat these patients for the same duration as patients with idiopathic VTE. We recommend treating patients with idiopathic VTE for at least 6 months. Ongoing studies will determine if more prolonged, or indefinite, anticoagulation is indicated for these patients.

E *First Episode of VTE with a Transient Risk Factor*

Subgroup analyses from recent studies suggest that as little as 4 weeks of treatment is adequate for patients who develop VTE in association with a transient risk factor such as recent surgery or immobilization in a plaster cast because they appear to

Duration of Anticoagulation in Venous Thromboembolism

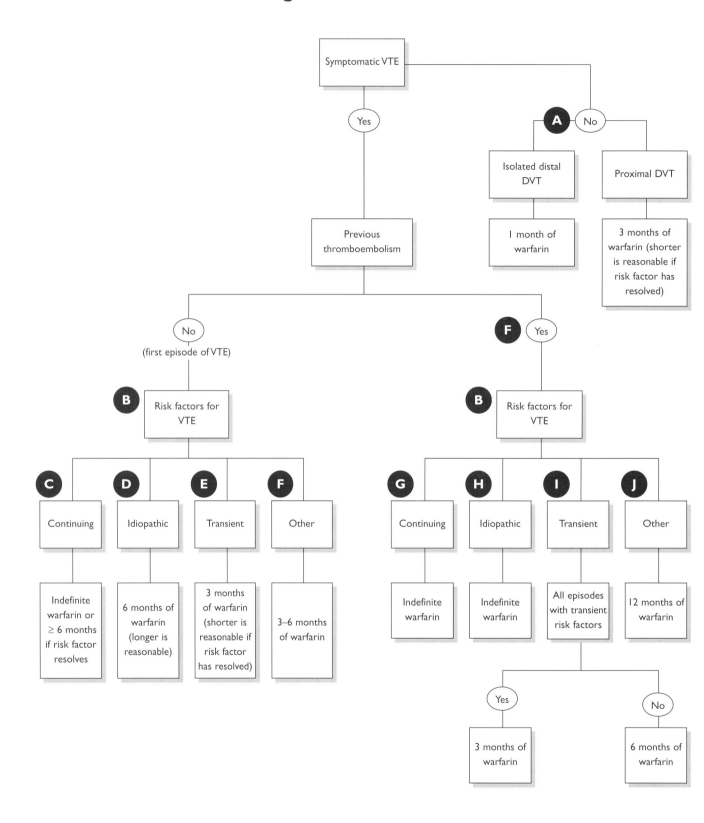

have a low risk of recurrence (less than 5% per year) when anticoagulants are stopped;[1,2,5,12] however, until confirmed by prospective studies, these patients should be treated for 3 months unless there are additional factors which preclude treatment beyond 4 weeks.

F *First Episode of VTE with Unclear Risk Factor Status*

Not all patients can be categorized as having "continuing," "idiopathic," or "transient" risk factor status. Patients may have VTE with immobilization due to an exacerbation of a chronic medical condition that will improve but will not completely resolve (e.g., respiratory or cardiac failure, rheumatoid arthritis). We generally treat such patients for 3 to 6 months.

G *Previous VTE and Continuing Risk Factors*

These patients (see Table 16.2) have a high risk of recurrence and should be anticoagulated indefinitely.

H *Previous VTE and an Idiopathic Recurrence*

These patients have a high risk of recurrence and generally should be anticoagulated indefinitely; however, if all previous episodes of VTE occurred secondary to a transient risk factor, 12 months of anticoagulation is a reasonable alternative.

I *Previous VTE and a Transient Risk Factor*

Despite a previous history of VTE, patients who have a recurrence secondary to a transient risk factor probably do not have a high long-term risk of recurrence, particularly if all previous episodes of VTE were also associated with a transient risk factor. If all previous episodes were associated with a transient risk factor, we treat these patients for 3 months. If any previous episodes were idiopathic, we treat patients for 6 months.

J *Previous VTE and Unclear Risk Factor Status*

As described in section F, these patients are likely to have an intermediate to high risk of recurrence. We treat them empirically for 12 months unless this decision is influenced by additional factors (see Table 16.1).

Bibliography

1. Research Committee of the British Thoracic Society. Optimum duration of anticoagulation for deep-vein thrombosis and pulmonary embolism. Lancet 1992;340:873–6.

2. Levine MN, Hirsh J, Gent M, et al. Optimal duration of oral anticoagulant therapy: a randomized trial comparing four weeks with three months of warfarin in patients with proximal deep vein thrombosis. Thromb Haemost 1995;74:606–11.

3. Schulman S, Rhedin A-S, Lindmarker P, et al. A comparison of six weeks with six months of oral anticoagulant therapy after a first episode of venous thromboembolism. N Engl J Med 1995;332:1661–5.

4. Prandoni P, Lensing AWA, Cogo A, et al. The long-term clinical course of acute deep venous thrombosis. Ann Intern Med 1996;125:1–7.

5. Hirsh J. The optimal duration of anticoagulant therapy for venous thrombosis. N Engl J Med 1995;332:1710–1.

6. Ridker PM, Miletich JP, Stampfer MJ, Goldhaber SZ, Lindpaintner K, Hennekens CH. Factor V Leiden and risks of recurrent idiopathic venous thromboembolism. Circulation 1995;92:2800–2.

7. Nachman RL, Silverstein R. Hypercoagulable states. Ann Intern Med 1993;119:819–27.

8. Hirsh J, Prins MH, Samama M. Therapeutic agents and their practical use in thrombotic disorders; approach to the thrombophilic patient for hemostasis and thrombosis: basic principles and clinical practice. In: Colman RW, Hirsh J, Marder VJ, Salzman EW, eds. Hemostasis and thrombosis: basic principles and clinical practice. 3rd edn. Philadelphia: J.B. Lippincott Co., 1993:1543–61.

9. Love PE, Santoro SA. Antiphospholipid antibodies: anticardiolipin and the lupus anticoagulant in systemic lupus erythematosus (SLE) and in non-SLE disorders. Ann Intern Med 1990;112:682–98.

10. Khamashta MA, Cuadrado MJ, Mujic F, Taub NA, Hunt BJ, Hughes GRV. The management of thrombosis in the antiphospholipid-antibody syndrome. N Engl J Med 1995;332:993–7.

11. Ginsburg KS, Liang MH, Newcomer L, et al. Anticardiolipin antibodies and the risk for ischemic stroke and venous thrombosis. Ann Intern Med 1992;117:997–1002.

12. Chesterman CN. After a first episode of venous thromboembolism—stop anticoagulant treatment after four to six weeks in patients with "reversible" risk factors. Br Med J 1995;311:700–1.

Chapter 17

Management of
Venous Thromboembolism
in Pediatric Patients

Paul Monagle

Anthony Chan

Unlike venous thromboembolism (VTE) in adults, VTE in pediatric patients is usually a complication of a primary illness or therapy. As survival rates for major childhood illnesses such as congenital heart disease and cancer improve, the incidence of VTE is increasing dramatically. In critically ill children, the diagnosis of VTE requires a high index of clinical suspicion. The epidemiology of VTE in pediatric and neonatal patients is significantly different than that of adults, as shown in Table 17.1.[1,2] Age-related changes in the hemostatic system are responsible for many differences, both in etiology and response to therapy. Throughout this chapter, we highlight the differences in epidemiology and physiology that have an impact on the management of pediatric patients with VTE. The management guidelines for VTE in adults are frequently extrapolated to VTE in pediatric patients although they may not be optimal in this population. Ongoing studies will likely result in specific guidelines for pediatric patients in the near future. This chapter discusses peripheral VTE only and does not include venous thromboembolism of the central nervous system or renal, hepatic, or other specific internal organs.

A Risk Factors

The majority of pediatric patients with VTE have multiple risk factors. In a large prospective study, only 4% of pediatric VTE was idiopathic, 12% of children had only one risk factor, and 84% had two or more risk factors. The most common risk factors for children are listed in Table 17.1. Upper limb VTE is more frequently associated with central venous lines (CVL) in children with cancer and congenital heart disease. The proportion of idiopathic VTE is increased in the lower limbs.

Table 17.1   Epidemiology of Pediatric and Adult VTE

	Adult	Child (1 month–18 years)	Neonate
Incidence	0.1% population	0.0007% population	0.24% NICU admissions
Site of thrombus	> 95% lower limb	~ 40% upper limb ~ 60% lower limb	> 90% abdominal
Associated conditions	33% idiopathic 33% transient risk factors 33% continuing risk factors	33% CVL-related 23% cancer 21% surgery/trauma 15% congenital heart disease 4% idiopathic	> 90% umbilical vein catheter related

Long-term parenteral nutrition using CVL is a particularly high-risk situation. In neonates, the single most important risk factor is umbilical vein catheterization. Homozygous protein C and S deficiencies and maternal systemic lupus erythematosus are rare causes of VTE.

B Presentation of VTE in the Upper Venous System

In the upper venous system, the most common presentation is CVL dysfunction. Other signs and symptoms include superior vena cava syndrome, upper limb swelling, facial swelling, and collateral vessel dilatation, which is particularly visible over the upper chest wall. Many patients are outpatients with gradual onset of symptoms. Pleural effusions and chylothorax may occur, especially in neonates. Venous thromboembolism can also present as stroke with paradoxical emboli in children with a right-to-left shunt due to congenital heart disease.

C Presentation of VTE in the Lower Venous System

In the lower limbs, idiopathic VTE may present with pain, swelling, redness, or disuse of a limb in young children. Usually, CVL-related VTE presents with CVL dysfunction. A high index of suspicion is required as many pediatric patients with lower limb CVLs are critically ill with a variety of diseases that may mask or simulate the presence of VTE.

D Investigation of VTE in the Upper Venous System

Ultrasound has not been validated as a replacement for venography in the upper venous system. Linograms (contrast injected through the CVL) frequently under-estimate the presence and extent of thrombosis. The gold standard for the diagnosis of upper system VTE is venography. Failure to use venography can lead to a missed diagnosis, which can have major consequences (Figure 17.1).

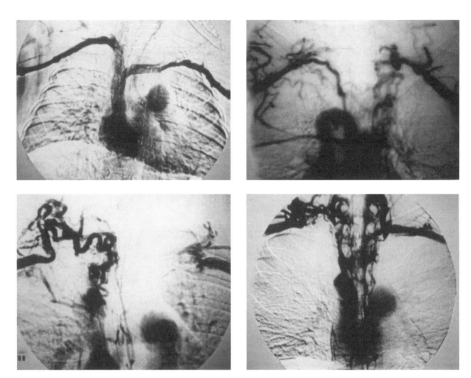

Figure 17.1   Four bilateral venograms of patients receiving home total parenteral nutrition. The *upper left* venogram is normal whereas the other three show varying degrees of venous occlusion with collateral circulation. All patients had normal linograms.

E   *Investigation of VTE in the Lower Venous System*

In contrast to the upper venous system, the lower limbs (iliac to popliteal veins) can usually be adequately visualized by duplex ultrasound. However, because there are no studies to validate this approach in pediatric patients, venography is recommended in pediatric patients with suspected intra-abdominal thrombi and in those with equivocal lower limb duplex ultrasounds. In neonates, ultrasound frequently provides good visualization of intra-abdominal vessels and is useful for sequential examinations.

F   *Congenital Prothrombotic States*

Venous thromboembolism in pediatric patients is frequently associated with multiple causative factors, a fact that is often ignored. Most pediatric patients with VTE should be investigated for a congenital prothrombotic state, regardless of the presence of acquired risk factors. A family history is important but is often negative. Proteins C and S, antithrombin, activated protein C resistance, factor V_{Leiden}, lupus anticoagulant, and antiphospholipid antibodies should be assessed. For neonates, investigation of the parents may be more reliable due to the difficulty in the interpretation of test results in neonates. All results should be compared to age-appropriate reference ranges.[3]

G *Acute Management*

Anticoagulation with unfractionated heparin (UFH) and oral anticoagulants (OACs) remains the mainstay of therapy for VTE in pediatric patients. Target ranges are extrapolated from recommendations in adults. Dose requirements are age-dependent, and validated nomograms for UFH and OAC therapy in pediatric patients are listed in Tables 17.2 and 17.3. Oral anticoagulant therapy is particularly difficult to monitor in infants due to poor venous access, vitamin K supplementation of standard infant formula, the frequency of intercurrent illness, and common use of other drugs that interfere with OAC. Home monitoring with whole blood prothrombin time monitors may decrease the trauma of blood taking and improve monitoring and safety. The usual duration of therapy is 5 to 10 days of standard heparin (SH) followed by 3 to 6 months of OAC. These recommendations, which reflect adult guidelines, should be individualized on the basis of ongoing risk factors and concurrent disease processes.

The use of low-molecular-weight heparin (LMWH) has an increasing importance in pediatric patients because of the minimal monitoring required, compared to UFH and OAC; this is especially helpful in small pediatric patients, in whom phlebotomy can be a major procedure. Enoxaparin and reviparin are currently the only LMWHs that have been evaluated in dose-finding studies performed in children (Table 17.4). Duration of therapy is usually the same as for UFH and OAC.

Embolectomy and thrombolytic therapy are usually reserved for life-threatening occlusive thrombi and are usually performed/administered in conjunction with anticoagulation. Low-dose thrombolytic therapy is frequently used to restore CVL

Table 17.2   Pediatric Protocol for Unfractionated Heparin Administration

I.	Loading dose: heparin 75 U/kg IV over 10 minutes
II.	Initial maintenance dose: 28 U/kg/hr for infants younger than 1 year
III.	Initial maintenance dose: 20 U/kg/hr for children older than 1 year
IV.	Adjust heparin to maintain therapeutic aPTT (e.g., 60 to 85 seconds assuming this reflects an antifactor Xa level of 0.30 to 0.70)

APTT (seconds)	Bolus (U/kg)	Hold (minutes)	% Rate Change	Repeat aPTT
< 50	50	0	+10	4 hr
50–59	0	0	+10	4 hr
60–85	0	0	0	Next day
86–95	0	0	-10	4 hr
96–120	0	30	-10	4 hr
> 120	0	60	-15	4 hr

V.	Obtain blood for aPTT 4 hr after administration of the heparin loading dose and 4 hr after every change in the infusion rate
VI.	When aPTT values are therapeutic, a daily CBC and aPTT

Table 17.3   Pediatric Protocol for Warfarin to Maintain an INR between 2.0 and 3.0

I.   Day 1: if the baseline INR is less than 1.2 : Dose = 0.2 mg/kg, maximum 10 mg
II.   Loading days 2 to 4: If the INR is:

INR	Action
1.1–1.3	Repeat loading dose
1.4–3.0	50% of loading dose
3.1–3.5	25% of loading dose
> 3.5	Hold dose until INR < 3.5, then restart at 50% less than the previous dose

III.   Maintenance oral anticoagulation dosage guidelines:

INR	Action
1.1–1.4	Increase by 20% of dose
1.5–1.9	Increase by 10% of dose
2.0–3.0	No change
3.1–3.5	Decrease by 10% of dose
> 3.5	Hold dose until INR < 3.5, then restart at 20% less than the previous dose

patency (Table 17.5). Successful restoration of CVL patency is not equivalent to adequate treatment of associated VTE. The availability of other venous access sites and the expected intensity and duration of therapy for the primary disease are important factors to consider when deciding whether or not to remove a CVL.

Table 17.4   Pediatric Protocol for Low-Molecular-Weight Heparin Administration

I.   Dose: enoxaparin (Lovenox) (100 anti Xa units/mg)
        Age > 1 yr < 18 yr:
            Treatment dose: 1mg/kg subcutaneously 12 hourly
            Prophylactic dose: 0.5 mg/kg subcutaneously 12 hourly
        Age < 1 yr:
            Treatment dose: 1.5 mg/kg subcutaneously 12 hourly
            Prophylactic dose: 0.75 mg/kg subcutaneously 12 hourly

II.   Adjust the dose of LMWH according to the following for treatment dosage:

Anti-Xa	Hold Next Dose	Dose Change	Repeat Anti-Xa
< 0.35 u/ml	0	Increase by 25%	4 hours post next dose
0.35–0.49 u/ml	0	Increase by 10%	4 hours post next dose
0.5–1.0 u/ml	0	0	Weekly at 4 hours post dose
1.1–1.5 u/ml	0	Decrease by 20%	4 hours post next dose
1.5–2.0 u/ml	3 hr	Decrease by 30%	4 hours post next dose
> 2.0 u/ml	Until anti-Xa < 0.5 u/ml	Decrease by 40%	Repeat q 12 hours

Suspected Deep Vein Thrombosis

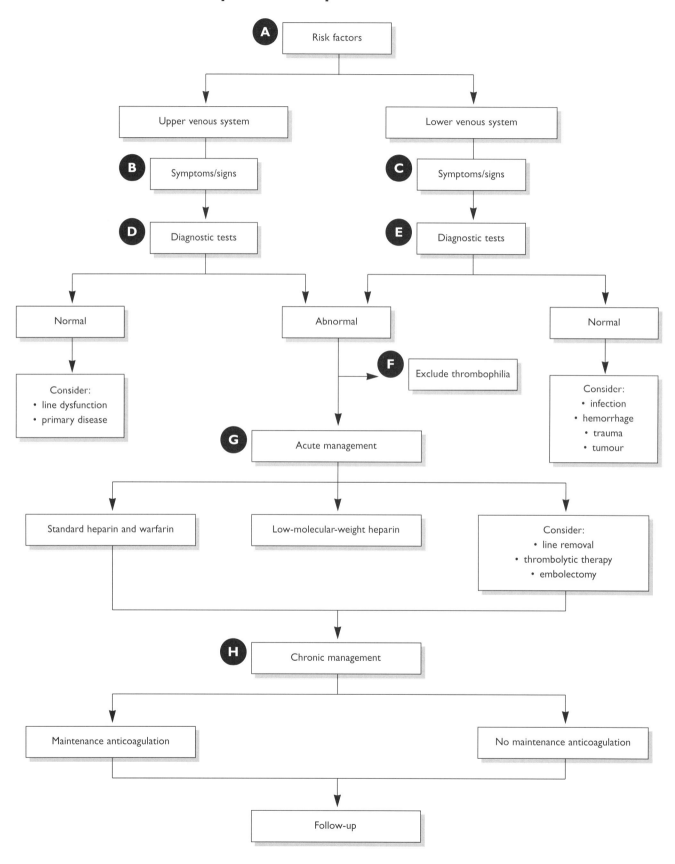

Table 17.5   Guidelines for Local Instillation of Urokinase

Treatment	Single-Lumen CVL	Double-Lumen CVL	SC Port
Urokinase	2 ml x 2–4 hr*	2 ml per lumen x 2–4 hr*	3 ml x 2–4 hr*
(5000 units/ml undiluted)	If unsuccessful in obtaining blood return, repeat above once in 24 hr		

*Note: After 2 to 4 hr instillation of each drug, withdraw drug. If possible, flush the catheter with 0.9% sodium chloride, attempt to aspirate blood.

H *Chronic Management*

The presence of ongoing risk factors, such as the continued presence of a CVL, may necessitate the need for long-term secondary prophylaxis. Current regimes, which are based on case series, include use of low-dose OACs (INR 1.5 to 2.0), and LMWH. When prothrombotic disorders are identified, family studies with appropriate counseling are required. The role of prophylaxis with anticoagulants depends on age, concurrent disease, and family history. All pediatric patients with VTE require long-term follow-up. The risks of recurrence and postphlebitic syndrome exist although the incidences have not been fully determined.[1]

Bibliography

1. Andrew M, David M, Adams M, et al. Venous thromboembolic complications (VTE) in children: first analysis of the Canadian Registry of VTE. Blood 1996;83:1251–7.
2. Schmidt B, Andrew M. Neonatal thrombosis: report of a prospective Canadian and international registry. Pediatrics 1995;96:939–43.
3. Andrew M, Paes B, Johnston M. Development of the hemostatic system in the neonate and young infant. Am J Pediatr Hematol Oncol 1990;12:95–104.

Additional Reading

Michelson A, Bovill E, Andrew M. Antithrombotic therapy in children. Chest 1995;108(4)(Suppl): 506–22.

Chapter 18

HEPARIN-INDUCED THROMBOCYTOPENIA

Theodore E Warkentin

Heparin-induced thrombocytopenia (HIT) is an immunohematologic syndrome characterized by thrombocytopenia and a high risk for thrombosis.[1,2] It is caused by an IgG antibody (HIT-IgG) that recognizes a multimolecular complex of heparin and platelet factor 4 (PF4) on the platelet surface. The resulting immune complex interacts with the platelet Fc receptors, leading to potent platelet activation. Formation of procoagulant, platelet-derived microparticles[3] and, possibly, activation of endothelium via cross-reactivity of the pathogenic IgG for complexes of PF4 and endothelial heparan sulfate also contribute to the risk for thrombosis. A recent study found that a low-molecular-weight heparin preparation (enoxaparin [Lovenox®]) was less likely to cause HIT than an unfractionated heparin preparation in a postoperative orthopedic patient population.[1] Recent evidence suggests that certain common treatment approaches, such as substituting warfarin for heparin during acute HIT, can lead to *worsening* of thrombosis, e.g., syndrome of warfarin-induced venous limb gangrene complicating HIT.[4,5] Recent treatment approaches that emphasize inhibition of factor Xa (danaparoid)[6-8] or thrombin (hirudin)[9] are effective.

A History and Physical

The history should focus on determining the timing of the onset of thrombocytopenia in relation to heparin use. Typically, in HIT the platelet count begins to fall 5 to 8 days after starting heparin (first day of heparin use = day zero) although thrombocytopenia may not occur until a few days later. An important exception is, an immediate fall in the platelet count following heparin use can also indicate HIT, particularly when the patient has *recently* been exposed to heparin (within 3 months). The history and physical examination should also focus on signs and symptoms suggestive of thrombosis, as both venous and arterial thrombosis are strongly associated with HIT.[1] Evidence suggesting alternate explanations for the thrombocytopenia should be sought, including fever or chills (septicemia), recent surgery or blood transfusions (hemodilution), shock or vital organ dysfunction (multiorgan system failure), among others. The clinician must consider HIT in thrombocytopenic patients receiving heparin who develop abdominal pain or hypotension, as acute adrenal failure secondary to bilateral adrenal hemorrhagic infarction occurs in about 1 to 2% of patients with HIT.

The development of painful, erythematous plaques or frank necrosis at heparin injection sites beginning 5 to 8 days after starting subcutaneous heparin injections can indicate HIT (see Figure 18.3). However, only approximately 10 to 20% of patients who generate HIT-IgG during subcutaneous heparin therapy develop this complication.

B *Diagnostic Testing for HIT*

There are two general classes of diagnostic assays: (1) *functional assays*, based on detecting activation of normal donor platelets in the presence of patient serum (or plasma) and therapeutic concentrations of heparin, and (2) *antigen assays*, based on detecting patient antibody against the pathogenic heparin/PF4 complex. Each type of assay has certain limitations. One assay, which measures the release of radioactive serotonin from washed platelets, has been clinically validated: a positive assay was strongly associated with the development of HIT in a clinical trial of heparin use.[1] However, many patients who form HIT-IgG while receiving heparin do not develop thrombocytopenia or thrombosis.[1] Unfortunately, few medical centers provide rapid, reliable diagnostic testing for HIT. Thus, the clinician usually must make initial diagnostic and therapeutic decisions based on clinical judgment.

C *Other Laboratory Tests*

The clinician should perform investigations for other possible causes for thrombocytopenia, including: (1) review of the peripheral blood film for evidence of septicemia, microangiopathy, platelet clumping, or bi- or pancytopenia; (2) blood cultures (thrombocytopenia in hospitalized patients often indicates microbial invasion of the blood); and (3) tests for disseminated intravascular coagulation (DIC). Although most HIT patients will have elevated D-dimer levels (either because of thrombosis or DIC), only about 5% will have low fibrinogen levels.

D *Consider Other Common Causes of Thrombocytopenia in Patients Receiving Heparin*

Most patients who receive heparin have other common causes for acute thrombocytopenia. These include intensive care unit patients (septicemia, multisystem organ failure, DIC), patients with acute MI (the combination of streptokinase and heparin often causes transient thrombocytopenia), early postoperative patients (hemodilution with blood products and other fluids), and patients with cancer-associated thrombosis who often have DIC.

E   Evaluate for Thrombosis

Deep venous thrombosis (DVT) and pulmonary embolism occur commonly in patients with HIT.[1,2] Indeed, a large series of serologically confirmed HIT patients observed more patients with pulmonary embolism than all arterial thrombotic events combined.[2] The clinician should have a very high index of suspicion for thrombosis in HIT patients (Figure 18.1) and investigate suggestive symptoms and signs with appropriate objective studies.

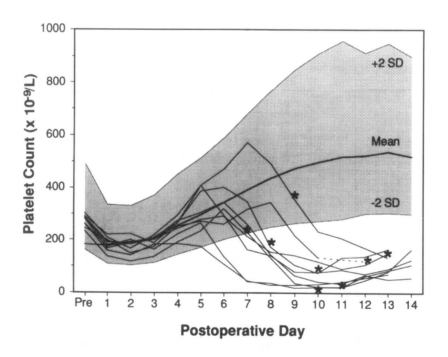

Figure 18.1   Typical temporal platelet count profile of heparin-induced thrombocytopenia. The bold line indicates the mean, and the shaded area the mean ± two standard deviations (SD), for the platelet count range of the reference (HIT antibody negative) patient population (n = 367). Note that there is a uniform early postoperative platelet count fall (maximal postoperative days 1 to 3), followed by return to baseline (approximately day 5), followed by platelet counts higher than baseline (with maximal values at days 11 to 14). The nine solid lines correspond to the serial platelet counts of nine patients with serologically confirmed heparin-induced thrombocytopenia. Asterisks indicate the occurrence of thrombotic complications in the patients with heparin-induced thrombocytopenia. A dotted line is shown for one patient because the platelet count was not available on the day that thrombosis developed. (Reprinted with permission from: Warkentin TE, Levine MN, Hirsh J, et al. Heparin-induced thrombocytopenia in patients treated with low-molecular-weight heparin or unfractionated heparin. N Engl J Med 1995;332:1330–5. Copyright 1995 by Massachusetts Medical Society.)

F *High Risk for Thrombosis*

Patients who present with isolated HIT, i.e., HIT initially recognized because of thrombocytopenia without HIT-associated thrombosis, have a high risk for thrombosis (approximately 50% over the next 30 days) (Figure 18.2).[2] Thus, this author recommends alternate therapeutic-dose anticoagulation in patients with suspected HIT, especially if other prothrombotic risk factors are present (e.g., postoperative patients). However, objective testing for thrombosis (e.g., Doppler ultrasound studies) must be performed prior to committing the patient to longer-term anticoagulation. This treatment strategy is unproven.

G *Definite Indication for Anticoagulation Therapy*

Some HIT patients with isolated thrombocytopenia nevertheless have definite indications for alternative anticoagulation (e.g., atrial fibrillation, surgery requiring cardiopulmonary bypass).

H *Adjunctive Treatments for Thrombosis*

Limbs compromised by acute arterial occlusion can sometimes be salvaged by surgical thromboembolectomy or thrombolytic therapy. Inferior vena cava filters are sometimes useful in patients with HIT and DVT who cannot be treated with anticoagulants.

I *Alternative Anticoagulants to Treat HIT*

An agent that inhibits thrombin generation, either indirectly via factor Xa inhibition (e.g., danaparoid) or directly via thrombin inactivation (lepirudin, argatroban), is recommended to treat HIT.

Danaparoid sodium (Orgaran®) is a heterogeneous mixture of anticoagulant glycosaminoglycans, predominantly heparan sulfate (~84%) and dermatan sulfate (~12%). Its anticoagulant effect is mediated via (1) a subfraction of heparan sulfate with high antithrombin affinity (responsible for antifactor Xa effect and half of the drug's minor antithrombin effect), (2) dermatan sulfate (minor antithrombin effect via interaction with heparan cofactor II), (3) other uncharacterized mechanisms. For patients of average body weight, we use the following regimen to achieve therapeutic anticoagulation (750 antifactor Xa unit ampules): a loading dose of 2250 U bolus, followed by 400 U/hr × 4 hr, then 300 U/hr × 4 hr, then a maintenance dose of 150 to 200 U/hr. This intravenous administration regimen generally will achieve a therapeutic anticoagulant level (0.5 to 0.8 anti-Xa U/mL), and thus laboratory monitoring is usually not necessary. A randomized, but nonblinded, clinical trial found danaparoid to be significantly more effective than dextran in the treatment of HIT-associated thrombosis.[6] Danaparoid also was more effective than ancrod in a retrospective historical cohort study.[7] Overall, danaparoid is effective—as defined by resolution of thrombocytopenia without new or progressive thrombosis—in at least 90% of HIT patients.[6–8] Approximately 10 to 40% of HIT sera show in vitro cross-reactivity with danaparoid; however, most of these patients do not develop clinical evidence for cross-reactivity when treated with this agent.[7] In my opinion, danaparoid therapy should not be delayed for performing in vitro cross-reactivity testing. Danaparoid is now available in Canada and the U.S., where it has been approved for use in DVT prophylaxis.

Recombinant hirudin (lepirudin [Refludan®]), a potent thrombin inhibitor derived from the medicinal leech, is approved to treat HIT-associated thrombosis in the United States and Europe. Lepirudin was effective in treating thrombosis in HIT patients, compared with historical controls.[9] The intravenous treatment regimen used in this study was a loading dose of 0.4 mg/kg bolus, followed by a maintenance dose of 0.15 mg/kg/hr, with dose-adjustments to maintain the aPTT 1.5 to 3.0 times the mean of the normal laboratory aPTT range.

Argatroban (Novostan®) is a synthetic direct thrombin inhibitor that has been used in an experimental protocol to treat HIT, both with and without thrombosis, in a multicenter cohort study in North America. The results of this study have not yet been published.

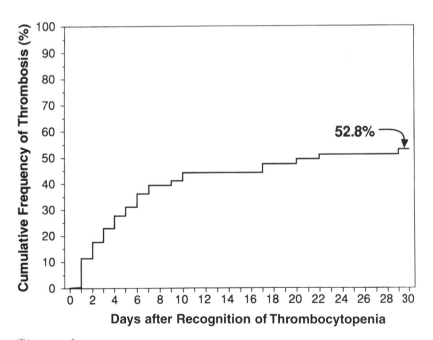

Figure 18.2   Cumulative frequency of thrombosis in heparin-induced thrombocytopenia patients presenting with isolated thrombocytopenia. Approximately 50% of heparin-induced thrombocytopenia patients initially recognized with isolated thrombocytopenia developed objective evidence for thrombosis during the subsequent 30-day period. (Reprinted by permission of the publisher from: Warkentin TE, Kelton JG. A 14-year study of heparin-induced thrombocytopenia. Am J Med 1996;101:502–7. Copyright 1996 by Excerpta Medica Inc.)

J   *Caution: Low-Molecular-Weight (LMW) Heparin, Warfarin, Ancrod*

Low-molecular-weight heparin preparations are essentially 100% cross-reactive in vitro with HIT serum. There is a high rate of treatment failure, i.e., persisting/ recurrent thrombocytopenia or new/progressive thrombosis, when used to treat HIT (estimated at 25 to 50%). This author does not recommend LMW heparin to treat HIT.

Warfarin is a vitamin K antagonist that has been used to treat HIT-associated thrombosis. However, we observed that warfarin use was associated with the development of venous limb gangrene in approximately 10% of patients who received warfarin for DVT complicating HIT.[4,5] This syndrome is characterized by acral (distal) necrosis complicating DVT despite palpable or Doppler-identifiable arterial pulses; pathology reveals thrombi in the smaller veins and venules. Typically, these patients have a *supra*therapeutic international normalized ratio level (INR ≥ 4.0) at the time of their tissue necrosis. Laboratory studies show severe reductions in protein C activity but persisting thrombin generation (as assessed by elevated thrombin-antithrombin complex levels) despite these elevated INR values. This syndrome can be avoided by gradually starting warfarin following platelet count recovery, or during adequate anticoagulation with agents that inhibit factor Xa or thrombin (e.g., danaparoid, lepirudin, argatroban).

Ancrod is a defibrinogenating snake venom that has been used to treat HIT, especially in Canada. However, this author does not recommend the use of ancrod

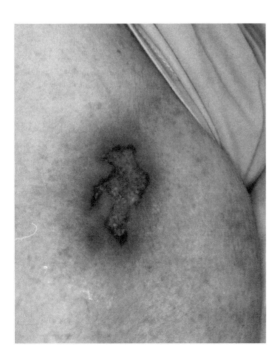

Figure 18.3   Heparin-induced skin necrosis at a heparin injection site on the left extensor surface of the upper arm. The platelet count fell from 701 to 127 x 10⁹/L in association with the onset of skin lesions. (Photograph provided courtesy of Dr. Wendy M. Nicholson and Dr. S. Louisy, Burlington, Ontario.)

Heparin-Induced Thrombocytopenia

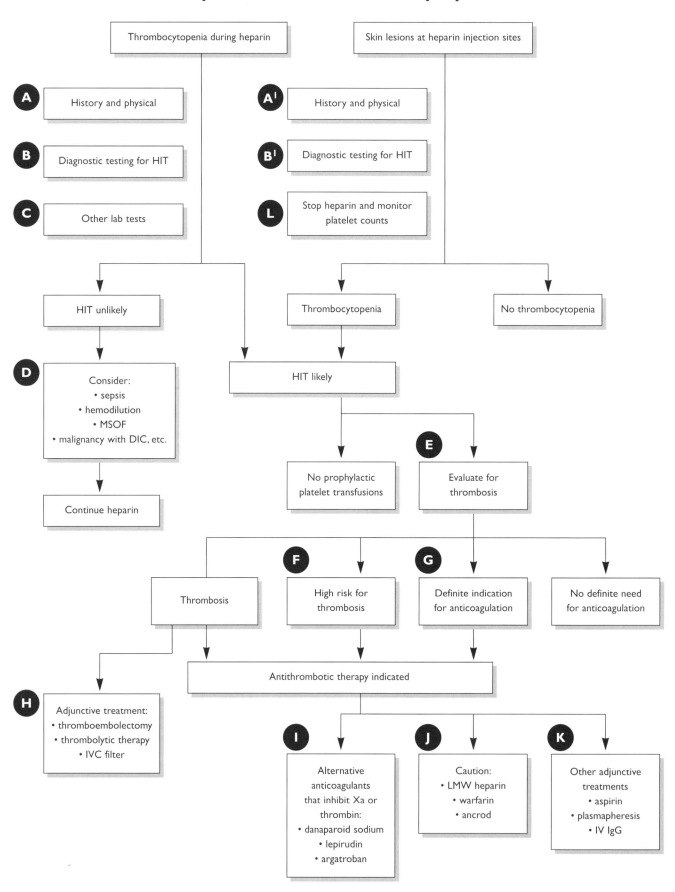

for the following reasons:[7] (1) ancrod does not inhibit, and may actually increase, thrombin generation in HIT; (2) the combination of ancrod and warfarin has been associated with several cases of warfarin-induced venous limb gangrene;[5] (3) ancrod was less effective than danaparoid in preventing new or progressive thrombosis in a historical comparative study in one medical community.

K *Other Adjunctive Treatments*

Some reports have indicated benefit with aspirin or other antiplatelet agents, high-dose intravenous gammaglobulin, and plasmapheresis. However, these therapies should be considered as adjuncts to primary therapy with danaparoid or a specific thrombin inhibitor.

L *Heparin-Induced Skin Lesions: Stop Heparin and Monitor Platelet Counts*

Most patients who develop heparin-induced skin lesions (Figure 18.3) do *not* develop thrombocytopenia. However, it is important to monitor the platelet count for a few days even after stopping the heparin injections because the platelet count fall can begin after the heparin has been stopped. Patients who develop heparin-induced skin lesions and thrombocytopenia have a particularly high risk for developing *arterial* thrombosis.[10]

Bibliography

1. Warkentin TE, Levine MN, Hirsh J, et al. Heparin-induced thrombocytopenia in patients treated with low-molecular-weight heparin or unfractionated heparin. N Engl J Med 1995;332: 1330–5.
2. Warkentin TE, Kelton JG. A 14-year study of heparin-induced thrombocytopenia. Am J Med 1996;101:502–7.
3. Warkentin TE, Hayward CPM, Boshkov LK, et al. Sera from patients with heparin-induced thrombocytopenia generate platelet-derived microparticles with procoagulant activity: an explanation for the thrombotic complications of heparin-induced thrombocytopenia. Blood 1994;84:3691–9.
4. Warkentin TE. Heparin-induced thrombocytopenia: IgG-mediated platelet activation, platelet microparticle generation, and altered procoagulant/anticoagulant balance in the pathogenesis of thrombosis and venous limb gangrene complicating heparin-induced thrombocytopenia. Transfus Med Rev 1996;10:249–58.
5. Warkentin TE, Elavathil LJ, Hayward CPM, Johnston MA, Russett JI, Kelton JG. The pathogenesis of venous limb gangrene associated with heparin-induced thrombocytopenia. Ann Intern Med 1997;127:804–12.

6. Chong BH. Low molecular weight heparinoid and heparin-induced thrombocytopenia (abstract). Aust NZ J Med 1996;26:331.

7. Warkentin TE. Danaparoid (Orgaran®) for the treatment of heparin-induced thrombocytopenia (HIT) and thrombosis: effects on *in vivo* thrombin and cross-linked fibrin generation, and evaluation of the clinical significance of *in vitro* cross-reactivity (XR) of danaparoid for HIT-IgG. Blood 1996;88(Suppl 1):626a.

8. Magnani HN. Heparin-induced thrombocytopenia (HIT): an overview of 230 patients treated with Orgaran (Org 10172). Thromb Haemost 1993;70:554–61.

9. Greinacher A, Völpel H, Pötzsch B. Recombinant hirudin in the treatment of patients with heparin-induced thrombocytopenia (HIT) (abstract). Blood 1996;88(Suppl 1):281a.

10. Warkentin TE. Heparin-induced thrombocytopenia, skin lesions, and arterial thrombosis: a new clinical syndrome. Can J Cardiol 1996;12(Suppl E):151E.

Additional Reading

Aster RH. Heparin-induced thrombocytopenia and thrombosis (editorial). N Engl J Med 1995; 332:1374–6.

Greinacher A. Antigen generation in heparin-associated thrombocytopenia: the nonimmunologic type and the immunologic type are closely linked in their pathogenesis. Semin Thromb Hemost 1995;21:106–16.

Warkentin TE, Kelton JG. Interaction of heparin with platelets, including heparin-induced thrombocytopenia. In: Bounameaux H, ed. Low-molecular-weight heparins in prophylaxis and therapy of thromboembolic diseases. New York: Marcel Dekker, 1994:75–127.

Warkentin TE, Chong BH, Greinacher A. Heparin-induced thrombocytopenia towards consensus. Thromb Haemost 1998;79:1–7.

Warkentin TE. Heparin-induced skin lesions. Br J Haematol 1996;92:494–7.

Chapter 19

PERIOPERATIVE MANAGEMENT
OF ANTICOAGULANTS

Clive Kearon

Perioperative management of orally anticoagulated patients is guided by the risk of thromboembolism and bleeding associated with different anticoagulant strategies. The risk of thromboembolism and associated morbidity depends on the indication for anticoagulation: if and how long before patients have had a previous episode of thromboembolism, and whether or not surgery increases the risk of thromboembolism.[1] The risk of preoperative bleeding is generally low but is high following major surgery. Because the risk of thromboembolism and bleeding are often influenced by the surgical procedure, anticoagulant management needs to be considered separately for the preoperative and postoperative periods.

PREOPERATIVE ANTICOAGULATION

A Indications for Warfarin

To assess the risks associated with temporarily stopping anticoagulants, the consequences, as well as the absolute risk, of a thromboembolic event need to be considered. Arterial thromboembolism often results in death (~ 40%) or major disability (~ 20%) whereas venous thromboembolism (VTE) rarely presents as sudden death (~ 5 to 10%), and major disability is also unusual (less than 5%) in patients with treated VTE.

B Arterial Indications for Anticoagulation

Primary prophylaxis of arterial thromboembolism is most commonly undertaken in patients with atrial fibrillation, valvular heart disease (native or prosthetic), and recent myocardial infarct. Secondary prophylaxis is undertaken after patients (with or without the above conditions) have had an arterial thromboembolic event (usually a stroke). Previous thromboembolism is a major risk factor for recurrence.[2,3]

C *Previous Arterial Thromboembolism*

These patients have a higher risk of embolism than patients without previous episodes; the period of subtherapeutic anticoagulation should therefore be kept to a minimum. In patients whose international normalized ratio (INR) is 2.0 to 3.0, it takes 4 days for it to spontaneously fall to less than 1.5, an intensity of anticoagulation at which increased intraoperative bleeding is not expected after anticoagulation is stopped.[4] Therefore, four daily doses of warfarin should be withheld preoperatively, and the INR should be measured the day before surgery to determine if a small dose of vitamin K is needed to accelerate the reversal of anticoagulation. We generally give 1 mg of vitamin K subcutaneously if the INR is more than 1.7 the day prior to surgery, and repeat the INR the morning of surgery. If necessary, plasma can then be given prior to surgery if the INR is still not acceptable to the surgeon (i.e., INR 1.3 to 1.7, 1 unit; INR 1.7 to 2.0, 2 units); however, administration of blood products should generally be avoided for elective surgery.

D *No Previous Arterial Thromboembolism*

The risk of thromboembolism after discontinuing anticoagulation is lower in patients who have not had a previous episode. Warfarin can be withheld for five doses to ensure that coagulation has returned to normal prior to surgery; however, in patients with prosthetic heart valves who have a higher risk of thromboembolism, only four doses of warfarin should be withheld. Since the usual intensity of anticoagulation is higher in patients with mechanical heart valves (i.e., INR 2.5 to 3.5), a small dose of vitamin K is required more often in these patients the day before surgery.

E *Last Episode of Arterial Thromboembolism within 1 Month*

The risk of recurrent arterial thromboembolism is highest within a month of an acute event (about 0.5% per day).[3] To minimize the possibility of preoperative embolism, intravenous heparin should be administered when the INR drops to less than 2.0. Stopping intravenous heparin 6 hours prior to surgery should be adequate for the activated partial thromboplastin time (aPTT) to return to normal.

F *Venous Indications for Anticoagulation*

The main venous indication for anticoagulation is prevention of recurrent VTE. An exception occurs in selected patients with hereditary hypercoagulable states (e.g., antithrombin, protein C, protein S deficiencies, and a strong family history of thromboembolism).

G *Interval since Last VTE Event*

The risk of recurrent venous thromboembolism declines rapidly with the duration of anticoagulation.[5]

H *Last VTE Event within 1 Month*

These patients have a very high risk of recurrent VTE if anticoagulants are stopped. Therefore, if feasible, surgery should be deferred until the patients have received 1 to 3 months of anticoagulation. If this is not feasible, preoperative thromboembolic risk should be minimized by administering intravenous heparin when the INR is less than 2.0 (see section E).

I *Last VTE between 1 and 3 Months*

These patients have a moderately high risk of recurrent VTE if anticoagulants are stopped. Warfarin should only be withheld for four doses to minimize this period of high risk (see section C).

J *Last VTE More Than 3 Months*

These patients have a much lower risk of recurrent VTE than those who have been treated for less than 3 months.

K *Low Risk of VTE in the Absence of Immobilization*

Immobility greatly increases the risk of VTE. If patients are hospitalized prior to surgery, additional VTE prophylaxis should be administered once the INR is less than 1.8. Prophylactic regimens for high-risk surgical patients (i.e., 3000 U of low-molecular-weight heparin, SQ, bid) are suitable[6] (see Chapter 2). The risk of VTE in these patients is probably not high enough to use intravenous heparin preoperatively.

L *Last VTE between 1 and 3 Months, Preoperative Immobilization*

The risk of recurrent VTE is high enough in these patients that intravenous heparin should be administered while the INR is less than 2.0 (see section E).

M *Last VTE within 2 Weeks*

These patients have the highest risk of recurrence. The risk of pulmonary embolism is small if intravenous heparin is withheld for 24 hours or less, namely, 6 hours preoperatively and 12 to 18 hours postoperatively, and if the duration of surgery is short. Consequently, patients undergoing minor surgery who do not have a high risk

Preoperative Anticoagulation

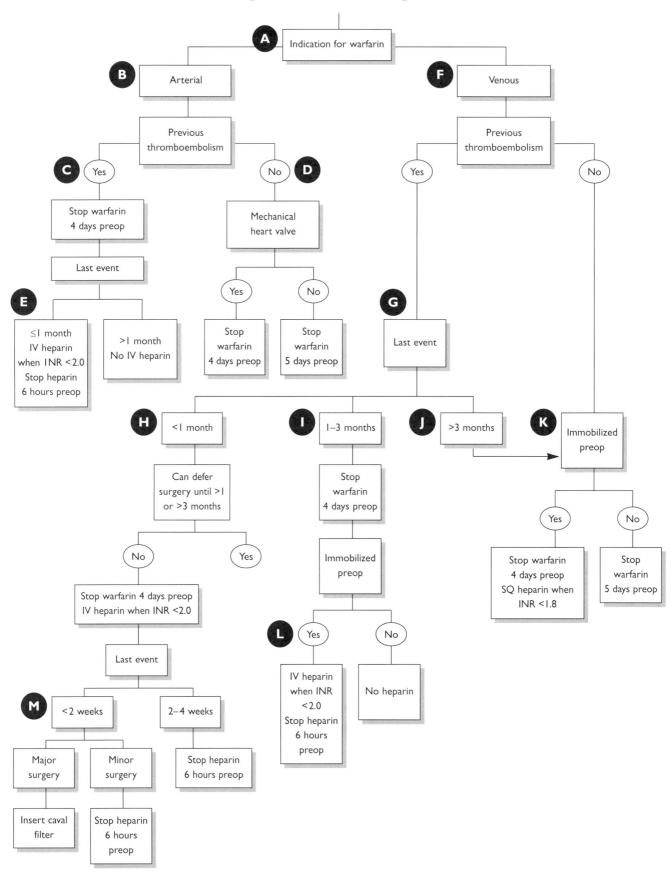

Postoperative Anticoagulation

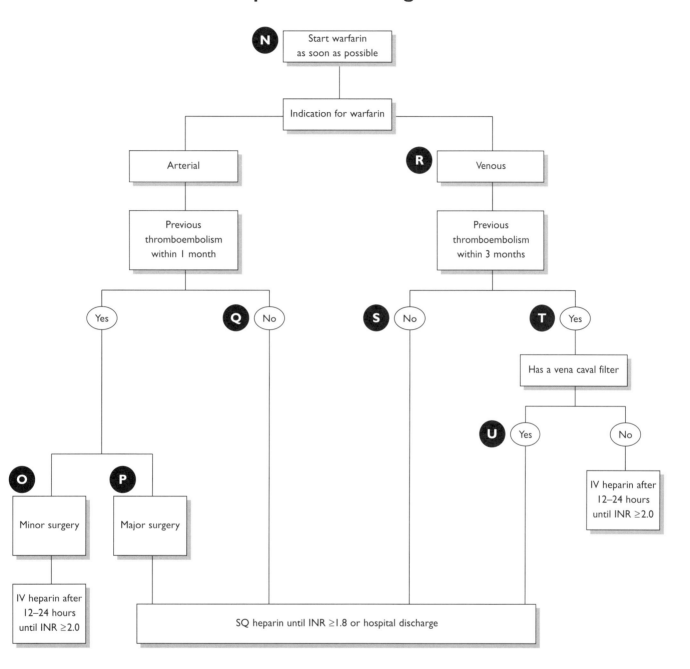

SQ (subcutaneous) heparin as recommended for patients at high risk for postoperative VTE (e.g., low-molecular-weight heparin, 3000 U twice daily)

for postoperative bleeding can be managed with pre- and postoperative intravenous heparin. Patients undergoing major surgery and/or those who have a high risk of postoperative bleeding should have a vena caval filter inserted preoperatively or intraoperatively.

POSTOPERATIVE ANTICOAGULATION

N *Start Warfarin as Soon as Possible*

If coagulation has previously returned to normal, there is a 24-hour delay after warfarin is restarted before the INR begins to increase. Thus, warfarin should be restarted as soon as possible after surgery in all patients who do not have additional invasive procedures planned. In patients who are having a minor procedure associated with a low risk of bleeding, warfarin can be restarted shortly before surgery.

O *Previous Arterial Thromboembolism within a Month of Minor Surgery*

The risk of recurrence is sufficiently high within a month of acute arterial thromboembolism that intravenous heparin is warranted until the INR reaches 2.0, provided the risk of bleeding is not very high. Intravenous heparin should be started 12 hours after surgery, without a loading bolus, at about 18 units per kilogram per hour.[7] For the anticoagulant response to stabilize (no bolus), the first aPTT measurement should be performed after 12 hours.

P *Previous Arterial Thromboembolism within a Month of Major Surgery*

Despite a high risk of recurrent arterial thromboembolism while the INR is subtherapeutic, intravenous heparin is not recommended shortly after major surgery as the risk of bleeding will likely outweigh the antithrombotic benefit. Subcutaneous unfractionated heparin or low-molecular-weight heparin, given in doses recommended for VTE prophylaxis of high risk patients (see section K) is safe and should be given until the INR reaches 1.8. This is likely to occur prior to discharge in patients who have had major surgery.

Q *No Previous Arterial Thromboembolism within a Month of Surgery*

This includes patients without previous arterial thromboembolism and those with thromboembolism that has occurred more than a month previously. The risk of thromboembolism is not high enough in these patients to warrant postoperative intravenous heparin. Subcutaneous heparin (section P) should be used in inpatients but the benefits of subcutaneous heparin may not be large enough to delay discharge or to justify its use after discharge.

R Postoperative VTE

Surgery is a major risk factor for VTE, and the risk of thrombosis is much higher postoperatively than it is preoperatively (may increase 100-fold).[1] For this reason, the need for antithrombotic prophylaxis is much greater postoperatively than it is preoperatively.

S No Thromboembolism within 3 Months

Provided there have been no previous episodes of thromboembolism, or the last episode was more than 3 months ago, postoperative intravenous heparin is not indicated. Subcutaneous heparin is recommended in doses used for VTE prophylaxis of high-risk patients. If patients are discharged before their INR has reached 1.8, and if they can receive subcutaneous injections at home, this is recommended in the highest-risk patients. Restarting warfarin may induce a transient hypercoagulable state in patients with protein C or protein S deficiency, so patients with these conditions should receive subcutaneous heparin until the INR is 2.0 or greater for 2 days.

T Thromboembolism within 3 Months of Surgery

These patients have a very high risk of postoperative recurrent venous thromboembolism and intravenous heparin is recommended until the INR is 2.0 or greater.

U Thromboembolism within 3 Months of Surgery with Vena Caval Filter

Although patients with a vena caval filter are at high risk of recurrent VTE, they are protected from pulmonary embolism, and consequently, intravenous heparin can be avoided in the early postoperative period.

Bibliography

1. Kearon C, Hirsh J. Management of anticoagulation before and after elective surgery. N Engl J Med 1997;336:1506–11.
2. Atrial Fibrillation Investigators. Risk factors for stroke and efficacy of antithrombotic therapy in atrial fibrillation: analysis of pooled data from five randomized trials. Arch Intern Med 1994;154:1449–57.

3. Cerebral Embolism Task Force. Cardiogenic brain embolism. Arch Neurol 1986;43:71–84.

4. White RH, McKittrick T, Hutchinson R, Twitchell J. Temporary discontinuation of warfarin therapy: changes in the international normalized ratio. Ann Intern Med 1995;122:40–2.

5. Coon WW, Willis PW. Recurrence of venous thromboembolism. Surgery 1973;73:823–7.

6. Clagett GP, Anderson FA, Heit J, Levine MN, Wheeler HB. Prevention of venous thromboembolism. Chest 1995;108(Suppl):312S–34S.

7. Raschke RA, Reilly BM, Guidry JR, Fontana JR, Srinivas S. The weight-based heparin dosing nomogram compared with a "standard care" nomogram. Ann Intern Med 1993;119:874–81.

Chapter 20

HEPARIN RESISTANCE

Patrick Brill-Edwards

Unfractionated heparin is effective in treating patients with venous thromboembolism (VTE) provided that an adequate anticoagulant effect is achieved.[1] The anticoagulant response to heparin varies among patients,[2–4] so it is important to use an appropriate initial dose; a bolus of 5000 U heparin followed by a starting infusion rate of 30,000 to 35,000 U/24 hours[5–11] achieves a suitable anticoagulant effect for most patients. Monitoring with a test such as the activated partial thromboplastin time (aPTT) is necessary to ensure an adequate anticoagulant effect is achieved and also to reduce the likelihood of an excessive effect, which may increase the risk of bleeding. Several studies[3,5,7] have demonstrated that the use of a nomogram to adjust the heparin dose improves the likelihood of obtaining a therapeutic anticoagulant effect. The therapeutic range for aPTT results targets a minimum and maximum anticoagulant effect, and this range is unique to each reagent and laboratory system.[12]

Despite large daily doses of heparin, however, the aPTT may remain subtherapeutic. The term used to describe such patients is "heparin resistance," and it has been defined as a subtherapeutic aPTT despite daily heparin doses of more than 40,000 U.[1,4,13] The aPTT response to heparin can be impaired by increased levels of factor VIII, which can prevent the usual heparin dose-related prolongation of the aPTT, whereas heparin assay results are not affected by factor VIII.[14,15] The result is a dissociation of aPTT results and heparin assay results, with aPTT results being subtherapeutic while the heparin assay results are therapeutic.[4] The dissociation of aPTT and heparin assay results due to elevated factor VIII levels may be present in 50% of heparin-resistant patients.[4]

Increased factor VIII levels are often responsible for the dissociation of aPTT and heparin level results but are not the only cause of the increased dose requirements seen in heparin-resistant patients. In the only randomized control clinical trial of patients with heparin resistance, Levine and colleagues compared heparin dosage according to aPTT results to dosage according to anti-factor Xa heparin levels. The dose of heparin required in the heparin level group was not as high as the aPTT group (40,000 vs. 45,000 U/24hr). The need for such an increased heparin dose in the former group could not be explained by increased factor VIII levels because heparin levels are not affected by increased levels of factor VIII. Subsequent studies by Young and associates[16–18] have demonstrated that nonspecific binding of heparin to plasma proteins accounts for the increased dose requirements that are characteristic of patients labelled as heparin-resistant. Of these plasma proteins, vitronectin plays an important role in nonspecific binding of heparin.[19] Factor VIII, vitronectin, and other plasma proteins are often elevated in patients with inflammatory diseases and in animal models of acute inflammation.[19] Heparin-resistant patients have increased heparin requirements because nonspecific binding to plasma proteins decreases the amount of heparin available in plasma to exert an anticoagulant effect via antithrombin III. However, some of these patients may also exhibit a dissociation of aPTT and heparin level results due to concomitantly high factor VIII levels.

Measurement of factor VIII levels and other plasma proteins is not practical in the clinical setting, and there is no evidence that such measurements aid in the management of heparin-resistant patients. There are several strategies that can be employed when treating patients with heparin resistance.

A *Need for an Adequate Heparin Dose*

An adequate initial dose of heparin is necessary to minimize recurrent VTE.[20] Since a large heparin dose requirement is a feature of heparin resistance, use of an adequate initial dose of heparin allows for early detection of affected patients. Although a bolus of 5000 U followed by an infusion of 30,000 to 35,000 U may be reasonable as a starting point,[5–11] there is evidence that the initial heparin dose should be adjusted for weight.[5] In a randomized trial of two dose nomograms, patients were randomized to a 5000 U bolus followed by 1000 U/hr or an 80 U/kg bolus followed by an infusion of 18 U/kg/hr. At 24 and 48 hours, a statistically significant difference in the proportion of patients in or above the therapeutic range occurred in the group receiving the weight-based nomogram compared with those receiving a standard dose (85% vs. 42%, and 84% vs. 52%, respectively). There were no major bleeding episodes in the weight-based nomogram group despite the superior anticoagulant effect. A weight-based nomogram allows for an optimal dose of heparin for each individual.

Management of Suspected Heparin Resistance

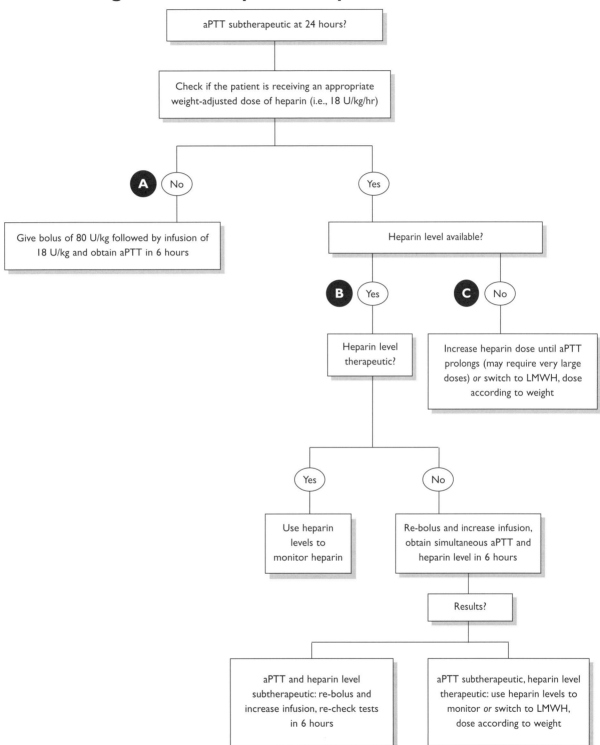

B *Use of Heparin Levels*

When heparin resistance is encountered, it is optimal to monitor the heparin effect using heparin levels. In a randomized trial of VTE patients with heparin resistance,[4] heparin effect was monitored by the aPTT in one group and by anti-factor Xa heparin levels in the other group. There was no statistically significant difference in the rates of recurrent VTE or bleeding between the two groups. However, the group monitored according to heparin levels required a smaller mean daily dose of heparin (approximately 4000 U less per day). Fifty per cent of the patients in the study with a subtherapeutic aPTT result demonstrated a dissociation of aPTT results from heparin levels (subtherapeutic aPTT with when anti-factor Xa heparin level was therapeutic), and this impairment in prolongation of the aPTT was linked to elevated factor VIII levels. It is likely that use of anti-factor Xa heparin levels to monitor patients with heparin resistance results in a lower mean daily dose because heparin levels are not affected by increased levels of factor VIII, and therefore increased doses of heparin are not required to overcome the impaired aPTT response.

C *Management When Heparin Levels Are Unavailable*

When heparin resistance is diagnosed and heparin levels are not available, it is reasonable to consider the use of low-molecular-weight heparins (LMWHs). Low-molecular-weight heparins do not bind to plasma proteins well[16–18] and therefore are superior with respect to bioavailability[21] compared with unfractionated heparin. There is ample clinical evidence indicating that LMWHs are safe and effective when given according to body weight,[22–25] and this can be done without monitoring the anticoagulant effect. Alternatively, unfractionated heparin can be continued with aPTT monitoring.

Bibliography

1. Ginsberg JS. Management of venous thromboembolism. N Engl J Med 1996;335:1816–28.
2. Hirsh J, van Aken W, Gallus AS. Heparin kinetics in venous thromboembolus. Circulation 1976;53:691–5.
3. Cruickshank MK, Levine MN, Hirsh J, Roberts RS, Siguenza M. A standard heparin nomogram for the management of heparin therapy. Arch Intern Med 1991;151:333–7.
4. Levine MN, Hirsh J, Gent M, et al. A randomized trial comparing activated thromboplastin time with heparin assay in patients with acute venous thromboembolism requiring large daily doses of heparin. Arch Intern Med 1994;154:49–56.
5. Raschke RA, Reilly BM, Guidry JR, Fontana JR, Srinivas S. The weight-based heparin dosing nomogram compared with a "standard care" nomogram. Ann Intern Med 1993;119:874–81.

6. Hull RD, Raskob GE, Hirsh J, et al. Continuous intravenous heparin compared with intermittent subcutaneous heparin in the initial treatment of proximal vein thrombosis. N Engl J Med 1986;315:1109–14.

7. Hull RD, Raskob GE, Rosenbloom D, et al. Heparin for 5 days as compared with 10 days in the initial treatment of proximal venous thrombosis. N Engl J Med 1990;322:1260–4.

8. Brandjes DPM, Heijboer H, Buller HR, de Rijk M, Jagt H, ten Cate JW. Acenocoumarol and heparin compared with acenocoumarol alone in the initial treatment of proximal-vein thrombosis. N Engl J Med 1992;327:1485–9.

9. Prandoni P, Lensing AWA, Buller HR, et al. Comparison of subcutaneous low-molecular-weight heparin with intravenous standard heparin in proximal deep-vein thrombosis. Lancet 1992;339:441–5.

10. Pini M, Pattacini C, Quintavalla R, et al. Subcutaneous vs intravenous heparin in the treatment of deep venous thrombosis—a randomized clinical trial. Thromb Haemost 1990; 64:222–6.

11. Simonneau G, Charbonnier B, Decousus H, et al. Subcutaneous low-molecular-weight heparin compared with continuous intravenous unfractionated heparin in the treatment of proximal deep vein thrombosis. Arch Intern Med 1993;153:1541–6.

12. Brill-Edwards P, Ginsberg JS, Johnston M, Hirsh J. Establishing a therapeutic range for heparin therapy. Ann Intern Med 1993;119:104–9.

13. Anand S, Brimble S, Ginsberg JS. Management of iliofemoral thrombosis in a pregnant patient with heparin resistance. Arch Intern Med 1997;157:815–6.

14. Edson VR, Krivit V, White JG. Kaolin partial thromboplastin time: high levels of procoagulants producing short clotting times or masking deficiencies of other procoagulants or low concentrations of anticoagulants. J Lab Clin Med 1967;70:463–70.

15. Chiu HM, Hirsh J, Yung WL, Regoeczi E, Gent M. Relationship between the anticoagulant and antithrombotic effects of heparin in experimental venous thrombosis. Blood 1977; 49:171–84.

16. Young E, Cosmi B, Weitz JI, Hirsh J. Comparison of the non-specific binding of unfractionated heparin and low-molecular-weight heparin (enoxaparin) to plasma proteins. Thromb Haemost 1993;70:625–30.

17. Young E, Prins M, Levine MN, Hirsh J. Heparin binding to plasma proteins, an important mechanism for heparin resistance. Thromb Haemost 1992;67:639–43.

18. Young E, Wells PS, Holloway S, Weitz JI, Hirsh J. Ex-vivo and in-vitro evidence that low-molecular-weight heparins exhibit less binding to plasma proteins than unfractionated heparin. Thromb Haemost 1994;71:300–4.

19. Young E, Podor TJ, Venner T, Hirsh J. Induction of the acute-phase reaction increases heparin-binding proteins in plasma. Aterioscler Thromb Vasc Biol 1997;17:1568–74.

20. Anand S, Ginsberg JS, Kearon C, Gent M, Hirsh J. The relation between the activated partial thromboplastin time response and recurrence in patients with venous thrombosis treated with continuous intravenous heparin. Arch Intern Med 1996;156:1677–81.

21. Hirsh J, Levine MN. Low-molecular-weight heparin. Blood 1992;79:1–17.

22. Levine MN, Gent M, Hirsh J, et al. A comparison of low-molecular-weight heparin administered primarily at home with unfractionated heparin administered in the hospital for proximal deep-vein thrombosis. N Engl J Med 1996;334:677–81.

23. Koopman MMW, Prandoni P, Piovella F, et al. Treatment of venous thrombosis with intravenous unfractionated heparin administered in the hospital as compared with subcutaneous low-molecular-weight heparin administered at home. N Engl J Med 1996;334:682–7.

24. The Columbus Investigators. Low-molecular-weight heparin in the treatment of patients with venous thromboembolism. N Engl J Med 1997;337:657–62.

25. Simonneau G, Sors H, Charbonnier B, et al. A comparison of low-molecular-weight heparin with unfractionated heparin for acute pulmonary embolism. N Engl J Med 1997; 337:663–9.

Chapter 21

SCREENING FOR THROMBOPHILIC STATES

Mark A Crowther

Jeffrey S Ginsberg

Venous thromboembolism (VTE) occurs annually in 1 in 10,000 patients under the age of 40, and in 1 in 1000 patients over the age of 65.[1] In the majority of cases, VTE occurs in the setting of an identifiable risk factor for thrombosis, such as recent surgery. However, VTE does occur unexpectedly in otherwise well outpatients. Thorough investigation of these patients with "idiopathic" thromboembolism frequently will reveal an inherited or acquired condition that predisposes to VTE.[2–4] These prothrombotic states, which have been termed the "thrombophilias," predispose to both first and recurrent episodes of thrombosis.

In any medical condition, the usefulness of a screening test is maximal when its results will lead directly to a change in patient care. Thus, screening patients for thrombophilia presupposes that the detection of an abnormality will alter management in a meaningful way. Although the utility of screening patients for thrombophilia has not been directly addressed in methodologically sound studies, it is likely that the presence of a predisposition for thrombosis in an otherwise well outpatient could alter that patient's management. For example, the presence of activated protein C resistance would lead us to advise a patient against the use of the oral contraceptive pill.[5]

A *Should One Suspect Thrombophilia?*

Screening for a thrombophilic state should be performed in all patients less than 60 years of age who present with a first episode of idiopathic VTE. We do not screen patients older than 60 who have idiopathic VTE nor do we screen those with VTE in the setting of a clear-cut risk factor for thrombosis, such as recent orthopedic surgery or metastatic cancer. Patients with VTE whose only risk factor is the birth control pill, estrogen replacement therapy, or pregnancy should probably be screened for thrombophilia. However, screening should be performed after the pregnancy is completed or the hormonal therapy has been stopped; the high levels of estrogen in such patients can influence the results of thrombophilic testing (see below).[6]

Patients with recurrent VTE, even in the setting of a risk factor, should be screened, as should patients who develop VTE in unusual sites (e.g., cerebral venous sinuses, mesenteric or hepatic veins).[7,8] Finally, patients with recalcitrant superficial phlebitis, warfarin-induced skin necrosis, and those with a strong family history of thrombosis should also be screened.[4,9]

Thrombosis occurs frequently in patients who have more than one risk factor: this situation can occur, for instance, if a patient with a known congenital deficiency of an anticoagulant protein undergoes a surgical procedure which is associated with a high risk of VTE.

B *Screening Tests for Thrombophilia*

Testing for thrombophilia is best performed after the completion of anticoagulant therapy because both acute thrombosis and anticoagulant therapy alter the results of laboratory tests for thrombophilia. However, it is often convenient to obtain plasma samples from patients with newly diagnosed VTE before anticoagulants are administered. If testing performed at this time is abnormal, the finding should be confirmed after anticoagulants have been discontinued.

Warfarin reduces the plasma levels of protein C, protein S, and prothrombin. As a result, levels of these proteins should only be measured after the patient has been off warfarin for a minimum of 7 days. Heparin therapy reduces antithrombin levels[10] while both heparin and warfarin interfere with testing for the lupus anticoagulant and activated protein C resistance. Antithrombin and protein S levels are reduced during pregnancy and the postpartum period; therefore, testing for these deficiencies should be performed 6 or more weeks after delivery.[11] Genetic testing (for factor V_{Leiden}, metabolic causes of hyperhomocystinemia, or abnormalities in the prothrombin gene) is not affected by anticoagulants or the presence of acute thrombosis.

Some patients with suspected thrombophilia are thought to have a very high risk of recurrent thrombosis. In these patients, simply stopping warfarin for 5 to 7 days prior to testing to allow protein C and S levels to return to the normal range might be associated with recurrent thrombosis. In such patients, self-administered unfractionated heparin or low-molecular-weight heparin can be started on the day following discontinuation of warfarin and continued until the evening prior to testing. Heparin and warfarin are then restarted immediately after the testing is performed, and the heparin is stopped when the international normalized ratio (INR) has been therapeutic for 2 consecutive days.

The most common congenital thrombophilic state is activated protein C resistance (APCR), which is found in 16 to 30% of patients with acute idiopathic VTE.[3] More than 90% of patients with APCR have a specific genetic mutation, factor V_{Leiden}. This mutation slows APC-mediated inactivation of factor V. An acquired form of APCR can be found in pregnant patients and in patients with antiphospholipid antibodies (see below).[12,13] The frequency of APCR varies widely amongst different ethnic groups: it occurs in about 5% of a mixed population derived predominately from Europe.[14] The risk of recurrent thrombosis in patients with APCR after discontinuation of warfarin is not known.

Antithrombin is a plasma protein that acts as an anticoagulant by inactivating thrombin and factor Xa. Antithrombin deficiency is found in 3 to 6% of patients with acute idiopathic VTE.[4] Antithrombin deficiency is commonly divided into three types: Type I is a quantitative deficiency of antithrombin, Type II is a qualitative abnormality of antithrombin's ability to inactivate clotting factors, and Type III is due to a mutation that reduces the ability of antithrombin to bind with heparin.[15] In those patients with antithrombin deficiency who suffer venous thrombosis, most will have their first thrombotic event by the age of 50. Thrombosis often occurs in association with a transient risk factor, such as pregnancy.[16] Acquired antithrombin deficiency occurs in patients with sepsis, with disseminated intravascular coagulation, during pregnancy, and in patients receiving l-asparaginase.

Protein C is a naturally occurring anticoagulant protein that produces its anticoagulant effect by degrading activated coagulation factors V and VIII. Protein C deficiency is found in 2 to 5% of patients presenting with a first episode of idiopathic VTE.[2,4] The majority of patients with heterozygous protein C deficiency who have an episode of VTE will do so by the age of 60[16] while many patients with homozygous protein C deficiency present in the neonatal period with purpura fulminans. Protein C deficiency is usually classified into two types: Type I is characterized by reduced antigenic and functional protein C levels while Type II is characterized by normal antigenic levels of protein C with reduced functional activity.[17] Both Type I and Type II deficiency are associated with a thrombophilic state. Acquired protein C deficiency is found in patients with liver disease, in patients who are vitamin K deficient, and in patients who are taking warfarin.

Protein S is a cofactor for the anticoagulant effect of protein C. In the circulation, approximately 60% of protein S is inactivated as a result of binding to C4b-binding protein. Reduced levels of both the total and free (unbound) fractions of protein S are associated with an increased risk of VTE.[16] Homozygous protein S deficiency can cause purpura fulminans. Acquired protein S deficiency is found in patients with liver disease, in patients with antiphospholipid antibodies, and in patients who are vitamin K deficient or are receiving warfarin.

Recently, the association between elevated basal levels of prothrombin and a thrombophilic state have been confirmed. Many patients who have both VTE and basal prothrombin levels > 1.5 U/L have a mutation in the prothrombin regulatory sequence. The mechanism of thrombophilia in these patients is unclear; however, it is possible that this finding explains the prothrombotic state of 10 to 20% of patients with idiopathic VTE.[18] In addition, there is a statistical association between elevated basal plasma levels of coagulation factor VIII and thrombosis.[19] The significance of this finding is not clear.

Patients with malignancy have a high risk of VTE. Malignancy predisposes to thrombosis through a variety of mechanisms. For example, patients frequently have reduced mobility, tumors may directly compress or invade blood vessels, and some tumor cell types (such as adenocarcinoma) release tissue thromboplastin. Additionally, it is likely that some chemotherapeutic agents disrupt endothelial function, further increasing the risk of thrombosis.

Any patient with malignancy who presents with a history suggestive of VTE, or clinical signs or symptoms of VTE, should be thoroughly evaluated using accurate diagnostic testing. Because of the high risk of recurrent thrombosis, many patients with malignancy who have had one episode of thrombosis remain on life-long warfarin therapy. Additionally, patients with malignancies such as prostate cancer can have recurrent VTE in spite of therapeutic warfarin doses: such patients require higher intensity warfarin or long-term subcutaneous heparin or low-molecular-weight heparin.

Other common acquired conditions predisposing to VTE are the antiphospholipid antibody (APLA) syndromes. Antiphospholipid antibodies are a heterogeneous group of antibodies directed against anionic phospholipids in concert with cell-surface glycoproteins. Antiphospholipid antibodies are usually divided into two classes: anticardiolipin antibodies and the lupus anticoagulant. Antiphospholipid antibodies may be transient (seen after viral infection or in patients receiving certain medications), or persistent. Persistent antiphospholipid antibodies are associated with a high risk of VTE. The mechanism of thrombosis in these patients is unclear: reduced protein C activity, reduced free protein S levels, and endothelial cell dysfunction have all been proposed. Antiphospholipid antibody syndromes are associated with a high risk of recurrent VTE, and some patients with APLA suffer recurrent VTE while receiving "therapeutic" doses of warfarin.

Elevated serum levels of homocysteine (an amino acid) are associated with both arterial and venous thromboembolism.[20] Congenital hyperhomocystinemia occurs as a result of deficiencies of one of several enzymes involved in homocysteine metabolism. The most common abnormalities are deficiencies of the cystathionine β-synthase (CβS) or methylenetetrahydrofolate reductase (MTHFR) genes. Dietary deficiencies of folic acid, or vitamins B_6 or B_{12} are associated with hyperhomocystinemia, particularly in patients with mild deficiencies of CβS or MTHFR. Patients with mild hyperhomocystinemia will have an exaggerated increase in their serum homocysteine levels after receiving an oral loading dose of the amino acid methionine when compared with patients who do not have hyperhomocystinemia.[20] Patients in whom this abnormal response may be seen include those with mild deficiencies of CβS or MTHFR, or in patients with deficiencies of vitamins B_6, B_{12}, or folate.

A rare cause of thrombophilia is paroxysmal nocturnal hemoglobinuria (PNH). Paroxysmal nocturnal hemoglobinuria is associated with aplastic anemia and frequently presents with acute venous thrombosis (often Budd-Chiari syndrome). Other conditions that have been described in association with thrombophilia include heparin cofactor II deficiency, and abnormalities of plasminogen, fibrinogen, and plasminogen activator inhibitor 1 (PAI-1). The clinical significance of these abnormalities is not clear; thus, routine screening for these abnormalities cannot be recommended.

C *Abnormal Results on the Thrombophilia Screen*

The aim of treatment with oral anticoagulants is to reduce the risk of recurrent VTE to an acceptable level, without an excess risk of bleeding. Warfarin therapy (with a target INR of 2.0 to 3.0) reduces the risk of recurrent thrombosis by about 90%; however, it is associated with an annual risk of major or life-threatening hemorrhage of 1 to 2%.[21] The risk of hemorrhage rises substantially with increasing age.[22] Therefore, for most conditions, warfarin is discontinued after 3 to 6 months, and the patient is watched closely for clinical evidence of recurrent thrombosis.

In patients with a thrombophilic disorder, the risk of recurrent thromboembolism is probably high after warfarin is stopped.[23] Thus, long-term warfarin is often recommended to prevent recurrence in these patients. In patients who have had more than one previous episode of VTE, warfarin should be continued for life. We do not use long-term warfarin in patients with known thrombophilic disorders who have not had a thrombotic event. We advise the patient of the signs and symptoms of VTE and tell them to seek medical attention promptly should they occur. In addition, we counsel patients to avoid situations that put them at high risk of thromboembolism. For example, we advise patients with activated protein C resistance to avoid the use of estrogen-containing oral contraceptive medications.[24]

Patient with Objectively Diagnosed Venous Thromboembolism

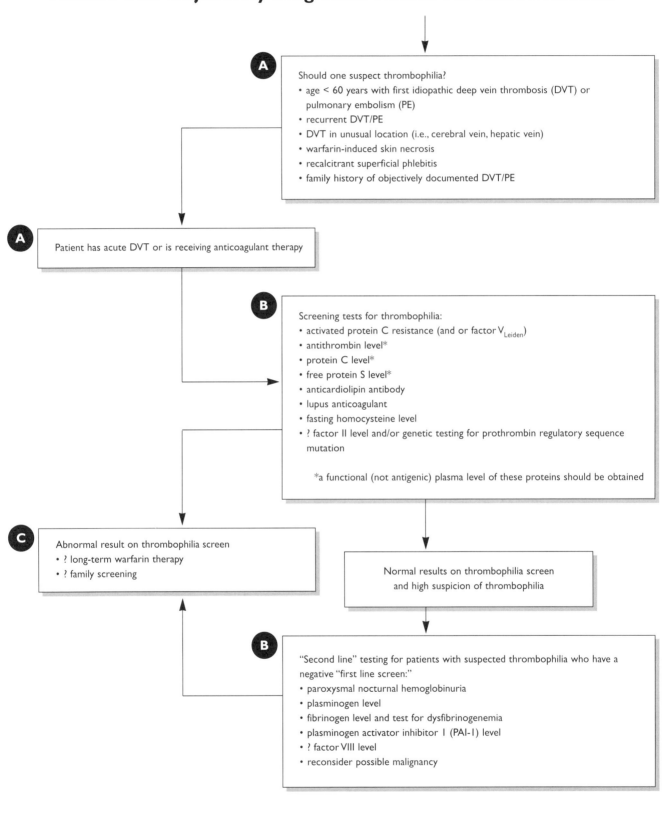

A Should one suspect thrombophilia?
- age < 60 years with first idiopathic deep vein thrombosis (DVT) or pulmonary embolism (PE)
- recurrent DVT/PE
- DVT in unusual location (i.e., cerebral vein, hepatic vein)
- warfarin-induced skin necrosis
- recalcitrant superficial phlebitis
- family history of objectively documented DVT/PE

A Patient has acute DVT or is receiving anticoagulant therapy

B Screening tests for thrombophilia:
- activated protein C resistance (and or factor V$_{Leiden}$)
- antithrombin level*
- protein C level*
- free protein S level*
- anticardiolipin antibody
- lupus anticoagulant
- fasting homocysteine level
- ? factor II level and/or genetic testing for prothrombin regulatory sequence mutation

   *a functional (not antigenic) plasma level of these proteins should be obtained

C Abnormal result on thrombophilia screen
- ? long-term warfarin therapy
- ? family screening

Normal results on thrombophilia screen and high suspicion of thrombophilia

B "Second line" testing for patients with suspected thrombophilia who have a negative "first line screen:"
- paroxysmal nocturnal hemoglobinuria
- plasminogen level
- fibrinogen level and test for dysfibrinogenemia
- plasminogen activator inhibitor 1 (PAI-1) level
- ? factor VIII level
- reconsider possible malignancy

All patients should receive appropriate thromboembolic prophylaxis during times of increased risk of thrombosis. Patients with a thrombophilic disorder should also receive prophylaxis; however, in some cases (such as the postpartum period in patients with antithrombin deficiency), intensified prophylaxis, often with therapeutic doses of warfarin, should be considered. Additionally, intensified pre-discharge screening for VTE may be justified in these patients.

Treatment with a fast-acting parenteral anticoagulant, in concert with warfarin, is required in all patients with acute venous thromboembolism. Because of a potential hypercoagulable state due to the early fall in the level of protein C, coupled with near-normal levels of factors II and X in the first 72 hours of warfarin therapy, the parenteral anticoagulant should be continued for a minimum of 4 days, irrespective of the INR value.[25] This is particularly important in patients with known protein C or S deficiency, in whom premature discontinuation of the parenteral anticoagulant can be associated with warfarin-induced skin necrosis. Some patients with cancer or antiphospholipid antibodies have a high risk of recurrence, even when receiving warfarin with a target INR of 2.0 to 3.0. If recurrent thromboembolism occurs in spite of warfarin, these patients should receive either warfarin (with or without aspirin) with a target INR of 3.0 to 4.0, or long-term parenteral anticoagulation with heparin or a low-molecular-weight heparin.[26]

Bibliography

1. Ridker PM, Glynn RJ, Miletich JP, et al. Age-specific incidence rates of venous thromboembolism among heterozygous carriers of factor V Leiden mutation. Ann Intern Med 1997;126:528–31.

2. Koster T, Rosendaal FR, Briet E, et al. Protein C deficiency in a controlled series of unselected outpatients: an infrequent but clear risk factor for venous thrombosis (Leiden Thrombophilia Study). Blood 1995;95:2756–61.

3. Manten B, Westendorp RG, Koster T, Reitsma PH, Rosendaal FR. Risk factor profiles in patients with different clinical manifestations of venous thromboembolism: a focus on the factor V Leiden mutation. Thromb Haemost 1996;76:510–3.

4. Mateo J, Oliver A, Borrell M, Sala N, Fontcuberta J. Laboratory evaluation and clinical characteristics of 2,132 consecutive unselected patients with venous thromboembolism—results of the Spanish Multicentric Study on Thrombophilia (EMET-Study). Thromb Haemost 1997;77:444–51.

5. Vandenbroucke JP, Koster T, Briet E, Reitsma PH, Bertina RM. Increased risk of venous thrombosis in oral-contraceptive users who are carriers of factor V Leiden mutation. Lancet 1994;344:1453–7.

6. Faught W, Garner P, Jones G, Ivey B. Changes in protein C and protein S levels in normal pregnancy. Am J Obstet Gynecol 1995;95(1 Pt 1):147–50.

7. Pelletier S, Landi B, Piette JC, et al. Antiphospholipid syndrome as the second cause of non-tumorous Budd-Chiari syndrome. J Hepatol 1994;21:76–80.

8. Daif A, Awada A, al-Rajeh S, et al. Cerebral venous thrombosis in adults. A study of 40 cases from Saudi Arabia. Stroke 1995;26:1193–5.

9. Koeleman BP, Reitsma PH, Allaart CF, Bertina RM. Activated protein C resistance as an additional risk factor for thrombosis in protein C-deficient families. Blood 1994;84:1031–5.

10. Harbourne T, Nicolaides AN. The effect of operation and subcutaneous heparin on plasma levels of antithrombin III. Thromb Res 1986;43:657–62.

11. Aillaud MF, Pouymayou K, Brunet D, et al. New direct assay of free protein S antigen applied to diagnosis of protein S deficiency. Thromb Haemost 1996;75:283–5.

12. Schlit AF, Col-De BC, Moriau M, Lavenne-Pardonge E. Acquired activated protein C resistance in pregnancy. Thromb Res 1996;84:203–6.

13. De Stefano V, Mastrangelo K, Paciaroni K, et al. Acquired activated Protein C resistance in patients with lupus anticoagulants. Thromb Haemost 1995;74:797–8.

14. Lee DH, Henderson P, Blajchman M. Prevalence of factor V Leiden in a Canadian blood donor population. Can Med Assoc J 1996;155:285–9.

15. Blajchman MA. An overview of the mechanism of action of antithrombin and its inherited deficiency states. Blood Coagul Fibrinolysis 1994;5(Suppl 1):S5–11; discussion S59.

16. De Stefano V, Finazzi G, Mannucci PM. Inherited thrombophilia: pathogenesis, clinical syndromes, and management. Blood 1996;87:3531–44.

17. Miyata T, Zheng YZ, Sakata T, Tsushima N, Kato H. Three missense mutations in the protein C heavy chain causing type I and type II protein C deficiency. Thromb Haemost 1994;71:32–7.

18. Hillarp A, Svensson PJ, Dahlback B. Prothrombin gene mutation and venous thrombosis in unselected outpatients. Thromb Haemost 1997;78(Suppl):378–9.

19. Koster T, Blann AD, Briet E, Vandenbroucke JP, Rosendaal FR. Role of clotting factor VIII in effect of von Willebrand factor on occurrence of deep-vein thrombosis. Lancet 1995;345:152–5.

20. Fermo I, Vigano' DS, Paroni R, Mazzola G, Calori G, D'Angelo A. Prevalence of moderate hyperhomocysteinemia in patients with early-onset venous and arterial occlusive disease. Ann Intern Med 1995;123:747–53.

21. Cortelazzo S, Finazzi G, Viero P, Galli M, Remuzzi A, Parenzan LBT. Thrombotic and hemorrhagic complications in patients with mechanical heart valve prosthesis attending an anticoagulation clinic. Thromb Haemost 1993;69:316–20.

22. Anonymous. Bleeding during antithrombotic therapy in patients with atrial fibrillation. The Stroke Prevention in Atrial Fibrillation Investigators. Arch Intern Med 1996;156:409–16.

23. Simioni P, Prandoni P, Lensing A, et al. The risk of recurrent venous thromboembolism in patients with an Arg506->Gln mutation in the gene for factor V (factor V Leiden). N Engl J Med 1997;336:399–403.

24. Bloemenkamp KW, Rosendaal FR, Helmerhorst FM, Buller HR, Vandenbroucke JP. Enhancement by factor V Leiden mutation of risk of deep-vein thrombosis associated with oral contraceptives containing a third-generation progestagen. Lancet 1995;346:1593–6.

25. Harrison L, Johnston M, Massicotte MP, Crowther M, Moffat K, Hirsh J. Comparison of 5-mg and 10-mg loading doses in initiation of warfarin therapy. Ann Intern Med 1997;126:133–6.

26. Rosove MH, Brewer PM. Antiphospholipid thrombosis: clinical course after the first thrombotic event in 70 patients. Ann Intern Med 1992;117:303–8.

Chapter 22

DIAGNOSIS AND MANAGEMENT OF UPPER LIMB DEEP VEIN THROMBOSIS

Alberto Cogo

Upper limb deep vein thrombosis (DVT) comprises a minority (~ 5%) of all episodes of DVT. This probably accounts for the paucity of information currently available on its pathogenesis, diagnosis, and management. Most of the information in this chapter comes from a recent article in which a large series of consecutive patients with clinically suspected upper limb DVT were investigated.[1]

A Clinically Suspected Upper Limb DVT

Upper limb DVT should be suspected when swelling, pain, functional disability, skin discoloration, and distended superficial veins (as a single pattern or in combination) of the upper extremity or shoulder occur. The clinical suspicion is increased by the presence of specific risk factors, such as central venous catheters, previous episodes of venous thrombosis, known thrombophilia, estrogen use, cancer, and unusual muscular exercise ("effort thrombosis").[1–4] Sometimes, upper limb DVT arises spontaneously and in otherwise healthy patients.

B Is Pulmonary Embolism Suspected?

The prevalence of both symptomatic and asymptomatic pulmonary embolism in patients with upper limb DVT is relatively high (30% or higher).[1,5,6] Pulmonary embolism should be promptly investigated if compatible symptoms and/or signs are seen on presentation.

C Give Full-Dose Heparin

If an accurate diagnostic test cannot be rapidly performed, it is reasonable to start anticoagulant treatment. In fact, the hazard of withholding effective treatment in a potentially fatal disease (due to its strong association with pulmonary embolism) is greater than that of using heparin, with its associated hemorrhagic complications, while waiting for a definitive diagnostic test.

D *Perform an Objective Diagnostic Test*

Clinical manifestations of upper limb DVT are nonspecific, and the prevalence of the disease among symptomatic patients is less than 50%.[1] Therefore, definitive management decisions should be based only on the results of accurate objective diagnostic tests. Contrast venography, the reference standard test, is costly and invasive and, therefore, should be performed only if noninvasive procedures are not available or their results are indeterminate. Among noninvasive tests, real-time B-mode ultrasonography and color Doppler devices are both accurate and reproducible.[6] However, since color Doppler is more expensive and time consuming, and requires considerable expertise for its execution, real-time B-mode ultrasonography should be regarded as the first-choice alternative to contrast venography. The positive and negative predictive values of both B-mode ultrasonography and color Doppler are sufficently high to guide management decision. However, since the safety of withholding anticoagulants in symptomatic patients with negative noninvasive test results on the day of presentation has never been investigated in a properly designed trial, it seems reasonable to repeat the test within 1 week, or to perform contrast venography, if symptoms persist and/or a clear alternative diagnosis is not reached.

On venography, the diagnosis of DVT is made in the presence of a constant intraluminal filling defect involving one or more segments from the brachial to the subclavian veins. Other findings, such as nonvisualization of a venous segment despite repeated contrast injection or abrupt termination of the contrast column, might be due to technical artifacts and are not definitive for DVT. The single criterion of vein compressibility (compression ultrasonography) is used with real-time B-mode ultrasonography. With color Doppler, the presence of deep vein thrombosis is indicated by the absence of color signal within the lumen of the vein, even after manual distal limb compression, or by direct visualization of an intraluminal filling defect. Noninvasive diagnostic test results can be inconclusive mainly because one or more venous segments, commonly the subclavian vein, are not visualized.

E *Give Full-Dose Heparin Followed by Oral Anticoagulants*

In a recent cohort study, consecutive symptomatic patients with upper limb DVT were treated with full-dose unfractionated heparin followed by oral anticoagulants (target INR: 2.0 to 3.0). During the first 3 months of follow-up, recurrent thromboembolic events and bleeding complications were rare.[1] The efficacy and safety of more invasive approaches, such as thrombolytic therapy or thrombectomy, have never been investigated in properly designed trials. Therefore, these modalities should not be routinely performed; rather, they should be reserved for selected patients (e.g., those with extensive DVT and very low risk of bleeding).

F *Decide the Duration of Secondary Prophylaxis*

The optimal duration of antithrombotic therapy after a first episode of upper limb DVT has not been investigated in rigorous trials and, therefore, the recommendations provided are empiric. Nevertheless, to prevent recurrences, it seems reasonable to use oral anticoagulants (target INR: 2.0 to 3.0) in all patients for at least 3 months. At this time, we decide whether or not to stop anticoagulants by determining the presence or absence of risk factors for thrombosis. If the DVT was triggered by a transient risk factor (recent trauma, central venous catheter) that has been removed, oral anticoagulants are discontinued after 3 months. If the DVT is idiopathic (i.e., no acquired or inherited risk factor is identified), secondary prophylaxis is continued for at least 1 year. After stopping secondary prophylaxis, all patients are instructed to return promptly if signs or symptoms of recurrent thrombosis appear. In patients with a permanent risk factor (untreatable cancer, inherited thrombophilia) secondary prophylaxis with oral anticoagulants is continued life long.

G *Clinically Suspected Recurrent Upper Limb DVT*

After a first episode of upper limb DVT, the long-term recurrence rate is substantial (approximately 8% after 2 years).[1] When patients present with a clinically suspected recurrent upper limb DVT, contrast venography should be performed since the utility of noninvasive procedures has not been demonstrated in this setting. Recurrent thrombosis is confirmed by the presence of a new intraluminal filling defect.

H *Consider Post-thrombotic Syndrome*

Late sequelae of upper extremity DVT can occur; however, the exact incidence and clinical course of upper-limb post-thrombotic syndrome are currently unknown. Moreover, no standardized approach exists for the management of post-thrombotic syndrome. If symptoms are severe, we advise patients to use a graduated compression sleeve covering the entire limb. Intermittent pneumatic compression therapy with an intermittent compression pump may provide some relief in patients with breakthrough persistent symptoms.

Clinically Suspected Upper Limb Deep Vein Thrombosis (DVT)

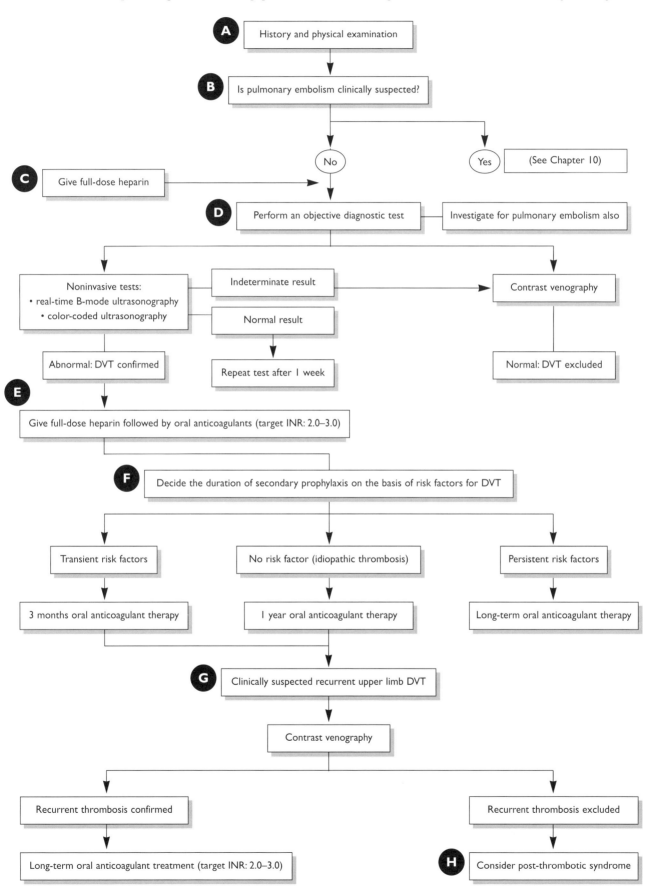

Bibliography

1. Prandoni P, Polistena P, Bernardi E, et al. Upper extremity deep-vein thrombosis: Risk factors, diagnosis and complication. Arch Intern Med 1997;157:57–62.

2. Clagett GP, Eberhart RC. Artificial devices in clinical practice. In: Colman RW, Hirsh J, Marder VJ, Salzman EW, eds. Hemostasis and thrombosis. Philadelphia: J.P. Lippincott Company, 1995.

3. De Maeseneer M, De Hert S, Van Schil P, Schoofs E. Deep venous thrombosis of the upper extremity: case reports and review of the literature. Acta Chir Belg 1989;89:253–61.

4. Hill SL, Berry RE. Subclavian vein thrombosis: a continuing challenge. Surgery 1990;108:1–9.

5. Monreal M, Lafoz E, Ruiz J, Valls R, Alastrue A. Upper extremity deep venous thrombosis and pulmonary embolism: a prospective study. Chest 1991;99:280–3.

6. Black MD, French GJ, Rasuli P, Bouchard AC. Upper extremity deep venous thrombosis. Underdiagnosed and potentially lethal. Chest 1993;103:1887–90.

Chapter 23

DIAGNOSIS AND MANAGEMENT OF PORTAL VEIN THROMBOSIS

Stephen J Skehan

Gervais Tougas

Thrombosis of the portal vein, with or without involvement of splenic or mesenteric veins, is an uncommon condition which usually occurs in association with recognized precipitating factors. Its diagnosis requires a high index of suspicion since portal vein thrombosis is often asymptomatic until complications of chronic portal hypertension, such as esophageal variceal hemorrhage, occur. With the availability of noninvasive techniques including Doppler ultrasonography and computed tomography, portal vein thrombosis can now be readily diagnosed without resorting to more invasive approaches, such as mesenteric angiography. Earlier diagnosis and aggressive therapy including thrombolysis, anticoagulation, or surgery when indicated, now provide for effective treatment in acute portal vein thrombosis. In those patients with established portal hypertension, initial control and prevention of variceal bleeding through improved endoscopic techniques, such as sclerotherapy and the rubber-band ligation of varices, have decreased the need for surgery with its significant mortality and high morbidity.

A *Situation Predisposing to Portal Vein Thrombosis*
The following summarizes the conditions that predispose to portal vein thrombosis:
1. Decreased intrahepatic venous flow
    cirrhosis (any cause)
    hepatocellular carcinoma
    portal fibrosis, idiopathic portal hypertension, hepatoportal fibrosis
    liver transplantation
2. Neoplasia
    through portal vein invasion or extrinsic compression
    pancreas, lung, stomach, biliary tract, genitourinary system

3. Infection

   especially in children (umbilical sepsis)

   appendicitis, biliary tract sepsis, peritonitis, septicemia

4. Inflammation

   pancreatitis, inflammatory bowel disease

5. Myeloproliferative disorders

6. Hypercoagulable states

   inherited (antithrombin, protein C or S deficiencies)

   acquired (drugs, pregnancy, connective tissue disorders)

7. Trauma and iatrogenic causes

   blunt trauma

   abdominal surgery and splenectomy (including laparoscopic surgery)

   splenorenal or portocaval shunt

   liver transplantation

   transhepatic variceal obliteration

B *Clinical Presentation*

Acute portal vein thrombosis is most often asymptomatic unless mesenteric venous return is also compromised. Hematemesis, increased abdominal girth, ascites, and abdominal pain are the most common symptoms associated with portal vein thrombosis. Hematemesis is the consequence of ruptured esophageal varices resulting from

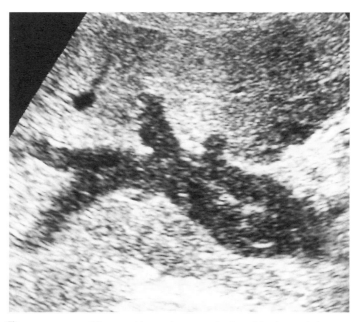

Figure 23.1 Ultrasound image demonstrating branching, hypoechoic material completely filling the lumen of the portal vein in a patient with hepatocellular carcinoma.

longstanding portal hypertension. As with any variceal hemorrhage, bleeding is often very severe. Occasionally, melena can be the first manifestation of variceal bleeding. Gastric and even intestinal varices can sometimes develop and bleed as well.

When symptomatic, acute portal vein thrombosis can present with abdominal pain, which is the result of extension of the thrombus into the mesenteric veins with resultant bowel ischemia. If prolonged, intestinal ischemia can also result in intestinal bleeding.

In cirrhotic subjects, the first manifestation of portal vein thrombosis might be a rapid increase of abdominal girth due to worsening ascites. This might be particularly true in patients who develop spontaneous bacterial peritonitis.

C *Diagnosis: Ultrasound*

This technique is inexpensive, rapid, and reliable (Figure 23.1). If the sonographer is confident that appearances are normal, portal vein thrombosis can be ruled out.

An arterial signal detected within the thrombus using Doppler techniques is highly specific (95% or higher) for malignant thrombus (Figure 23.2).

Ultrasound is also excellent for assessing secondary or associated features of portal vein thrombosis (e.g., splenomegaly, ascites, hepatic neoplasms, varices, and retrograde flow in the splenic and superior mesenteric veins).

The technique is technically difficult in many patients due to body habitus, ascites, overlying bowel gas, and a small high liver.

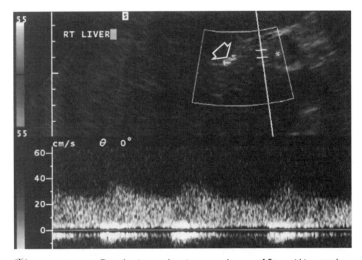

Figure 23.2   Doppler image showing several areas of flow *within* portal venous thrombus (*) in a patient with hepatocellular carcinoma (different patient from Figure 23.1). The normal hepatic artery (arrow) lies anterior to the portal vein (above it on the image). The waveform at the bottom of the image, which is clearly arterial, comes from the cursor placed within the malignant thrombus and not from the hepatic artery.

D *Diagnosis: Computed Tomographic (CT) Portography*

Spiral CT, now available in most centers is not dependent on body habitus although patients must be able to hold their breath for 15 to 20 seconds. It is associated with a relatively high contrast load (which is given via an arm vein) and is, therefore, unsuitable for patients with renal failure and/or contrast allergy.

Three-dimensional reconstructions can be very helpful to show anatomy (Figures 23.3A and B).

Neovascularisation and identification of thrombus greater than 23 mm in diameter in the main portal vein are good indicators of a malignant thrombus.

E *Diagnosis: Angiography/Magnetic Resonance Imaging (MRI)*

Diagnostic studies can occasionally not be obtained with either CT or ultrasound. In such cases, indirect portography in the late stages of coeliac and superior mesenteric artery injections should demonstrate the portal vein (Figures 23.4A and B). Direct portography using a splenic puncture can be used as a last resort to delineate the portal vein.

Several different sequences such as spin-echo, gradient-echo, and phase-contrast cine-MRI have been shown to be accurate for diagnosing portal vein thrombosis. Current limitations include the availability of facilities, relatively long scanning times, and a susceptibility to artifacts. All of these limitations are likely to be overcome in the near future, and MRI will probably become a first- or second-line investigation.

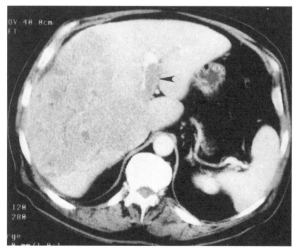

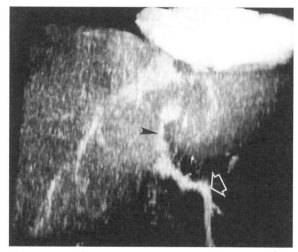

Figure 23.3a   Axial CT image through the liver in the same patient as Figure 23.2. Thrombus is seen to partially occlude the left portal vein (arrow) while the right portal vein fails to enhance at all due to complete thrombosis. The large hypoattenuating area in the right lobe is due to a combination of tumor and hypoperfusion.

Figure 23.3b   Three-dimensional CT image (maximum intensity projection) in the same case, showing the normal superior mesenteric vein and main portal vein (white arrow), with focal narrowing of the left branch (black arrowhead) and complete absence of the right branch. Contrast in the heart is seen above the left lobe of the liver. The other enhancing structures in the liver are the hepatic veins.

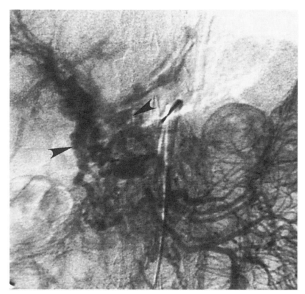

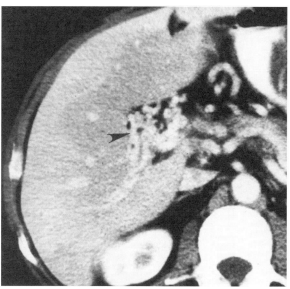

Figure 23.4a   Venous phase of superior mesenteric angiogram in a patient with cavernous transformation of the portal vein, demonstrating a leash of tortuous vessels (between arrowheads) instead of a normal single portal vein. (Courtesy of Dr. John Rawlinson, McMaster University.)

Figure 23.4b   Corresponding axial CT image from the same patient, again clearly showing multiple small portal vessels (arrowhead), with no normal portal vein.

F *Management: Thrombolysis*

Although controlled randomized trials are lacking, most experts recommend initial thrombolytic therapy with streptokinase or urokinase in patients with acute, benign portal vein thrombosis who do not have evidence of intestinal ischemia, followed by an intravenous heparin infusion with subsequent oral anticoagulation.

G *Management: Portal Hypertension*

The treatment of chronic portal vein thrombosis, including that associated with cavernous transformation or partial recanalization, is essentially the treatment of portal hypertension and its complications. Anticoagulation has no role in this setting. Prophylactic endoscopic sclerotherapy or rubber-band ligation of varices are used to prevent bleeding episodes. The same treatment is used for acute variceal bleeding, in addition to aggressive resuscitation measures and correction of coagulopathy.

H *Management: Uncontrolled Acute Bleeding*

Emergency surgery (shunt or esophageal transection) is to be avoided, if at all possible, in this setting as it is associated with greater than 30% mortality.

Diagnosis of Portal Vein Thrombosis

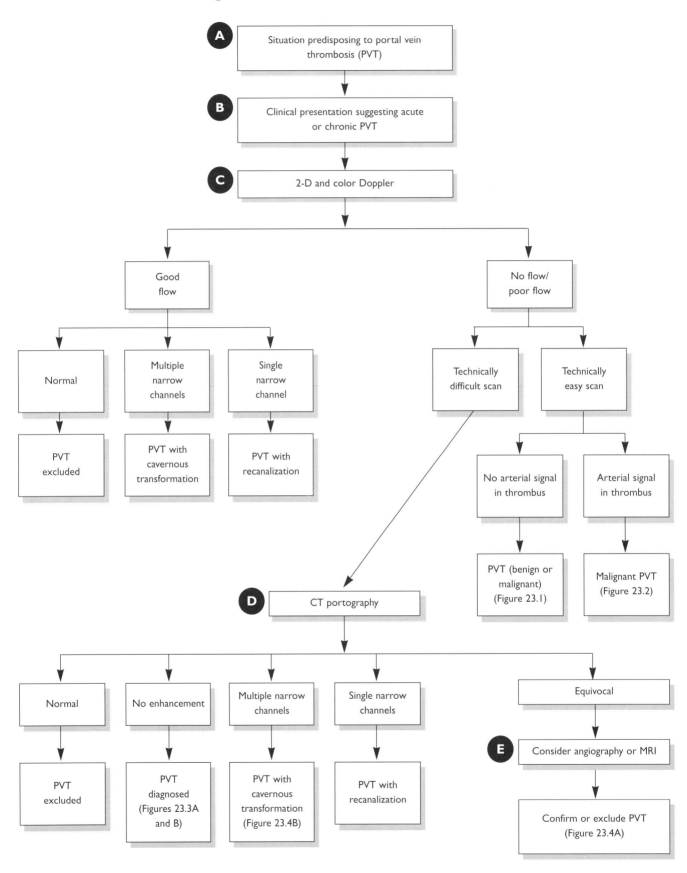

Management of Portal Vein Thrombosis

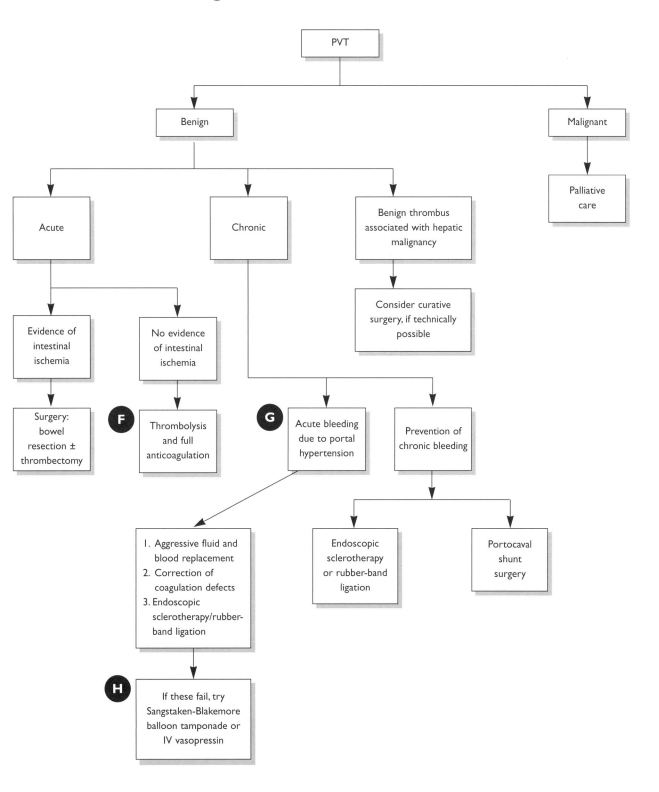

Additional Reading

Cohe J, Edelman RR, Chopra S. Portal vein thrombosis: a review. Am J Med 1992;92:173–82.

Merkel CM, Bolognesi S, Bellon D, et al. Long-term follow-up study of adult patients with non-cirrhotic obstruction of the portal system: comparison with cirrhotic patients. J Hepatol 1992;15:299–303.

Olafsson S, Blei AT. Diagnosis and management of ascites in the age of TIPS. Am J Roentgenol 1995;165:9–16.

Seu P, Shackleton CR, Shaked A, et al. Improved results of liver transplantation in patients with portal vein thrombosis. Arch Surg 1996;131:840–5.

Tublin ME, Dodd III GD, Baron RL. Benign and malignant portal vein thrombosis: differentiation by CT characteristics. Am J Roentgenol 1997;168:719–23.

Bach AM, Hann LE, Brown KT, et al. Portal vein evaluation with US: comparison to angiography combined with CT arterial portography. Radiology 1996;201:149–54.

Tessler FN, Gehring BJ, Gomes AS, et al. Diagnosis of portal vein vein thrombosis: value of colour Doppler imaging. Am J Roentgenol 1991;157:293–6.

Parvey HR, Raval B, Sandler CM. Portal vein thrombosis: imaging findings (pictorial essay). Am J Roentgenol 1994;162:77–81.

Chapter 24

Diagnosis and Management of Cerebral Venous Thrombosis

Robert J Duke

Thrombosis of cerebral veins and dural sinuses is under-recognized. The clinical spectrum of presentation is extremely broad but cerebral venous thrombosis (CVT) should be suspected in an atypical stroke-like presentation, or isolated intracranial hypertension, especially in clinical settings predisposing to thrombosis (Table 24.1). Less frequently, a specific clinical syndrome such as that of cavernous sinus thrombosis is present. The clinical features are generally nonspecific and require neuroradiological investigations to confirm the diagnosis, and laboratory tests are needed to identify predisposing hypercoagulable states.

A Initial Neuroimaging Examination

When CVT is suspected, CT scan with and without contrast injection is the first neuroimaging examination to carry out, both to rule out other conditions and to confirm CVT. Three abnormalities are considered direct signs of CVT: the cord sign, the dense triangle sign, and the delta (or empty) triangle sign. The cord sign, visible on unenhanced CT scans, represents the visualization of a thrombosed cortical vein; it is extremely rare, and its diagnostic value is debated. The dense triangle sign reflects spontaneous sagittal sinus thrombosis but is rarely present. The empty delta sign, the most frequent direct sign, appears after contrast injection and reflects the opacification of collateral veins in the parasagittal sinus wall, contrasting with the non-enhanced clot inside the sinus. It is present only when thrombosis affects the posterior third of the sagittal sinus. Computed tomography scan can also be useful in demonstrating cavernous sinus thrombosis. Indirect and nonspecific abnormalities are more frequent, including intense contrast enhancement of the falx cerebri and tentorium, and cerebral infarction, often with petechial hemorrhages and associated hematomas.[1]

Table 24.1   Clinical Situations in which CVT Should Be Suspected

Clinical setting
Regional trauma
Regional sepsis
Pregnancy, puerperium, or "the pill"
Dehydration
Malignancy
Inherited or acquired thrombophilic state
Neurological presentation
Isolated intracranial hypertension
Atypical stroke (seizures, hemorrhagic component, unusual locations)
Cavernous sinus thrombosis (painful ophthalmoplegia, proptosis, chemosis)

B Diagnosis and Follow-up of CVT by MRI

Magnetic resonance imaging (MRI) at present is the method of choice for diagnosis and follow-up of a CVT. In the very early stage, there is an absence of flow void, and the occluded vessels appear isointense on T1-weighted images and hypointense on T2-weighted images. A few days later, the absence of flow void persists but the thrombus becomes hyperintense, initially on T1- and then on T2-weighted images. Also, MRI offers the advantage of sometimes showing parenchymal lesions not visible on CT scan and in demonstrating an underlying cause such as an adjacent tumour or unsuspected mastoiditis.

C Reliability of Angiography

While angiography has remained the gold standard for evaluation of new methods, diagnosis of CVT relies on identification of partial or complete lack of filling of veins or sinuses. Anatomical variability in the anterior third of the superior sagittal sinus and of cortical veins can make interpretation difficult.

D Coagulation Tests

Investigation of patients with coagulation tests recommended in Table 24.2 identifies

Table 24.2   Coagulation Tests Recommended in Patients with CVT

Prothrombin time	Protein C activity
Activated partial thromboplastin time	Protein S activity
Anticardiolipin antibodies	Activated protein C resistance (APC-R)
Lupus anticoagulant	Factor V_{Leiden} mutation if APC-R is equivocal
Antithrombin activity	

Table 24.3   Treatment of Cerebral Venous Thrombosis

A.	**Treatment of underlying predisposing factor**
	(e.g., sepsis, dehydration, estrogen)
B.	**Nonspecific symptomatic**
	(e.g., anticonvulsants, mannitol, steroids for ICP)
C.	**Antithrombotic**

	Heparin — immediate: bolus 3000 U
	    aPTT adjusted
	Fibrinolytics — IV or local infusion. Unproven.
	    Consider in rapidly-progressive major venous sinus thrombosis
	Warfarin — recommend 3 to 6 mo; longer if thrombophilia identified

hypercoagulable states in 15 to 20% of cases. The most frequent abnormality identified is activated protein C resistance, as a result of a point mutation in the coagulation factor V (Arg^{506} Gln), also termed Factor V_{Leiden}.[2] Almost invariably, such varieties of thrombophilia are associated with other predisposing factors, suggesting that while these abnormalities should be looked for in patients with CVT, their presence should not deter the search for other potential causes. It is recommended that these tests be performed twice: once just before heparin is started, and again in 6 months, after anticoagulation therapy has been discontinued in most patients (see Chapter 21).

E   *Treatment of CVT*

The treatment of CVT is outlined in Table 24.3. There is good evidence to suggest that heparin is not only effective but also safe, even in the presence of intracerebral hemorrhage.[3] Its safety in septic CVT has not been established nor has its efficacy in isolated cortical vein thrombosis. The role, if any, for thrombolytic agents remains uncertain. Selective catheterization of dural venous sinuses with infusion of urokinase has been reported to be successful and safe even in patients with pre-existing hemorrhage. The duration of heparin therapy is not standardized but by analogy with deep vein thrombosis, conversion to oral anticoagulants after 1 week of heparin therapy is customary. Warfarin therapy for 3 to 6 months is advised, except where there is a known thrombotic tendency, in which case treatment is prolonged indefinitely.

Clinical Suspicion of Cerebral Venous Thrombosis

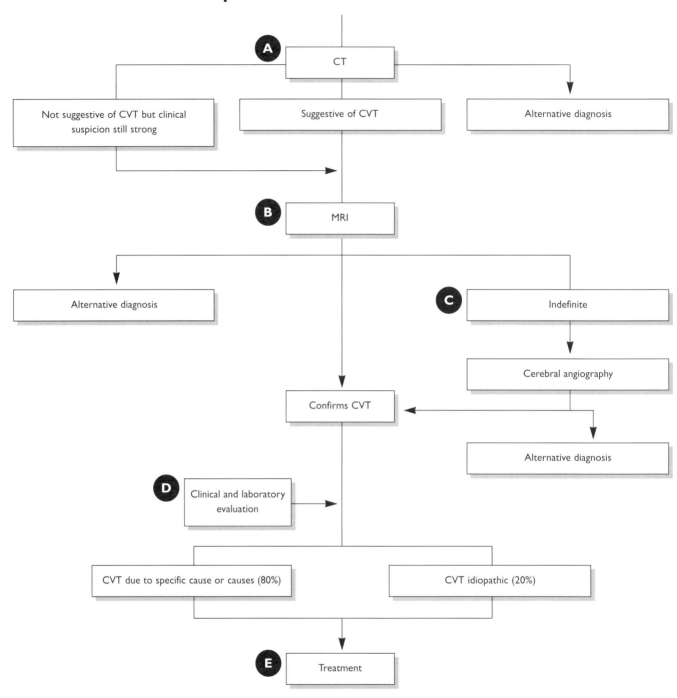

Bibliography

1. Einhaupl KM, Villringer A, Meister W, et al. Heparin treatment in sinus venous thrombosis. Lancet 1991;338:597–600.
2. Jacobs K, Moulin T, Bogousslavsky J, et al. The stroke syndrome of cortical vein thrombosis. Neurology 1996;47:376–81.
3. Brey RL, Coull BM. Cerebral venous thrombosis. Role of activated protein C resistance and factor V gene mutation. Stroke 1996;27:1719–20.

Additional Reading

Ameri A, Bousser M-G. Cerebral venous thrombosis. Neurol Clin 1992;10(1):87–111.

Chapter 25

PARADOXICAL EMBOLIZATION: DIAGNOSIS AND MANAGEMENT

Michael D Ezekowitz

Most systemic emboli arise from sources in the left-sided cardiac chambers or from an arterial location. Systemic embolization may also arise from the venous circulation or the right heart chambers. This phenomenon is termed "paradoxical embolization." The gist of the paradox lies in the fact that the embolic material is not filtered from the circulation by the pulmonary capillaries. Instead, it transits to the systemic circulation through a defect or connection between the right and left heart. Documentation of this phenomenon has been either by pathologic demonstration, transesophageal echo or, most commonly, by a presumptive diagnosis based on a constellation of clinical observations and predisposing conditions.

The diagnosis is based on the presence of four criteria (Table 25.1): 1) the presence of systemic embolization, 2) communication between the right and left heart circulation that bypasses the pulmonary capillaries, 3) physiologic conditions predisposing to right-to-left shunting, and 4) the embolic source.

A Acute Arterial Occlusion

The patient may present with an embolic stroke, acute pain in the limb, acute abdominal pain due to mesenteric ischemia, or symptoms related to acute arterial obstruction. Direct diagnosis is difficult and often based on a combination of clinical presentation and relevant radiologic procedures.

B Right-to-Left Communication

When a paradoxical embolism is suspected, it is important to search for communications between the right and left heart circulation that bypass the pulmonary capillaries. These are: a) manifest cardiac defects, b) potential intracardiac shunts, such as a patent foramen ovale, and c) pulmonary arterious malformations.

In addition to a communication, a physiologic condition predisposing to right and left shunt should be sought: a) chronic pulmonary hypertension, b) acute pulmonary hypertension, c) transient elevation of right heart pressures, in excess of left heart pressures, e.g., Valsalva's maneuver, coughing etc., and d) right-to-left flow across a patent foramen ovale.

Congenital cardiac conditions with the potential for right-to-left shunting are listed in Table 25.2.

Diagnosis of a patent foramen ovale or other congenital abnormalities. This usually rests on transthoracic, two-dimensional echocardiography or transesophageal echocardiography. Using the latter technique, the atria are easily visualized as is the intra-atrial septum. In cases where there is doubt, a transesophageal echocardiogram or a transthoracic echocardiogram is performed during a Valsalva maneuver, using color Doppler; flow across a patent foramen ovale can be visualized. In addition, a bubble study can be performed. The shunting can also be provoked by a Valsalva maneuver. Bubbles are then seen on the left side of the heart.

C Embolic Source

The presence of one or more of the following is a potential embolic source:

a) The presence of an intravascular systemic venous tumor or thrombus.
b) A right heart chambered tumor, thrombus, or a vegetation in the right-sided cardiac valves.
c) Deep venous thrombosis.

Table 25.1 Criteria for the Diagnosis of Paradoxical Embolization

Embolic source

Systemic venous thrombosis
Intravascular systemic venous tumor (e.g., renal cell carcinoma, hepatocellular carcinoma)
Thrombus or tumor (e.g., atrial myxoma) within the right heart chambers
Vegetations of the right-sided cardiac valves

Communication between the Right and Left Heart Circulation that Bypasses the Pulmonary Capillaries

Manifest cardiac defects (e.g., atrial septal defect, ventricular septal defect, patent ductus arteriosus)
Potential intracardiac shunt (e.g., patent foramen ovale)
Pulmonary arteriovenous malformations (e.g., hereditary hemorrhagic telangiectasia syndrome)

Physiologic Conditions Predisposing to Right-to-Left Shunting

Chronic pulmonary hypertension
Acute pulmonary hypertension (e.g., pulmonary embolism)
Transient elevation of right heart pressures in excess of left heart pressures (e.g., Valsalva release, coughing)
Aberrant flow redirection across a patent foramen ovale

Systemic Arterial Embolization

Table 25.2   Cardiac Conditions with Right-to-Left Shunting

Interatrial communications
   a. Primum (partial atrioventricular canal defect) atrial septal defect
   b. Secundum atrial septal defect
   c. Sinus venous atrial septal defect
   d. Patent foramen ovale
Anomalous systemic venous drainage
Left superior vena cava to left atrium
Patent ductus arteriosus
Ventricular septal defects (with right ventricular systolic hypertension)
Complete atrioventricular canal defects
Tetralogy of Fallot
Aortopulmonary window
Postsurgical conditions
   a. Atrial septal defect with periprosthetic patch leak
   b. Ventricular septal defect with periprosthetic patch leak
   c. Fenestrated Fontan repair

D *Management*

The treatment involves anticoagulation for venous thrombosis, removal, if possible, of an intracardiac tumor, and treatment of endocarditis (as the most unusual cause). Endocarditis should also be considered in patients who have a prosthetic device in the right atrium such as a pacemaker lead or a chronic venous access catheter. For selected patients, correction of the communication should be performed. Factors predisposing to paradoxical embolization include pulmonary hypertension for which a reversible cause should be sought.

Diagnosis and Management of Suspected Paradoxical Embolism

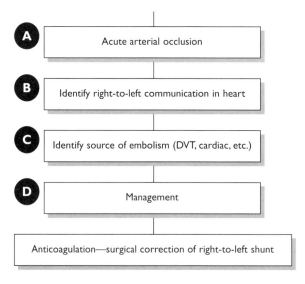

Additional Reading

1. Ezekowitz MD, ed. Cardiac sources of systemic embolization—diagnosis and management. Marcel Dekker, Inc., 1994.
2. Harvey JR, Teague SM, Anderson JL, Voyles WF, Thadani U. Clinically silent atrial septal defects with evidence for cerebral embolization. Ann Intern Med 1986;105:695–7.
3. Langholz D, Louis EK, Konstadt SN, Rao TLK, Scanlon PJ. Transesophageal echocardiographic demonstration of distinct mechanisms for right to left shunting across a patent foramen ovale in the absence of pulmonary hypertension. J Am Coll Cardiol 1991;18:1112–7.
4. Loscalzo J. Paradoxical embolism: clinical presentation, diagnostic strategies, and therapeutic options. Am Heart J 1986;112:141–5.
5. Louis EK, Konstadt SN, Rao TLK, Scanlon PJ. Transesophageal echocardiographic diagnosis of potential interatrial shunting across the foramen ovale in adults without prior stroke. J Am Coll Cardiol 1993;21:1231–7.

Chapter 26

BLEEDING AND UNFRACTIONATED HEPARIN

Said A Ibrahim

C Seth Landefeld

A *Bleeding and Heparin*

Bleeding is the most common complication of heparin therapy. The average daily risk of fatal bleeding from heparin is about 0.05% while that of major or minor bleeding is 0.8% and 2%, respectively. In general, low-dose subcutaneous heparin that is routinely used for prophylaxis against thromboembolic disorders carries a minimum risk of bleeding. The large doses of heparin used routinely for treatment of thromboembolic disorders and in cardiac surgery probably account for the majority of anticoagulant-related bleeding in hospitalized patients. Morbidity and mortality associated with heparin-induced bleeding depend mainly on the severity and the site of bleeding.[1–3] Although the soft tissues, such as surgical wounds, the gastrointestinal tract, and the urinary tract systems, account for the majority of sites of anticoagulant-related bleeding, intracranial bleeding (which accounts for about 2% of all heparin-induced bleeding) is the most feared because of the associated mortality risk.[3]

Heparin binds and potentiates the anticoagulant effect of antithrombin III. Heparin-antithrombin III complex binds to thrombin as well as factor Xa, IXa, and XIa, thereby inhibiting the coagulation cascade. This is the source of heparin's therapeutic effect—and a mechanism by which heparin causes bleeding.[1]

B *Contributing Factors*

When presented with a patient bleeding on heparin, the severity of the bleed should be evaluated; in addition, contributing factors should be considered. Patients receiving nonsteroidal anti-inflammatory agents have a higher risk for bleeding from heparin. Patients with an elevated prothrombin time (PT) (who are not on warfarin) may have malnutrition and vitamin K deficiency that contribute to their risk of bleeding. One should always search for such correctable issues.[4]

C *Severity of the Bleeding*

Any bleeding from heparin should be evaluated to determine whether it is life threatening. A life-threatening bleed is defined as one that either results in a significant volume loss—with or without hemodynamic compromise—or bleeding into a critical site, such as the intracranial space, the pericardial space, the adrenals, or the intraocular space.[3,5]

D *Life-Threatening Volume Loss*

Volume loss that results in significant hemodynamic compromise should first be treated by stopping the infusion of heparin, which should be followed by volume repletion. If the patient responds to these initial measures and stops bleeding, the clinician should monitor the patient for further volume loss. Heparin can sometimes be restarted if the etiology of the bleeding has been reversed and the patient's risk for thrombotic disorder remains high. If heparin is restarted, the best approach may be to lower the dose of heparin and aim for the lower limit of the therapeutic range as measured by the activated partial thromboplastin time (aPTT). Patients who continue to bleed after the above measures have been taken should be treated with intravenous protamine if their aPTT remains elevated. Protamine neutralizes heparin by forming a covalent complex. A dose of 1 mg of protamine reverses the anticoagulant effect of 100 units of heparin. The side effects of protamine include flushing, hypotension, bradycardia, and bronchospasm.[6,7]

E *Bleeding into a Critical Site*

Patients who bleed into a critical site such as the intracranial space should have their heparin infusion stopped immediately. The aPTT should be checked; if it is elevated, protamine should be administered in the above-mentioned dose. For patients with CNS bleeds, an immediate neuroradiologic evaluation should be done and a neurosurgical consultation obtained. Similarly, patients with intraocular bleeding should be evaluated by ophthalmology.

F *The aPTT is ≥ 80 Seconds*

When the heparin-induced bleeding is not life threatening or is minor in nature, one should first check the aPTT. If the aPTT is ≥ 80 seconds, the heparin infusion should be stopped for an hour and restarted at a lower dose, provided the bleeding has resolved and the original thrombotic risk is unchanged. Aiming for a lower range of the therapeutic aPTT is advised. If the patient has sustained a significant volume loss, it would be wise to replete the volume with either blood or fluids.

G *The aPTT is <80 Seconds*

If the aPTT is <80 seconds, local measures may be adequate for treating the bleed —e.g., local pressure on the bleeding vessel. Because the risk of recurrent bleeding or subtle bleeding has not been eliminated, however, the patient should be closely monitored. Patients who continue to bleed after all local conservative measures have been taken should have their heparin infusion stopped and appropriate alternative therapy used.[8]

H *Prevention of Bleeding on Heparin*

Prevention is the best defense against heparin-induced bleeding. However, not all heparin-related bleeding can be prevented. This is, in part, related to the complex pharmacologic properties of heparin in the unstable internal milieu of the hospitalized patient. On an individual patient basis, however, the risk of bleeding from heparin can be estimated and potentially reduced by identifying modifiable risk factors.[2,9,10] If the estimated risk of bleeding exceeds that of the benefits, an alternative intervention should be considered. Using some of the known independent risk factors for heparin-induced bleeding, a risk index score can be constructed for inpatients requiring heparin therapy.[2,5] This risk index can then be used on an individual basis to estimate the probability of bleeding due to heparin (or combined heparin and Coumadin therapy) during the hospital stay (Table 26.1). The major independent risk factors that have been previously used and validated for this purpose are: 1) the presence of four comorbid conditions: cardiac disease, liver dysfunction, renal insufficiency, poor general condition; 2) heparin activity measured by aPTT result >80 seconds; 3) age ≥60; and 4) worsening liver dysfunction. The frequency of major bleeding from heparin is about 3%, 16%, and 19% for patients in the low-, moderate-, and high-risk categories, respectively.[3,11] This objective method of risk estimation allows the clinician to calculate the risk of heparin for specific indications and may also allow for the recognition of risk factors that could be modified prior to treatment.

I *Indications for Treatment*

To assess the benefit of treatment, you should ask whether the indication for treatment is strong, i.e., is the evidence of efficacy and safety supported by data from randomized clinical trials? Examples of strong indications are the treatment and prophylaxis of venous thromboembolic disorders or acute arterial embolism. On the other hand, there are clinical situations in which evidence of the efficacy of heparin is weak—e.g., the use of heparin in peripheral vascular disease or stroke in evolution.[12]

J   Level of Risk

As shown in Table 26.1 the risk of bleeding from heparin can be categorized as high, medium, or low. Risk estimation should be done for all patients who are about to be treated with heparin.

K   Strong Indication—High Risk

Patients who have a strong indication for treatment but fall into the high-risk category (e.g., those with an acute embolism) should be evaluated for an alternative therapy. For instance, inferior vena cava (IVC) filters can be used to minimize the risk of recurrent embolism. It is, however, important to remember that IVC filters carry some risk of complications such as recurrent embolism.

Table 26.1   Estimating the Risk of Bleeding from Heparin

Independent Risk Factors	Risk Scores
Number of Comorbid Conditions*	
1	1
2	2
3 or 4	3
Age (years)	
60–79	1
≥ 80	2
aPTT Ratio	
2.0–2.9	1
≥ 3.0	2
Hepatic disease (worsening)	2

*Comorbid conditions: cardiac disease, renal insufficiency, hepatic dysfunction, poor general health

Index Risk Score	Risk Category	Frequency of Bleeding
0–2	Low	3%
3–4	Moderate	16%
≥ 5	High	19%

Adapted from Landefeld, et al, Am J Med 1990;89:570,573.

L *Strong Indication—Medium and Low Risk*

Patients who have a strong indication for heparin therapy but fall into the medium- or low-risk categories should have their risk reduced. Evaluate the patient's medication list and eliminate NSAIDs if they are not being used for another strong indication. For example, many elderly patients with osteoarthritis are routinely treated

Approach to a Patient Who Bleeds While Receiving Heparin

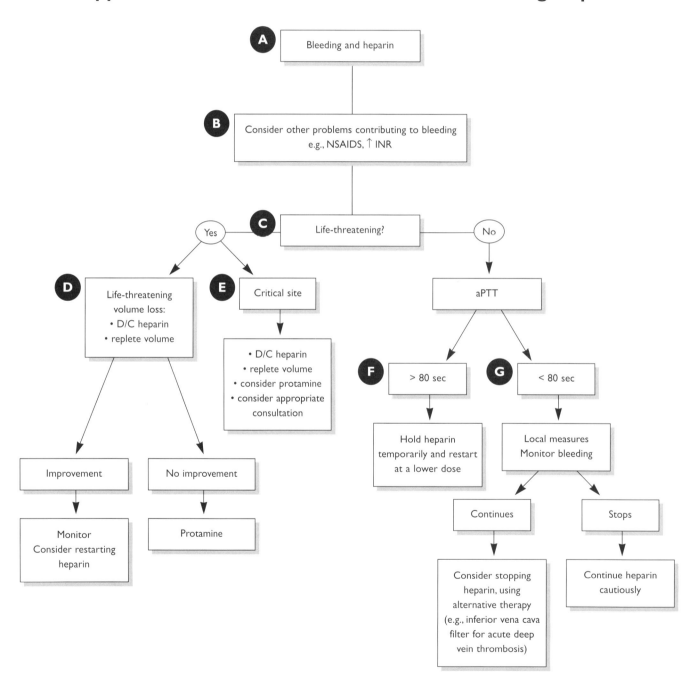

with NSAIDs when they could just as well be treated with acetaminophen. Surgical patients with bleeding lesions who need to be heparinized can have their risk reduced by treating the lesion first. Other means of reducing the patient's risk of bleeding include monitoring the patient's aPTT closely, minimizing the duration of heparin therapy, and using low-molecular-weight heparins.[4]

Bleeding is a major side effect of heparin therapy. Various independent risk factors have been identified and used to predict a patient's risk of bleeding from heparin. The mechanism of heparin-induced bleeding is mainly related to heparin's anticoagulant effect, which also accounts for its therapeutic effect. Although intracranial bleeding is the most feared complication of heparin, the gastrointestinal and the urinary tract systems, in addition to the soft tissues, account for the majority of heparin-induced bleeding sites. Prevention is the best strategy against bleeding from heparin. Once major bleeding occurs, however, heparin should be discontinued and its effect reversed using protamine. Fortunately, the majority of heparin-related bleeding tends to be minor in nature and responds to simple measures.

Figure 2

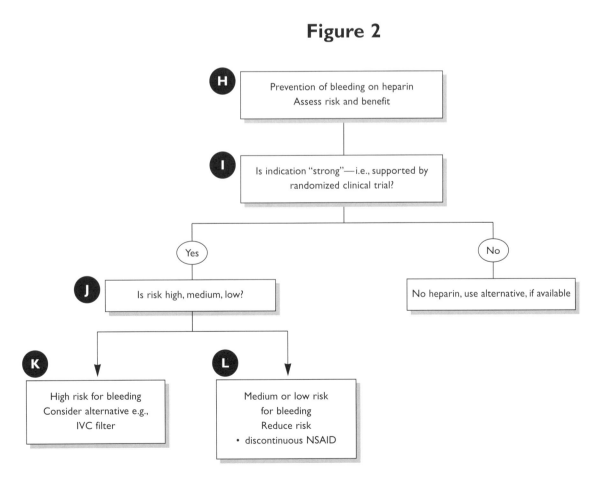

Bibliography

1. Hirsh J. Heparin. N Engl J Med 1991;324(22):1565–74.

2. Landefeld CS, McGuire E, Rosenblatt MW. A bleeding risk index for estimating the probability of major bleeding in hospitalized patients starting anticoagulant therapy. Am J Med 1990;89:569–78.

3. Landefeld CS, Beyth RJ. Anticoagulant-related bleeding: clinical epidemiology, prediction, and prevention. Am J Med 1993;95:315–28.

4. Landefeld CS, Anderson PA. Guideline-based consultation to prevent anticoagulant-related bleeding. Ann Intern Med 1992;116:829–37.

5. Landefeld CS, Anderson AP, Goodnough TL, et al. The bleeding severity index: validation and comparison to other methods for classifying bleeding complications in medical therapy. J Clin Epidemiol 1989;42:711–8.

6. Penner AJ. Managing the hemorrhagic complications of heparin therapy. Hematol Oncol Clin North Am 1993;7:1281–9.

7. Wolzt M, Weltermann A, Neiszpaur-Los M, et al. Studies on the neutralizing effects of protamine on unfractionated and low molecular weight heparin (Fragmin) at the site of activation of the coagulation system in man. Thromb Haemost 1995;73:439–43.

8. Prandoni P, Lensing AW, Buller HR, et al. Comparison of subcutaneous low molecular weight heparin with intravenous standard in proximal deep vein thrombosis. Lancet 1992;339:441–5.

9. Alexander WM, Hershel J. Predictors of bleeding during heparin therapy. JAMA 1980;244:1209–12.

10. Landefeld CS, Flatley M, Weisbergh M, Cook EF, Goldman L. Identification and preliminary validation of predictors of major bleeding in hospitalized patients starting anticoagulant therapy. Am J Med 1987;82:703–13.

11. Hershel J, Slone D, Borda TI, Shapiro S. Efficacy and toxicity of heparin in relation to age and sex. N Engl J Med 1968;279:284–6.

12. Levine M, Raskob EG, Landefeld CS, Hirsh J. Fourth ACCP consensus conference on antithrombotic therapy. Chest 1995;108(4):276s–90s.

Chapter 27

BLEEDING AND WARFARIN

Rebecca J Beyth

C Seth Landefeld

Bleeding is the main complication of warfarin therapy. Although most warfarin-related bleeding is not life threatening and does not result in permanent morbidity, intracerebral hemorrhage and death do occasionally occur. It is estimated that annually 1 to 5% of patients treated with long-term anticoagulant therapy will suffer a bleeding event that warrants hospitalization. The risk of warfarin-induced bleeding is influenced primarily by the intensity of the anticoagulant effect as measured by the International Normalized Ratio (INR), patient characteristics, the length of therapy, and the concomitant use of drugs that interfere with hemostasis.[1] The intensity of the anticoagulant response to warfarin is affected by the dose of warfarin, the patient's intake of vitamin K, and other factors (e.g., liver dysfunction, concomitant medications) that alter the pharmacokinetics and pharmacodynamics of warfarin.[2] Bleeding is about three times as likely in patients with an INR of 3.0 to 4.5 compared with those with an INR of 2.0 to 3.0. The risk of bleeding during warfarin therapy is also related to baseline patient characteristics other than the indication for therapy. Although studies have not consistently identified the same independent predictors of major bleeding, it is generally agreed that past history of gastrointestinal bleeding, serious comorbid conditions (e.g., renal insufficiency, anemia), and history of stroke are factors that increase the risk of bleeding from warfarin.[1,3–7] Whether age is a risk factor for warfarin-related bleeding remains unclear but older patients may benefit from close monitoring when they are treated with warfarin.[8] The cumulative risk of bleeding has been shown to be directly related to the length of warfarin therapy but the risk of bleeding also appears to vary during the course of anticoagulant therapy. Specifically, frequencies of bleeding have been noted to be higher early in the course of therapy.[4,6,9] Even though these factors or conditions may be present in any given patient, they should not be seen as absolute contraindications to warfarin therapy. Rather, they should be weighed against the benefits of warfarin in the context of individual patient preferences and values.

A *Strength of Treatment Indications*

Results from randomized clinical trials have shown that patients with venous thromboembolism (VTE) (i.e., deep vein thrombosis [DVT] or pulmonary embolus [PE]) should be treated initially with heparin and warfarin until the INR is consistently ≥ 2.0, when heparin may be stopped.[2,10] Long-term anticoagulant therapy should be continued for at least 3 months with prolongation of the prothrombin time to an INR of 2.0 to 3.0. Pooled analysis of five randomized primary prevention trials as well as evidence from a randomized secondary prevention trial show that long-term warfarin therapy (INR 2.0 to 3.0) should be strongly considered for all patients 65 years and older with atrial fibrillation, and for patients less than 65 years of age with other risk factors (e.g., prior TIA/stroke, hypertension, heart failure, diabetes, mitral stenosis, prosthetic heart valves, or thyrotoxicosis).[2,3] Although there is no data from randomized clinical trials, the evidence from nonrandomized trials is compelling enough to recommend life-long therapy with oral anticoagulants for all patients with mechanical prosthetic heart valves.[2,3,11,12] The prothrombin time should be prolonged to an INR 2.5 to 3.5 for tilting disks and bileaflet valves while patients with caged ball or caged disk valves should have a target INR as high as 4.0 to 4.9. It is recommended that patients with bioprosthetic valves in the mitral position be treated for the first 3 months after valve insertion with warfarin therapy at an INR of 2.0 to 3.0. Warfarin therapy is considered optional for patients with bioprosthetic valves in the atrial position who are in normal sinus rhythm. Following acute myocardial infarction (AMI), warfarin therapy is recommended for 2 to 3 months in patients who are considered to have an increased embolic risk or indefinitely if they have atrial fibrillation.[13] Long-term warfarin therapy is not routinely recommended in patients after femoropopliteal bypass and other vascular reconstructions.[14] There is firm evidence to recommend warfarin therapy for cardioembolic stroke but presently there is insufficient data to recommend oral anticoagulant therapy for patients with threatened stroke due to primary cerebrovascular disease.[2,15]

B *Risk Assessment*

The decision whether to initiate warfarin therapy in a particular patient hinges on the balance between the efficacy of warfarin in preventing a thromboembolic event and its likelihood of precipitating a hemorrhagic event. This situation is further complicated by the fact that there is no systematic and practical method for weighing risks and benefits, and the risks of both thromboembolic and hemorrhagic events vary over time. Patients considered at low risk for warfarin-related bleeding would be those < 65 years of age with no significant comorbid conditions (except for the indication for anticoagulant therapy) who do not require concomitant treatment with drugs that interfere with hemostasis. Medium-risk patients are those who have one or two risk factors for bleeding (such as a history of gastrointestinal bleeding and renal insufficiency) while high-risk patients would be those who possess three or more risk factors (e.g., an 80-year-old patient with a history of stroke, gastrointestinal bleeding, and recent myocardial infarction, and who develops a DVT). The estimated risk for major bleeding during warfarin therapy at 3 months has been reported to be 2% in low-risk patients, 5% in medium-risk patients, and 23% in high-risk patients.[4,6] While these risk factors need to be considered when starting warfarin therapy, they are not static; rather, the physician and the patient must continually re-evaluate the risks and benefits of warfarin therapy.

C *Alternative Therapies*

Among high-risk patients in whom the risk of warfarin-related bleeding outweighs its potential benefits, consideration should be given to the use of alternative therapies. For example, subcutaneous low-molecular-weight heparin, or unfractionated heparin, or an inferior vena cava interruption procedure are reasonable alternatives for treatment of a DVT in a medium- or high-risk patient. Likewise, aspirin rather than warfarin during the first 3 months after a bioprosthetic valve replacement in aortic position for high-risk patients may be prudent. Other steps, like avoiding aspirin or other drugs that interfere with hemostasis, may also help reduce the risk of bleeding in high-risk patients. Similarly, consideration of alternative antithrombotic agents along with risk reduction may be appropriate in certain patients. Also, if a trial of warfarin therapy determines that the patient is not able to comply with taking warfarin as prescribed, and the risk of bleeding is great, discontinuation of warfarin may be reasonable.

D *Risk Reduction*

For all patients starting long-term therapy with warfarin, an attempt should be made to minimize the risk of warfarin-related bleeding. The concomitant use of drugs that interfere with hemostasis, like aspirin or nonsteroidal anti-inflammatory agents, should be avoided. Closer and more frequent monitoring of the INR may be warranted in older patients, in patients considered at high risk for bleeding, or in patients in whom a drug that is known to potentiate the anticoagulant effect of warfarin is prescribed. Procedures that can be delayed or avoided until treatment with warfarin is complete also minimize the risk of bleeding. For patients who require a minimally invasive procedure (e.g., dental work or a superficial biopsy), a brief reduction in the INR (to approximately 1.3 to 2.0), with resumption to the normal dosage of warfarin immediately following the procedure, is recommended.

For patients in whom the risk of bleeding while on warfarin is high and the risk of thromboembolism without warfarin therapy is likewise high, discontinuation of warfarin 3 to 5 days prior to an operation with perioperative heparin therapy is safest. For patients between these two extremes, the risks and benefits of reduced warfarin, a short interruption in warfarin therapy, versus perioperative heparin need to be considered (see Chapter 19).[16]

E Warfarin-Related Bleeding

Contemporary rates of warfarin-related bleeding have been reported to range from 1 to 7% per year, depending on the indication for anticoagulant therapy and the criteria for classification of bleeding. Bleeding rates during long-term warfarin therapy are substantial with high-intensity therapy (INR > 3.0) and are lower with low-intensity therapy (INR 2.0 to 3.0). Although most bleeding is not life threatening, it does cause short-term morbidity and inconvenience to the patient, and may diminish quality of life. Prompt recognition of warfarin-related bleeding and early treatment of life-threatening bleeding can reduce associated morbidity.

F Other Factors Contributing to the Bleeding

When a patient presents with warfarin-related bleeding, other factors that may be contributing to the bleeding need to be considered. For example, if a patient presents with guaiac-positive stools while on warfarin therapy, it should be determined if the patient has also been using aspirin or other nonsteroidal anti-inflammatory drugs. Elimination of contributing causes may resolve or reduce the severity of the bleeding episode.

G Life-Threatening Bleeding

An initial step in the evaluation of a patient with warfarin-related bleeding is to determine whether or not the bleeding is life threatening. Life-threatening bleeding can be defined as that which leads to cardiopulmonary arrest, surgical or angiographic intervention, irreversible sequelae (e.g., acute MI), or at least two of the following: loss of 3 or more units of blood; systolic blood pressure < 90 mm Hg; or critical anemia (hematocrit ≤ 0.20).

H Life-Threatening Volume Loss

For bleeding that is life-threatening because of volume loss, warfarin should be discontinued and the intravascular volume repleted with intravenous fluids and blood as needed. If the bleeding stops, the INR should be monitored closely until it is safe to resume warfarin therapy if indicated, or an alternative therapy such as aspirin can be started. If the bleeding continues, the INR should be monitored, vitamin K should be administered subcutaneously or by slow intravenous infusion, and rapid reversal of the anticoagulant effect should be achieved with infusion of plasma or factor IX concentrate.

I *Life-Threatening Bleeding Sites*

If the site of bleeding is determined to be in a critical location (e.g., intracranial or pericardial), where the bleeding cannot be directly controlled or could result in devastating sequelae, warfarin should be discontinued and the INR monitored closely. Vitamin K and plasma or factor IX concentrate should be administered. Also, surgical consultation should be considered if it appears that surgical or angiographic intervention may be needed.

J *Non-Life-Threatening Bleeding with INR >3.0*

Patients who experience non-life-threatening bleeding while their INR is >3.0 may respond to a reduction in warfarin dosage. Warfarin can be held until the INR is in therapeutic range or vitamin K 1 mg orally or subcutaneously may be given if the INR is >4.5.[17]

Prevention of Bleeding on Warfarin: Assessing Risks and Benefits

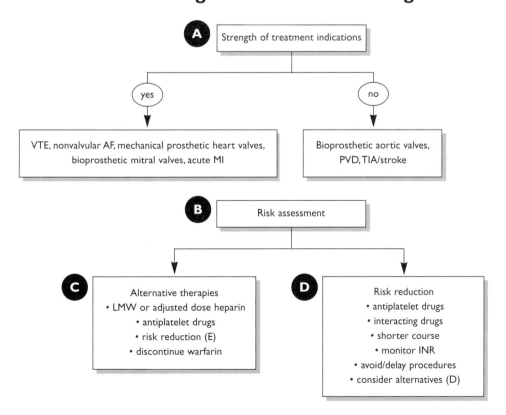

K *Non-Life-Threatening Bleeding with INR ≤3.0*

Bleeding that occurs when the INR is ≤3.0 is frequently associated with an obvious underlying cause or occult gastrointestinal or renal lesion. Local measures should be undertaken to control the bleeding and monitor the patient. If the bleeding stops, warfarin can be continued and diagnostic studies can be undertaken to determine the cause so that appropriate treatment (e.g, antiulcer therapy) may be instituted. If the bleeding continues, warfarin may need to be discontinued while a diagnostic workup is performed.

Management of Warfarin-Related Bleeding

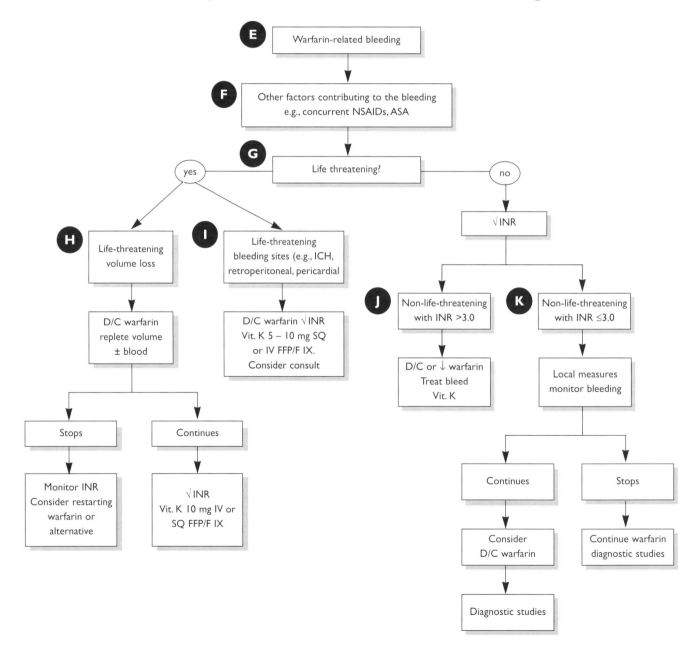

Bibliography

1. Landefeld CS, Beyth RJ. Anticoagulant-related bleeding: clinical epidemiology, risk estimation, and prevention. Am J Med 1993;95:315–28.

2. Hirsh J, Dalen JE, Deykin D, Poller L, Bussey H. Oral anticoagulants. Mechanisms of action, clinical effectiveness, and optimal therapeutic range. Chest 1995;108:231S–46S.

3. Atrial Fibrillation Investigators. Risk factors for stroke and efficacy of anti-thrombotic therapy in atrial fibrillation: analysis of pooled data from five randomized controlled trials. Arch Intern Med 1994;154:1449–57.

4. Beyth RJ, Landefeld CS. Prospective validation of a bleeding risk index for outpatients treated with warfarin. J Gen Intern Med 1995;10(Suppl):39.

5. Gitter MJ, Jaeger TM, Petterson TM, Gersh BJ, Silverstein MD. Bleeding and thromboembolism during anticoagulant therapy: a population-based study in Rochester, Minnesota. Mayo Clin Proc 1995;70:725–33.

6. Landefeld CS, Goldman L. Major bleeding in outpatients treated with warfarin: incidence and prediction by factors known at the start of outpatient therapy. Am J Med 1989;87:144–52.

7. Landefeld CS, Rosenblatt MW. Bleeding in outpatients treated with warfarin: relation to the prothrombin time and important remediable lesions. Am J Med 1989;87:153–9.

8. Beyth RJ, Landefeld CS. Anticoagulants in older patients. A safety perspective. Drugs Aging 1995;6:45–54.

9. Fihn SD, Callahan CM, Martin DC, McDonell MB, et al. The risk for and severity of bleeding complications in elderly patients treated with warfarin. Ann Intern Med 1996;124:970–9.

10. Hyers, TM, Hull RD, Weg JG. Antithrombotic thrombotic therapy for venous thrombo-embolic disease. Chest 1995;108:335S–51S.

11. Cannegieter SC, Rosendaal FR, Wintzen AR, et al. Optimal oral anticoagulant therapy in patients with mechanical heart valves. N Engl J Med 1995;333:11–17.

12. Eckman MH, Beshansky JR, Durand-Zaleski I, et al. Anticoagulation for noncardiac operations in patients with prosthetic heart valves. JAMA 1990;263:1513–21.

13. Cairns JA, Lewis HD, Meade TW, Sutton GC, Theroux P. Antithrombotic agents in coronary artery disease. Chest 1995;108:380S–400S.

14. Clagett GP, Krupski WC. Antithrombotic therapy in peripheral arterial occlusive disease. Chest 1995;108:431S–43S.

15. Cerebral Embolism Task Force. Cardiogenic brain embolism: the second report of the Cerebral Embolism Task Force. Arch Neurol 1989;46:727–41.

16. Sise HS, Moschos CB, Gauthier J, Becker R. The risk of interrupting long-term anticoagulant therapy. Rebound hypercoagulable state following hemorrhage. Circulation 1961;24:1137–42.

17. Shetty HG, Backhouse G, Bentley DP, et al. Effective reversal of warfarin-induced excessive anticoagulation with low dose vitamin K1. Thromb Haemost 1992;67:13–5.

Chapter 28

BLEEDING AND THROMBOLYTIC THERAPY

David R Anderson

Thrombolytic agents are the most potent form of antithrombotic therapy. They are the only drugs that exert their antithrombotic activity by actually dissolving blood clots and reducing the consequences of vessel obstruction. Not unexpectedly, the most common side effect of thrombolytic therapy is bleeding, which is both more frequent and more serious than with other forms of antithrombotic treatment. Use of thrombolytic therapy requires very careful consideration of the potential benefits and risks of this treatment to individual patients. In this chapter, we review the mechanisms of action of the thrombolytic agents, the risks of bleeding associated with their use, and the recommended management of bleeding complications.

Mechanism of Action of Thrombolytic Therapy

Thrombolytic agents exert their antithrombotic effect by converting plasminogen to the potent proteolytic enzyme, plasmin.[1,2] Plasmin causes thrombolysis by direct degradation of fibrin clots. Plasmin has a number of additional effects that may also be important to its antithrombotic activity. Plasmin degrades fibrinogen, the substrate for thrombus formation, and the procoagulant enzymes, factors Va and VIIIa. Plasmin causes the partial degradation of the platelet receptors glycoprotein Ib and glycoprotein IIb-IIIa, which are required for platelet adhesion and aggregation. Finally, plasmin degradation of fibrin results in the generation of fibrin degradation products, which may directly interfere with normal blood clot formation and make thrombi more susceptible to thrombolysis.

    Thrombolytic agents may be divided into two broad classes: those that are fibrin specific and those that are fibrin nonspecific.[1,2] Fibrin-specific agents have markedly enhanced thrombolytic activity upon binding to fibrin whereas they have very little thrombolytic activity when circulating free in the bloodstream in the absence of fibrin. As a result of these properties, fibrin-specific thrombolytic agents generate high concentrations of plasmin on the fibrin clot surface but little plasmin in the bloodstream distant from an area of thrombosis. A prototypical fibrin-specific thrombolytic agent is a tissue plasminogen activator.

Thrombolytic agents that lack fibrin specificity have no alteration in their thrombolytic activity in the presence of fibrin.[1,2] Streptokinase is the most commonly used nonfibrin-specific thrombolytic agent. Nonfibrin-specific thrombolytic agents cause plasmin generation throughout the bloodstream. Patients receiving nonfibrin-specific thrombolytic agents have a measurable systemic lytic state characterized by decreased levels of plasma fibrinogen and prolongation of coagulation tests such as the thrombin time and the activated partial thromboplastin time (aPTT). Fibrin-specific and nonspecific thrombolytic agents both cause generation of fibrin degradation products; however, the levels of these degradation products are much higher in patients receiving nonfibrin-specific agents.

The nonfibrin-specific thrombolytic drugs streptokinase and urokinase were the first thrombolytic agents used in clinical trials, and bleeding was found to be a frequent and serious complication.[3] It was hoped that through the absence of a systemic fibrinolytic effect, the more recently developed fibrin-specific thrombolytic agents would cause less bleeding than the nonfibrin-specific agents. However, large clinical trials comparing streptokinase and tissue plasminogen activator for the treatment of acute myocardial infarction have reported equivalent rates of serious bleeding complications, including intracerebral hemorrhage.[4] The explanation for this observation may be that fibrin-specific thrombolytic agents bind not only to intravascular thrombi where clot lysis is desirable but also to hemostatic plugs where clot lysis may be detrimental. It also suggests that, in itself, the "systemic" fibrinolytic effect generated by nonfibrin-specific thrombolytic agents does not significantly increase the risk of bleeding.

Selection of Patients for Thrombolytic Therapy

To minimize the risk of serious bleeding complications, the following groups were usually excluded from clinical trials evaluating thrombolytic therapy for the treatment of myocardial infarction and venous thromboembolism:[2] (a) patients with recent (in the previous 6 months) major internal bleeding; (b) patients who had undergone surgical procedures or biopsies in the previous 10 days; (c) patients with uncontrolled hypertension i.e., systolic blood pressure greater than 200 mm Hg, diastolic blood pressure greater than 100 mm Hg; (d) patients with an underlying bleeding diathesis (e.g., hemophilia); (e) patients with endocarditis or pericarditis; (f) patients with an aneurysm; or (g) patients with intracranial or intraspinal disease. In clinical practice, it is recommended that thrombolysis be avoided in these patients as well, except under exceptional circumstances.

Large clinical trials comparing thrombolytic therapy with a placebo or a non-thrombolytic control group following acute myocardial infarction have clearly demonstrated that thrombolysis increases the risk of major bleeding.[4] Major bleeding rates vary widely among studies, likely due to variations in bleeding criteria and the reporting of bleeding complications across studies. The most valid comparisons of bleeding risk come from comparing the relative rates of major bleeding using different thrombolytic treatment regimens within the large thrombolysis trials. Bleeding complications may develop from any site with thrombolytic therapy but they occur most commonly at the site of invasive procedures.[1,5] Intracerebral hemorrhage is the most serious bleeding complication associated with the use of thrombolytic therapy. Clinical trials involving patients treated for acute myocardial infarction have demonstrated the rate of intracerebral hemorrhage is ~ 0.5% with use of tissue plasminogen activator or streptokinase. Subgroup analyses of large acute myocardial infarction studies have demonstrated that the risk of intracerebral hemorrhage increases in older patients (> 70 years of age), patients with hypertension, patients with previous history of stroke, and patients with low body weight.[1]

Risk of bleeding with tissue plasminogen activator following acute myocardial infarction may relate to the dose of the lytic agent (a higher rate of intracerebral hemorrhage was observed with use of the 150 mg dose of tissue plasminogen activator compared to the standard 100 mg dose) and to the intensity of adjuvant intravenous unfractionated heparin therapy.[5] In contemporary thrombolytic trials for acute myocardial infarction, the recommended heparin dose following tissue plasminogen activator is a 5000 unit bolus followed by a continuous infusion of 1000 units per hour with subsequent doses adjusted using a standardized nomogram to maintain the aPTT at 60 to 85 seconds.[6]

Increased rates of major bleeding complications have been reported with the use of thrombolytic therapy for the treatment of deep vein thrombosis and pulmonary embolism. In a pooled analysis comparing streptokinase with heparin for the treatment of deep vein thrombosis, the rate of major bleeding was threefold higher with the use of thrombolytic therapy.[7] Similar increased bleeding rates were reported in a pooled analysis comparing thrombolytic therapy with heparin for the treatment of pulmonary embolism.[8] As with myocardial infarction, bleeding complications involving thrombolytic therapy for the treatment of deep vein thrombosis or pulmonary embolism most frequently occur at the sight of invasive procedures. However, more serious internal bleeding events including intracerebral hemorrhage have also been observed.

Since the clinical benefits of thrombolytic therapy are less evident for the treatment of pulmonary embolism and deep vein thrombosis than for acute myocardial infarction, very careful consideration must be given to using thrombolytic therapy for these former indications. Not only may thrombolytic therapy lead to serious bleeding complications in patients with deep vein thrombosis and pulmonary embolism but these bleeding complications may prevent or delay the use of parenteral anticoagulant therapy, which is of proven benefit for the treatment of these conditions.

Relationship between Bleeding Risk and Coagulation Laboratory Tests

Several studies have demonstrated a correlation between the results of coagulation studies and the risk of bleeding while receiving thrombolytic therapy.[1,2] However, tests such as the fibrinogen level, the thrombin time, the bleeding time, and the platelet count are not sufficiently predictive of bleeding risk to be useful in the prospective management of patients receiving thrombolytic therapy.

Treatment of Bleeding Complications on Thrombolytic Therapy

Patients developing major bleeding complications while receiving thrombolytic therapy require appropriate supportive care.[1,2,4,9] If bleeding occurs at the site of invasive procedures such as catheterization exit sites, local measures must be taken to control bleeding. For more severe bleeding complications, thrombolytic and adjuvant anticoagulant therapy may, at least temporarily, need to be discontinued and consideration should be given to using replacement blood products. Blood samples should be drawn for a manual fibrinogen level, an aPTT, and a platelet count. If the bleeding is severe, thrombolytic and adjuvant anticoagulant therapy should be discontinued. Patients receiving heparin with an elevated aPTT should receive protamine sulfate. One mg of protamine may be administered to neutralize each 100 units of heparin received over the past 4 hours. Eight to twelve units of cryoprecipitate may be administered for patients with hypofibrinogenemia in association with major bleeding. Platelet and fresh frozen plasma transfusions and use of an antifibrinolytic agent such as epsilon-aminocaproic acid should be considered for life-threatening bleeding or if bleeding continues despite stopping antithrombotic therapy.

Management for Patients with Bleeding from Thrombolytic Therapy

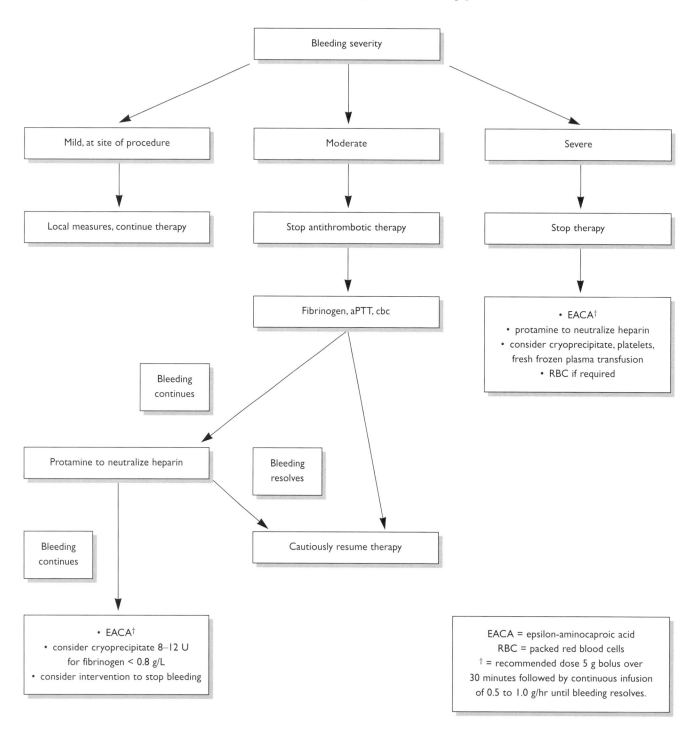

Bibliography

1. Hirsh J. Coronary thrombolysis: hemorrhagic complications. Can J Cardiol 1993;9:505–11.

2. Levine MN. Thrombolytic therapy for venous thromboembolism. Clin Chest Med 1995; 16:321–8.

3. Hyers TM, Hull RD, Weg JG. Antithrombotic therapy for venous thromboembolic disease. Chest 1995;108:335S–51S.

4. Levine MN, Goldhaber SZ, Gore JM, Hirsh J, Califf RM. Hemorrhagic complications of thrombolytic therapy in the treatment of myocardial infarction and venous thromboembolism. Chest 1995;108:291S–301S.

5. Bovill EG, Terrin ML, Stump DC, et al. Hemorrhagic events during therapy with recombinant tissue-type plasminogen activator, heparin and aspirin for acute myocardial infarction. Am Coll Phys 1991;115:256–65.

6. The Global User Of Strategies To Open Occluded Coronary Arteries (Gusto) IIb Investigators*. A comparison of recombinant hirudin with heparin for the treatment of acute coronary syndromes. N Engl J Med 1996;335:11:775–82.

7. Goldhaber SZ, Buring JE, Lipnick RJ, Hennekens CH. Pooled analyses of randomized trials of streptokinase and heparin in phlebographically documented acute deep vein thrombosis. Am J Med 1984;76:393–7.

8. Anderson DR, Levine MN. Thrombolytic therapy for the treatment of acute pulmonary embolism. Can Med Assoc J 1992;146:1317–24.

9. Sane DC, Califf RM, Topol EJ, Stump DC, Mark DB, Greenberg CS. Bleeding during thrombolytic therapy for acute myocardial infarction: mechanisms and management. Ann Intern Med 1989;111:1010–22.

PREVENTION AND MANAGEMENT OF POST-THROMBOTIC SYNDROME

Jeffrey S Ginsberg

Post-thrombotic syndrome (PTS) consists of pain, swelling, and, sometimes, ulceration of the leg after deep vein thrombosis.[1] The management of affected patients is severly hampered by the lack of a uniform definition and the paucity of useful data derived from properly designed trials. We tend to use a "symptomatic" definition, comprising persistent leg pain and swelling in a subject with previous deep vein thrombosis (DVT) that is typically best in the morning (or after a night of recumbent sleep) and progresses as the day goes on, combined with objective evidence of deep venous valvular incompetence derived from tests such as Doppler ultrasound, photoplethysmography, or air plethysmography. The use of this definition improves the specificity of the diagnosis of PTS.

   The results of a recent randomized trial in which patients with DVT were randomly allocated to graduated compression stockings or nothing suggests that the incidence and severity of PTS can be reduced with stocking therapy.[1] The results of this study should be confirmed before they are routinely adopted but they have the potential to change practice profoundly.

A *Typical Pain and Swelling in Patient with Previous DVT*
When a patient with previous DVT presents with leg pain and swelling, recurrent DVT must be excluded (see Chapter 6). To ensure that the symptoms are consistent with PTS, it is important to take a careful history. In addition, it is worthwhile to search for nonthrombotic causes of leg symptoms, such as a Baker's cyst.

B *Test for Venous Valvular Incompetence*
If the symptoms are "typical," a test for venous valvular incompetence should be performed, and if abnormal, PTS is diagnosed. We suggest examining for reflux

within the popliteal vein by Doppler (or "duplex" ultrasound), or performing photo-plethysmography or air plethysmography.

C *If the Diagnosis is Unclear, Explore Other Causes*

If the test(s) for venous valvular incompetence is (are) normal, PTS is less likely and the possibility of other conditions should be explored. If the investigations for other conditions are negative and the clinical presentation seems very likely to be PTS, it is reasonable to make a diagnosis of PTS and perform a trial of graduated compression stockings.

Prevention and Management of Post-thrombotic Syndrome

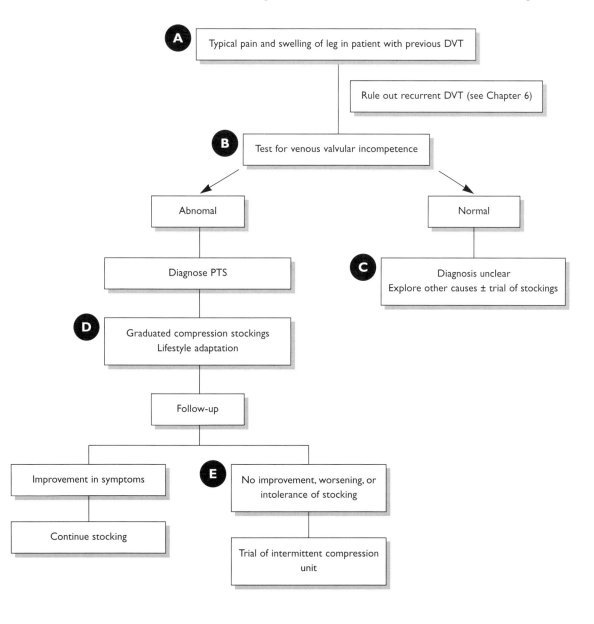

D *Graduated Compression Stockings and Lifestyle Adaptation*

If a diagnosis of PTS is made, the cornerstones of management involve lifestyle adaptation and the use of properly fitted graduated compression stockings. Lifestyle modifications include a number of maneuvers, including avoiding activities that make the problem worse and increasing activities that ameliorate the problem. For example, prolonged sitting or standing worsens the problem whereas physical exercise, like walking or swimming, is generally beneficial. Even with lifestyle modifications, all but the mildest of PTS still requires further therapy with graduated compression stockings. The key to appropriate stocking use is that they must fit properly without causing a tourniquet effect, and that they should be removed at night. Generally, below knee level stockings are adequate; however, if symptoms involve the thigh, a full-length stocking or pantyhose may be required.

E *No Improvement, Worsening, or Intolerance of Stockings*

In patients who do not improve with or who are intolerant of stockings, intermittent compression with an extremity pump is useful, particularly in those patients who have a lot of swelling.[2] We initiate the "pump" with home use on the affected leg twice a day for about 30 minutes. Subsequent to that, we recommend that patients vary the frequency, duration, and pressure of the pump to suit their individual needs.

Bibliography

1. Brandjes DPM, Buller HR, Heijboer H, et al. Randomised trial of effect of compression stockings in patients with symptomatic proximal-vein thrombosis. Lancet 1997;349:759–62.
2. Ginsberg JS, Brill-Edwards P, Kowalchuk G, Hirsh J. Intermittent compression units for the postphlebitic syndrome. Arch Intern Med 1989;149:1651–2.

Section 2

ARTERIAL THROMBOSIS

Chapter 30

Risk Stratification for Symptomatic Atherosclerosis

Sonia S Anand

Salim Yusuf

Vascular disease of the coronary, cerebral, and peripheral circulation is the most common noncommunicable disease in the western world. Early atherosclerosis is often evident in young adulthood and is the underlying pathology of all clinically significant vascular disease. The final common pathway for the majority of athero-sclerotic-based diseases is atherosclerotic plaque instability, rupture, and subsequent thrombus formation which leads to occlusion of a coronary, cerebral, or peripheral vessel. Compelling observational data from several landmark studies[1-3] suggest that tobacco use, elevation of cholesterol and blood pressure, and diabetes are important causal risk factors for clinical vascular disease. In individuals with symptomatic atherosclerosis, our approach to determining their prognoses and predicting their responses to risk factor modification is based upon the results of population-based studies, registries, and randomized controlled trials. Here we review the major risk factors for atherosclerotic clinical events, emphasize the importance of determining an individual's baseline risk of suffering these events in the future, and suggest strategies to minimize this risk.

A *History, Physical Examination, and Major Risk Factors*

A risk factor is one which is associated with an increased likelihood that disease will develop at a later time. Risk factors may be modifiable (e.g., smoking, hypertension, obesity) or nonmodifiable (age and gender) but both categories are important to consider when determining an individual's baseline risk. The contribution of one risk factor to the development of atherosclerosis may be increased by the presence of other risk factors for the same disease, a concept known as synergy. Data from most observational epidemiologic studies[4] reveal that the effects of multiple risk factors are additive and interactive. For example, individuals who have hypertension (systolic >140 mm Hg or diastolic > 90 mm Hg) and who have elevated cholesterol (cholesterol >5.2 mmol/L) are at twice the risk of suffering a vascular event, compared to individuals with a single risk factor (Figure 30.1). Understanding the multiplicativity of risk factors is essential when stratifying individuals for their risk of atherosclerosis. Therefore, to determine an individual's risk of future symptomatic atherosclerosis, the number and severity of risk factors must be considered. Longitudinal studies such as the Framingham study and the MRFIT screenees study allow prediction of future risk of coronary heart disease (CHD), stroke, and death, for up to 5 and 10 years. These approaches use age, sex, cholesterol, HDL-cholesterol, systolic blood pressure, cigarette smoking, diabetes, and ECG evidence of left ventricular hypertrophy (LVH) as risk predictors for symptomatic coronary disease. It should be noted, however, that in most observational studies a single measurement of a potential risk factor at baseline is correlated with future atherosclerotic disease. This approach likely underestimates the true impact of risk factors on the development of atherosclerosis due to random error with the initial measurement, a concept known as regression dilution bias.[5]

The workup in patients with known but stable atherosclerotic disease includes a detailed family history to screen for premature vascular disease (i.e., a relative with cardiovascular disease [CVD] <65 years of age), the patient's risk factor profile (e.g., smoking, diabetes, hypertension), previous vascular disease (e.g., myocardial infarction, stroke), and current symptoms (angina, TIAs, claudication). A physical examination to search for evidence of prior atherosclerotic disease, ankle-arm blood pressure, presence of carotid or renal bruits, clinical evidence of LVH, or risk factors such as elevations in blood pressure (systolic >140, diastolic >90 mm Hg), body mass index (BMI) (>26) and waist-to-hip ratio (abnormal would be >0.85 for

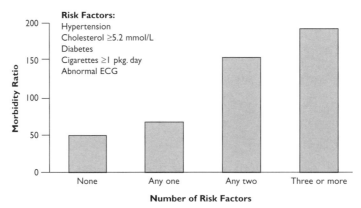

Figure 30.1   Coronary heart disease morbidity versus number of risk factors.

men, >0.90 for women) should also be performed. A baseline ECG is often informative to provide evidence of prior myocardial infarction (Q waves, S-T-T changes, conduction delays), or LVH. Many conditional probability models exist which give the 5- and 10-year estimates of the probability of a person developing CHD according to the major modifiable and nonmodifiable risk factors.[6] This initial assessment allows the clinician to determine the baseline risk of an individual prior to proceeding to other "high-tech" methods of risk stratification. Diagnostic tests such as exercise stress testing or angiography are usually not necessary, yet they often serve as useful adjuncts to the risk stratification process.

Tobacco.   Cigarette smoking is a powerful and independent causal factor for the development of CVD. During the 1990s tobacco consumption in the developed countries will cause about 30% of all deaths in the 35 to 69 years age group, making it the largest single cause of premature death.[7] The risk of CVD is increased two and a half to threefold in smokers compared with nonsmokers,[8] and again the relative impact of cigarette smoking is increased in younger age groups and less in older. However, there is encouraging evidence that preventive measures both before and after clinical manifestations of several diseases are worthwhile. Individuals who stop smoking before middle age subsequently avoid almost all the excess risk that they would have otherwise suffered, and even those who stop smoking in middle age (i.e., 35 years) are at significantly lower risk than those who continue to smoke. Although there is uncertainty about the effectiveness of clinical interventions to reduce smoking rates, a number of studies have demonstrated that physician counselling can change patient behaviour even when the advice is translated through relatively simple messages;[8] therefore, formal smoking cessation counselling should be offered routinely to all smokers. For those considered to be addicted, formal programs to deal with nicotine withdrawal and behavioral modification should be considered.

Dyslipidemia.   A vast body of epidemiologic studies have demonstrated a continuous and incremental relationship between serum cholesterol levels and CHD whereby the risk of CHD increases across the whole range of cholesterol values. A 10% difference in total cholesterol in middle age is associated with a 30% difference in the risk of CHD. This risk is more marked in younger individuals; at the age of 30 to 40, a 10% reduction in cholesterol equates to a 54% risk reduction whereas at the age of 60, it equates to a 27% difference. The proportionate gains in CHD reduction are related to the degree of cholesterol lowering, the duration of the intervention, and the age at which intervention is initiated. With the availability of the HMG-CoA reductase inhibitors, the degree of cholesterol lowering in trials of 5-years' duration is about 25%. Recent large randomized controlled trials in secondary prevention such as 4S (CARE and Post-CABG)[9–11] were able to demonstrate clear reductions (~20%) in total mortality with cholesterol lowering as they were largely confined to high-risk individuals. These trials support the conclusion that across a broad range of cholesterol values, cholesterol lowering therapies aimed at a reduction in total cholesterol of approximately 20 to 25% produce important (about 30%) reductions in cardiovascular events in patients with pre-existing vascular disease within the relatively short time frame of 5 years (mean time to event of only 2.5 years). Further, in all these trials, little impact of the cholesterol lowering therapy was observed within the first 2 years of treatment; the differences became more marked later, with survival curves continuing to diverge at the end of the trials. This suggests that longer treatment will lead to a much larger treatment benefit (perhaps as much as twofold) than that suggested by the 5-year trials.

Hypertension.   Prospective epidemiologic data demonstrate that increased risk of CVD (strokes, CHD, heart failure, and renal failure) due to elevated systolic or diastolic blood pressure is continuous and graded.[5] The Framingham data demonstrated a correlation between increasing blood pressure levels and CHD, and a progressive increase in cardiovascular risk with every increment of systolic pressure. It is estimated that for a middle-aged man, 20 mm Hg higher systolic BP is associated with 60% greater CVD mortality and a 40% higher all-cause mortality over 10 years.[3] Furthermore, observational studies predict that reductions of diastolic BP of 5 to 6 mm Hg result in a reduction in stroke of 34% and CHD of 20 to 25%. Observational studies also suggest that individuals conventionally believed to be normotensive may also potentially benefit from reductions in blood pressure if they have other risk factors (i.e., a patient whose systolic BP is between 130 to 160 may benefit). Randomized controlled trials suggest that both pharmacologic (e.g., diuretics and beta-blockers)[12,13] and nonpharmacologic therapies such as weight reduction, reduction of salt intake, and increased physical activity[6] are all effective in lowering blood pressure individually or in combination. A systematic review of 14 randomized control trials involving 37,000 hypertensive patients treated with beta-blockers or diuretics with a mean decrease in diastolic blood pressure of 5 to 6 mm Hg over 5 years, led to a highly significant 42% reduction in stroke incidence, and a 14% reduction in CHD.[5] Treatment of systolic hypertension in elderly patients also significantly reduces cardiovascular morbidity and mortality. Recently, the Dietary Approaches to Stop Hypertension (DASH) trial tested the effects of a high-fruit-and-vegetable, and low-fat diet compared to a standard diet in individuals with a systolic blood pressure of <160 mm Hg and diastolic pressure of between 80 and

95 mm Hg. Individuals who consumed at least eight servings of fruits and vegetables per day demonstrated an impressive 11-mm reduction in systolic blood pressure compared to the standard diet group.[12] Therefore, in both low-risk and higher-risk populations, it is important to recognize the continuous relationship between blood pressure and the risk of CHD and stroke. From a population perspective impressive reductions in hypertension and its sequelae can be achieved with nonpharmacologic interventions in lower-risk subgroups whereas in subgroups which are at high risk of future vascular events, more aggressive blood pressure reduction usually including the use of pharmacologic therapies should be sought. At present, the only drugs that have been shown to reduce mortality or morbidity in hypertension are diuretics and beta-blockers, with some suggestive data for ACE inhibitors.

Glucose intolerance. There is early evidence which suggests that glucose, like cholesterol and blood pressure, shares a continuous relationship with atherosclerosis.[14] Diabetics are at a much higher risk of CVD and death for any given level of the other major cardiovascular risk factors compared with nondiabetics, with a risk of cardiovascular death three times higher across all ages, even after adjustment for serum cholesterol, hypertension, and cigarette smoking.[15] Modest elevations of plasma glucose in a prediabetic range are associated with an increased risk of cardiovascular disease as this risk rises progressively with the level of postprandial glucose and appears to be "continuous" over a broad range of glucose levels. The link between elevated glucose levels, insulin, and associated dyslipidemia to atherosclerosis is complex, and the exact mechanism by which these factors are proatherogenic has not yet been elucidated. Currently our approach to risk factor modification in insulin-dependent diabetics is to maximize insulin use to achieve tight control of glucose as it is now clear that the progression of microvascular disease such as retinopathy, neuropathy, and nephropathy is slowed when this is achieved.[16] However, the extent to which tight metabolic control of hyperglycemia limits macrovascular disease has not yet been determined although preliminary evidence supports this hypothesis.[16,17] Opportunities for prevention of late-onset diabetes are greater because its development is associated with obesity, physical inactivity, and it usually has an adult onset. Whether or not tight control of glucose, in the setting of adult-onset diabetes, leads to a reduction in macrovascular complications is being addressed in ongoing clinical trials.

B Nonconventional Risk Factors

Apart from the major conventional risk factors for atherosclerosis (smoking, cholesterol, hypertension, diabetes), other risk factors such as obesity, lifestyle factors such as physical inactivity, and menopausal status in women should also be considered. Other less conventional risk factors such as elevated Lp(a), microalbuminuria, low HDL cholesterol, and hyperhomocystinemia should be considered in individuals who do not have any identifiable conventional risk factors, yet suffer premature vascular disease.

C Baseline Risk of Future Vascular Events

The baseline risk refers to the risk of an individual suffering a clinical manifestation of a disease (in this case atherosclerosis), and this risk may be low, moderate, or high. Each major risk factor (e.g., smoking, hypertension, elevated cholesterol) is independently and causally associated with the development of vascular disease, and it appears that these effects are at least additive when more than one risk factor is present (Figures 30.1 and 30.2). It is important to determine what this risk is so that the relative benefit of specific management strategies may be reasonably antici- pated. For example, an individual who has a 30% risk of developing a myocardial infarction in 1 year, compared to an individual with a 5% risk, will derive greater

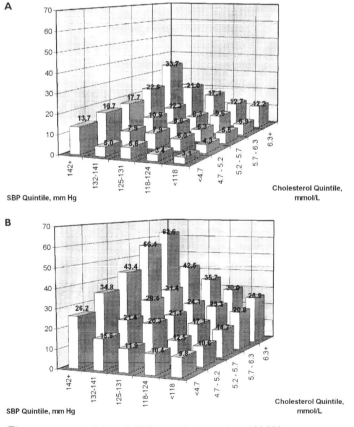

Figure 30.2   Adjusted CHD mortality rates (per 100,000 person years). A, nonsmokers; B, smokers.[15]

benefit from any treatment strategy (i.e., statins) which reduces this risk by 25%. The baseline risk in the first instance is reduced to 22.5% (absolute change = 7.5%) whereas in the second it is reduced from 5 to 3.75% (absolute change = 1.25%). The overall absolute risk reduction in a given individual will depend upon the age of initiation of treatment, the duration of intervention, and the inherent risk of future vascular event. However, it is shortsighted to believe that interventions used to lower risk will only be effective in those subgroups with high baseline risks such as the elderly. Although younger individuals have a lower baseline risk, they have a greater relative risk of suffering a vascular event over the long term; therefore, intervening with effective therapies, i.e., cholesterol reduction, will likely lead to a greater absolute risk reduction in this subgroup over the long term. All of these factors should be taken into account when decisions regarding the initiation, the type (pharmacologic vs. lifestyle), and duration (months, years, lifetime) of therapy are being considered.

D *Treatment Strategies*

Three complementary strategies should be considered. Primordial prevention refers to the prevention of the major risk factors themselves and is most effective when applied to the children of high-risk adult populations[18] or to populations that could develop risk factors (e.g., transition from a "rural" to an "urban" lifestyle in the developing countries). Primary prevention refers to an intervention to prevent disease before clinical symptoms of the disease have been manifested. On the other hand, secondary prevention refers to interventions to reduce risk factors after the manifestations of symptomatic atherosclerosis, such as angina, MI, or claudication. As the risk of future vascular events is higher in these patients, they stand to gain more from aggressive risk factor modification. However, as atherosclerosis represents a continuum of disease, any boundaries we impose on our approach to its modification are somewhat artificial, and it is much more useful to classify individuals as being low, moderate, or high risk to suffer symptomatic atherosclerotic disease in the future.

It is now clear that specific therapies aimed at atherosclerotic risk factor modification can result in decreased CHD mortality.[6] Targeting a single risk factor, as well as multifactorial approaches to risk factor modification lead to decreased morbidity and mortality from CHD, as evidenced by the 24% decline in CHD mortality witnessed over the past 30 years in North America, and an impressive 60% reduction in CHD mortality and stroke observed in Finland between 1972 and 1994.[19] It is estimated that approximately 75% of the decline in CHD mortality in Finland can be explained by risk factor changes.[19] Therefore, from a population perspective, strategies to reduce major conventional risk factors lead to impressive reductions in the overall burden of atherosclerotic disease. From an individual perspective, the current evidence has enabled clinicians to make confident therapeutic decisions to reduce the future risk of symptomatic atherosclerosis which include cholesterol reduction, blood pressure lowering, smoking cessation, and improved glucose control, weight loss, and physical activity. These complementary strategies are outlined in the following algorithm.

Apart from direct modification of causal factors to reduce the burden of vascular disease, higher-risk subgroups with symptomatic disease have also been shown to benefit from other pharmacologic therapies. Antiplatelet agents such as aspirin reduce the risk of future thromboembolic events in patients with angina, acute myocardial infarction (MI), transient ischemic attack (TIA), stroke, and peripheral vascular disease. The Antiplatelet Trialists' Collaboration involved 145 trials including 70,000 high-risk patients and 39,000 low-risk patients, and when all high-risk patients were examined together, use of antiplatelet therapy was associated with a 30% reduction in future MI and stroke, and a 17% reduction in vascular death.[20] When used in low-risk people (i.e., asymptomatic individuals), although the relative risk reductions are similar, the absolute reduction in clinically significant events is much lower. Current guidelines recommend that aspirin be used routinely in patients with stable and unstable angina, acute MI, TIA, previous atherothrombotic stroke, and peripheral vascular disease.[21] Other pharmacologic strategies which have been proven to be effective by well-controlled randomized clinical trials include the use of beta-blockers in post-MI and hypertensive patients, ACE inhibitors in patients with left ventricular dysfunction and diabetes, and other anticoagulants such as warfarin in post-MI patients. As well, effective preventive surgical treatments in high-risk patients with severe atherosclerosis include coronary artery bypass surgery with multivessel disease or disease of the left main coronary artery, and carotid endarterectomy in patients who have a high-grade symptomatic carotid stenosis. These approaches are considered in more detail elsewhere in the book.

Reductions in elevated blood pressure and cholesterol and cessation of cigarette smoking have clearly been shown to reduce the incidence of clinical vascular disease. Unfortunately, in the era of "high-tech" medical intervention, these efficacious strategies are often overlooked as prevention of disease by these means is often too intangible for individuals and physicians to accept. Although epidemiologic studies have provided much of our information around the probable success of risk factor modification and intervention, the recent era of well-controlled clinical trials have now provided evidence that has convinced most sceptics of the value of risk factor modification—especially in high-risk patients. Despite the substantial attention which has been focused on secondary prevention interventions, the greatest

Symptomatic Atherosclerosis (Angina, Post-MI, PVD, Stroke)

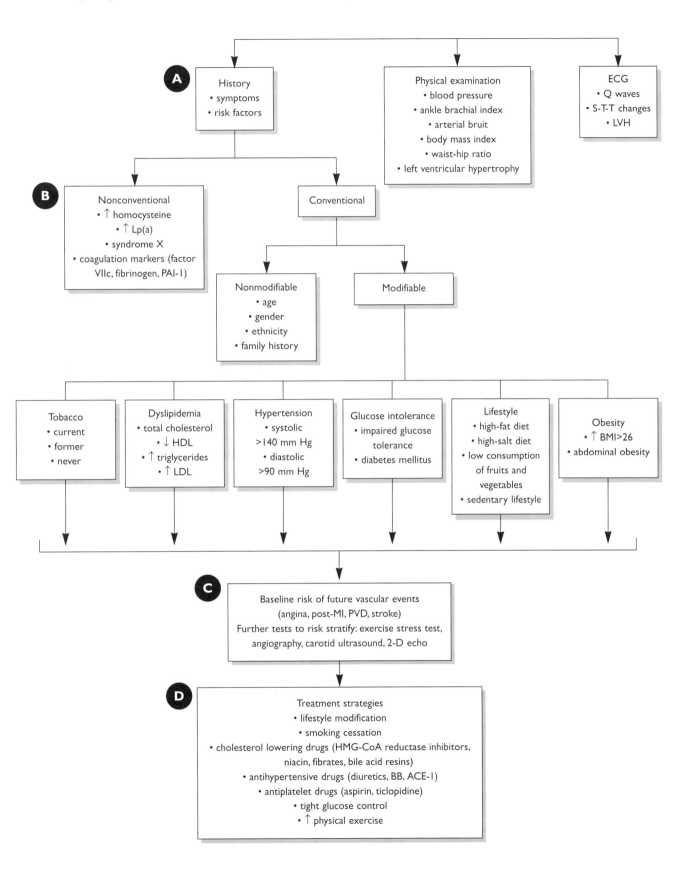

gains in reducing the prevalence of atherosclerosis occur by reducing the levels of atherosclerotic risk factors in the population as a whole.

Bibliography

1. Dawber TR, Meadors GF, Moore FEJ. Epidemiological approaches to heart disease: The Framingham Study. Am J Public Health 1951;41:279–86.

2. Menotti A, Keys A, Blackburn H, et al. Comparison of multivariate predictive power of major risk factors for coronary heart diseases in different countries: results from eight nations of the seven countries study, 25 year follow-up. J Cardiovasc Risk 1996;3:69–75.

3. Stamler J, Dyer AR, Shekelle RB, Neaton J, Stamler R. Relationship of baseline major risk factors to coronary and all-cause mortality, and to longevity: findings from long-term follow-up of Chicago cohorts. Cardiology 1993;82:191–222.

4. Pooling Project Research Group. Relationship of blood pressure, serum cholesterol, smoking habit, relative weight and ECG abnormalities to incidence of major coronary events. J Chron Dis 1978;31:201–306.

5. MacMahon S, Peto R, Cutler J, et al. Blood pressure, stroke, and coronary heart disease. Part 1, Prolonged differences in blood pressure: prospective observational studies corrected for the regression dilution bias. Lancet 1990;335:765–74.

6. Pearson TA. Primer in preventive cardiology. Dallas, Texas: American Heart Association, 1994.

7. Peto R, Lopez AD, Boreham J, Thun M, Heath C Jr. Mortality from tobacco in developed countries: indirect estimation from national vital statistics. Lancet 1992;339:1268–78.

8. Grundy SM, Greenland P, Herd A, et al. Cardiovascular and risk factor evaluation of healthy American adults. A statement for physicians by an Ad Hoc Committee appointed by the Steering Committee, American Heart Association. Use of computer simulation to explore analytical issues in nested case-control studies of cancer involving extended exposures: methods and preliminary findings. Circulation 1987;40(Suppl 2):201S–8S.

9. Anonymous. Randomised trial of cholesterol lowering in 4444 patients with coronary heart disease: the Scandinavian Simvastatin Survival Study (4S). Lancet 1994;344:1383–9.

10. Sacks FM, Pfeffer MA, Moye LA, Rouleau JL, Rutherford JD. The effect of pravastatin on coronary events after myocardial infarction in patients with average cholesterol levels. Cholesterol and Recurrent Events Trial investigators. N Engl J Med 1996;335:1001–9.

11. The Post Coronary Artery Bypass Graft Trial Investigators. The effect of aggressive lowering of low-density lipoprotein cholesterol levels and low-dose anticoagulation on obstructive changes in saphenous-vein coronary-artery bypass grafts. N Engl J Med 1997;336:153–62.

12. Sacks FM, Obarzanek E, Windhauser MM, et al. Rationale and design of the Dietary Approaches to Stop Hypertension trial (DASH). A multicenter controlled-feeding study of dietary patterns to lower blood pressure. Ann Epidemiol 1995;5:108–18.

13. Wassertheil-Smoller S, Applegate WB, Berge K, et al. Change in depression as a precursor of cardiovascular events. SHEP Cooperative Research Group (Systolic Hypertension in the Elderly). Arch Intern Med 1996;156(5):553–61.

14. Gerstein HC, Yusuf S. Dysglycaemia and risk of cardiovascular disease. Lancet 1996;347:949–50.

15. Stamler J, Vaccaro O, Neaton JD, Wentworth D. Diabetes, other risk factors, and 12-yr cardiovascular mortality for men screened in the Multiple Risk Factor Intervention Trial. Diabetes Care 1993;16:434–44.

16. Anonymous. The effect of intensive treatment of diabetes on the development and progression of long-term complications in insulin-dependent diabetes mellitus. The Diabetes Control and Complications Trial Research Group. N Engl J Med 1993;329:977–86.

17. Malmberg K, Ryden L, Efendic S, et al. Randomized trial of insulin-glucose infusion followed by subcutaneous insulin treatment in diabetic patients with acute myocardial infarction (DIGAMI study): effects on mortality at 1 year. J Am Coll Cardiol 1995;26:57–65.

18. Strasser T. Reflections on cardiovascular diseases. Interdisc Sci Rev 1978;3:225–30.

19. Vartiainen E, Puska P, Pekkanen J, Tuomilehto J, Jousilahti P. Changes in risk factors explain changes in mortality from ischaemic heart disease in Finland. BMJ 1994;309:23–7.

20. Antiplatelet Trialists' Collaboration. Collaborative overview of randomised trials of antiplatelet therapy: 1. Prevention of death, myocardial infarction, and stroke by prolonged antiplatelet therapy in various categories of patients. BMJ 1994;308:81–106.

21. Cairns J, Lewis D Jr, Meade TW, Sutton GC, Théroux P. Antithrombotic agents in coronary artery disease. Chest 1995;108:380S–400S.

Chapter 31

THROMBOLYSIS IN ACUTE MYOCARDIAL INFARCTION

Pierre Théroux

Acute myocardial infarction is one component of the "acute coronary syndromes." This terminology was introduced to regroup the clinical manifestations of rapidly developing coronary occlusion, most often precipitated by formation of an intra-coronary thrombus. An acute coronary syndrome is first recognized on clinical grounds; subsequent patient orientation and treatment is based on diagnostic procedures and most importantly on the 12-lead ECG. The symptoms of myocardial infarction are usually straightforward. At times, however, myocardial infarction may be silent with atypical manifestations, such as syncope, an unusual site for chest pain, fatigue, shortness of breath, or upper gastrointestinal symptoms. A 12-lead electrocardiogram should be obtained in all patients consulting for chest pain or equivalent symptoms, especially when the symptoms are not readily explainable by another cause.

A Administer ASA

Aspirin should be administered to all patients with documented or suspected acute coronary syndrome, unless contraindicated. The initial dose is 160 to 360 mg of a non-enteric presentation, ideally chewable. The efficacy of aspirin during the acute phase of an acute coronary syndrome has been documented in numerous trials in unstable angina, non-Q- and Q-wave myocardial infarction, and coronary artery bypass surgery.[1] There exist very few contraindications for this initial dose besides known allergy and bronchospasm; gastric intolerance is usually not a contraindication.

B S-T Segment Elevation

The diagnosis of myocardial infarction dictates consideration of reperfusion therapy. An electrocardiogram is usually the only confirmatory test required. Reports of CK values or of other markers of cell necrosis are not required. S-T segment elevation indicates transmural ischemia, the consequence of a complete coronary occlusion, with inadequate collateral circulation. Reperfusion therapy is aimed at stopping the evolving necrosis and limiting the size of infarction. Since necrosis grows exponentially with time, immediate action is required. The sooner thrombolysis is applied after the onset of symptoms, the greater is the reduction in mortality.[2]

C   *No S-T Segment Elevation*

A nondiagnostic initial ECG should be repeated when symptoms are evolving. More subtle changes of an early evolving infarction can also be present such as tall and symmetrical acute T waves in the anterior leads. Reciprocal S-T segment depression reinforces the indication of reperfusion therapy. S-T segment depression in leads V_1 and V_2 suggests a true posterior or high lateral wall infarction; leads L_2, L_3, and aV_F then often show some S-T changes. Recording the dorsal leads V_7, V_8, and V_9 increases the diagnostic yield. Thrombolysis is not indicated in the absence of S-T segment elevation or left bundle branch block; no benefit is then expected whereas the risk of serious bleeding persists. Thrombolysis may also precipitate an ischemic event in these patients.

D   *Alternative Diagnostic Procedures*

The ECG may occasionally be nondiagnostic in patients with otherwise very suggestive symptoms; examples are presence of a conduction defect such as left bundle branch block, a QRS complex triggered by a pacemaker, and others. Alternative diagnostic procedures may then be performed. A regional perfusion defect can be detected by a perfusion scan and regional wall motion abnormality by a 2-D echocardiogram or a left ventricular radionuclide scintigraphy. Systolic wall thinning on the echocardiogram is a reliable marker of severe transmural ischemia.

E   *Chest Pain Evolving for Less Than 12 Hours*

The indication for reperfusion therapy is chest pain evolving for less than 12 hours and presence of S-T *segment elevation* (≥1 mm in ≥2 contiguous leads) or of a new or presumably new *left bundle branch block*. Occasional patients may benefit from treatment applied 12 to 24 hours after onset of pain when some evidence exists that myocardium can be salvaged when a patient has evolving chest pain with persisting S-T segment elevation and no profound Q waves.[2]

F   *Rule Out Aortic Dissection or Pericarditis*

It is essential to rule out other causes for S-T segment elevation, and more specifically an aortic dissection or pericarditis as well as a nonatherosclerotic cause of myocardial infarction, such as chest wall trauma. This is achieved by clinical means. The

S-T segment is typically elevated in all ECG leads in acute pericarditis, with no mirror S-T segment depression in reciprocal leads. A dissecting aneurysm is suspected in inferior myocardial infarction when a murmur of aortic regurgitation, asymmetrical pulse, or severe dorsal pain is present. Patients with features of Marfan syndrome have an increased risk. An echocardiogram should be obtained when a dissection is suspected.

G Screen for Possible Contraindications

Consideration of thrombolysis requires rapid but well-oriented screening for the presence of possible contraindications. Most contraindications are related to the bleeding risk associated with clot lysis. Intracranial bleeding is the most dramatic complication that often results in death or severe disability. Factors associated with an increased risk of intracranial bleeding are a history of stroke or transient ischemic attack, advanced age, elevated systolic and diastolic blood pressure, lower body weight, and a history of hypertension. The contraindications are graded as strong, relative, or absent (Table 31.1). When a relative contraindication exists, the risk of severe bleeding is weighed against the potential benefit of treatment.

H Primary Angioplasty and Thrombolysis

Primary angioplasty and thrombolytic therapy are two valuable reperfusion strategies. Most patients will benefit from either one. Balloon angioplasty is associated with a high success rate, and a relatively low risk of bleeding, when it can be done

Table 31.1   Contraindications to Thrombolysis

Strong contraindications
Active internal bleeding
Suspected aortic dissection
Active intracranial disease
Any previous intracranial bleeding
Stroke or TIA within the previous 3 months
Recent head trauma
Pregnancy
Blood pressure >200 systolic, >120 diastolic
Trauma or surgery within the previous 2 weeks
Relative contraindications
Trauma or surgery within the previous 4 weeks
Previous stroke
Known bleeding diathesis
Blood pressure >180 systolic, or >100 diastolic

by an experienced operator within 1 hour after hospital admission. The multi-center GUSTO IIb trial reported a moderate advantage of primary angioplasty over thrombolysis in the primary outcome of death, nonfatal reinfarction, or nonfatal disabling stroke at 30 days (rate of 9.6% with angioplasty and 13.7% with t-PA, odds ratio, 0.67, p = .033). At 6 months, however, there was no significant difference in outcome between the two groups (13.3% vs. 15.7%, NS).[3] Patients with a large myocardial infarction, with hemodynamic compromise, or with a relative contraindication to thrombolysis are best referred to the catheterization laboratory when facilities are available; patients with a strong contraindication to thrombolysis should be transferred to a center with facilities for percutaneous interventions.

❚ *Thrombolytic Agents*

Four thrombolytic agents are currently approved for clinical use and many others are under investigation. Approved agents are streptokinase, anistreplase (APSAC), tissue plasminogen activator (t-PA), and reteplase (r-PA). Many major trials have been performed with these agents; their results have generated many debates[4–7] and have resulted in various consensus recommendations. All agree, however, that rapid administration of the lytic agent is more important than the choice of a specific agent. The GISSI-2 and ISIS-3 trials have not found an advantage of t-PA over streptokinase.[4,5] The GUSTO-1 trial, however, documented an absolute reduction of 1% in the risk of death at 30 days with a regimen of accelerated tissue plasminogen activator with intravenous heparin compared with streptokinase and intravenous or subcutaneous heparin (6.3% vs. 7.3%). The benefit of t-PA over streptokinase was statistically significant in the prespecified analyses of the subgroups of patients less than 75 years old, those with an anterior myocardial infarction, and those presenting less than 4 hours after onset of chest pain.[6] Anistreplase has an efficacy and safety profile similar to streptokinase. Reteplase in the GUSTO-2 trial was slightly inferior to t-PA but with overlapping confidence limits.[7] The choice of a thrombolytic agent is influenced by many factors and, not the least, cost-effectiveness considerations. In some countries, t-PA is administered in 75% of patients, and in others in 25%. Countries that are more selective usually reserve t-PA for patients younger than 75 years old and/or an anterior infarction and/or consulting relatively early after the onset of symptoms. Tissue plasminogen activator should be selected in patients who have received streptokinase or APSAC in the previous year, because of inhibiting antibodies developing against streptokinase, and probably be preferred in patients with a more extensive myocardial infarction. The dose of streptokinase is 1.5 million units over 30 to 60 minutes; of APSAC 30 U in 5 to 10 minutes; of t-PA 15 mg bolus, followed by 0.75 mg/kg in 30 minutes not to exceed 50 mg, then

Acute Coronary Syndromes: Suspected Myocardial Infarction

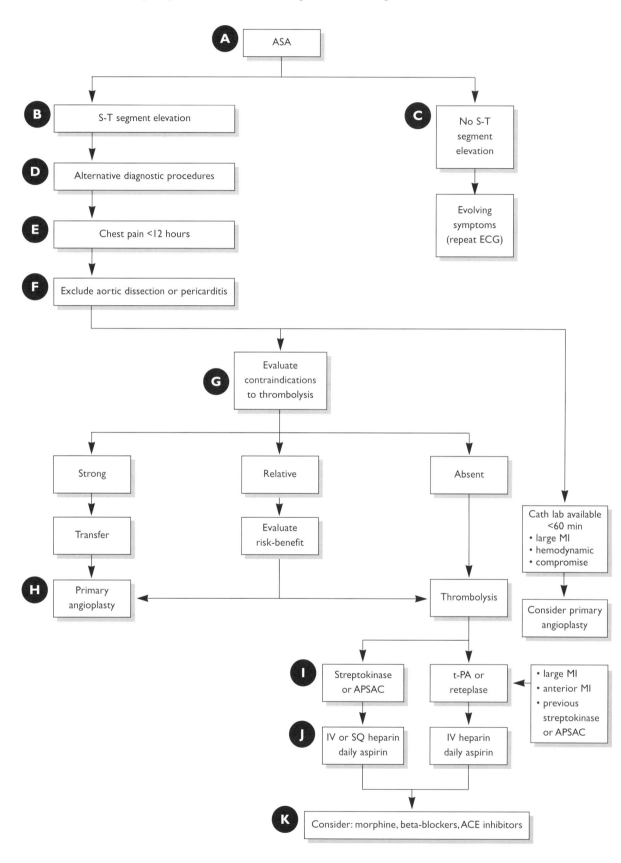

0.5 mg/kg over 60 minutes not to exceed 35 mg; the maximal dose is 100 mg. The dose of reteplase is 15 megaunits bolus followed after 30 minutes by another 15 MU bolus.

J *Intravenous Heparin*

Intravenous heparin is indicated with t-PA and with r-PA. The dose is 5000 unit bolus followed by an infusion of 1000 U per hour, with consideration for lower doses in older patients, females, and patients weighing <50 kg. The infusion rate is titrated after 12 hours to an optimal range for aPTT prolongation to 50 to 70 seconds. Heparin is optional with streptokinase and APSAC; it can be given subcutaneously or intravenously and initiated late or early after the start of the lytic agent (see Chapter 32).

K *Other Therapies*

Other therapies indicated routinely in the absence of contraindications are IV morphine for the relief of chest pain, IV and oral beta-blockade, and angiotensin converting enzyme inhibitors. Secondary prevention is discussed in Chapter 32. The global management of myocardial infarction also includes clinical detection of the success or failure of reperfusion, consideration of rescue angioplasty in selected patients, and risk stratification in the following days.

Bibliography

1. Antiplatelet Trialists' Collaboration. Collaborative overview of randomized trials of antiplatelet therapy I: Prevention of death, myocardial infarction, and stroke by prolonged antiplatelet therapy in various categories of patients. Br Med J 1994;308:81–106.
2. Fibrinolytic Therapy Trialists' (FTT) Collaborative Group. Indications for fibrinolytic therapy in suspected acute myocardial infarction: collaborative overview of early mortality and major morbidity results from all randomised trials of more than 1000 patients. Lancet 1994;343:311–22.
3. The GUSTO Angiographic Investigators. A clinical trial comparing primary coronary angioplasty with tissue plasminogen activator for acute myocardial infarction. N Eng J Med 1997;336:1621–8.
4. Gruppo italiano per lo studio della sopravivivenza nell'infarto miocardico. GISSI-2: A factorial randomised trial of alteplase versus streptokinase and heparin versus no heparin among 12,490 patients with acute myocardial infarction. Lancet 1990;336:65–71.
5. ISIS-3 (Third International Study of Infarct Survival) Collaborative Group. ISIS-3: a randomized comparison of streptokinase vs tissue plasminogen activator vs anistreplase and of aspirin plus heparin vs aspirin alone among 41,299 cases of suspected acute myocardial infarction. Lancet 1992;339:754–70.

6. The GUSTO Investigators. An international randomized trial comparing four thrombolytic strategies for acute myocardial infarction. N Engl J Med 1993;329:673–82.

7. The GUSTO Investigators. Results from the GUSTO-2 trial. Late-breaking clinical trials session at ACC'97.

Additional Reading

Report of the American College of Cardiology/American Heart Association Task Force on Practice Guidelines (Committee on Management of Acute Myocardial Infarction). Guidelines for the management of patients with acute myocardial infarction. Circulation 1996;94:2341–50.

Chapter 32

ANTITHROMBOTIC THERAPY FOR ACUTE MYOCARDIAL INFARCTION

Pierre Théroux

The initial approach to the diagnosis and treatment of myocardial infarction as part of the acute coronary syndromes is discussed in Chapter 31. Patients presenting with S-T segment elevation or new left bundle branch block are candidates for thrombolysis (see Chapter 31) with adjunctive antithrombotic therapy. Patients with S-T segment depression or with T-wave inversion are best managed with antithrombotic therapy. The diagnosis of myocardial infarction needs to be confirmed by an elevation of cardiac enzymes. Treatment, however, should not be delayed while awaiting laboratory results. Indeed, the diagnosis is most often made a posteriori when the results of the initial and follow-up blood samplings become available. The distinction between a non-Q-wave myocardial infarction and unstable angina is important for evaluation of prognosis but not for immediate management. Indeed, the general approach to management of an acute coronary syndrome is similar except for the indication of thrombolysis with S-T segment elevation. Therefore, the treatment tree in this chapter applies to patients with unstable angina as well as to patients with a non-Q-wave myocardial infarction.

A *Administration of Aspirin*

Aspirin should be given to all patients with the diagnosis of an acute coronary syndrome. It is administered when the diagnosis is suspected at a dose of 160 to 325 mg (two chewable tablets of 80 mg, or a single tablet of 325 mg orally) to achieve rapid inhibition of platelet aggregation.

B *Identification of S-T Segment Elevation*

Identification of S-T segment elevation or of a new left bundle branch block on the ECG dictates consideration of thrombolysis (Chapter 31). Thrombolysis should not be used in the absence of these findings since it may increase the rate of ischemic events.[1]

C Intravenous Heparin

Clinical studies and meta-analyses have documented that intravenous heparin adds significant protection against ischemic events in unstable angina and non-Q-wave myocardial infarction.[2–4] Heparin is therefore indicated, except when a contraindication exists. The dose recommended is a 5000 U bolus followed by an infusion at a rate of 1000 U per hour, titrated to achieve a prolongation of the activated partial thromboplastin time (aPTT) to 1.5 to 2.5 times control.

D Use of Low-Molecular-Weight Heparins

Recent trials with low-molecular-weight heparins suggest that these drugs are a reasonable alternative to heparin.[5–7] The advantages of low-molecular-weight heparins are the ease of administration, including the subcutaneous route once or twice daily, and the absence of a need for monitoring because of their predictable anticoagulant effect. Dalteparin has been evaluated in two trials. In one, the drug was compared with placebo and showed a significant reduction in cardiac events in the same range as that observed with unfractionated heparin.[5] In the second, a direct comparison of dalteparin to unfractionated heparin showed equivalence. The ESSENCE trial showed a significant advantage of enoxaparin compared with unfractionated heparin on the incidence of death, myocardial infarction (MI), and recurrent ischemia at 1 month. The difference in the composite endpoint of death and MI was not statistically significant between the two groups. Although total bleeding rates were increased with enoxaparin, major bleeding was not. The potential benefit of prolonged administration of enoxaparin and dalteparin after hospital discharge is now being evaluated in TIMI 11B and FRISC 2 trials.

E GPIIb/IIIa Antagonists

The GPIIb/IIIa antagonists represent a novel therapeutic approach. Whereas aspirin and other platelet inhibitors act indirectly through the inhibition of one of the many pathways to platelet aggregation, the GPIIb/IIIa inhibitors act directly on the platelet receptor to prevent fibrinogen binding and aggregation. Abciximab, a monoclonal antibody against the receptor, is already approved in high-risk coronary angioplasty. Two conclusive trials have documented their efficacy in unstable angina and non-Q-wave myocardial infarction when added to aspirin and to heparin. In the Platelet Receptor Inhibition for Ischemic Syndrome Management in Patients

Limited by Unstable Signs and Symptoms trial (PRISM-PLUS trial), the addition of tirofiban to standard treatment reduced the composite outcome of death, myocardial infarction, or refractory ischemia by 32% at 1 week and by 19% at 6 months. The reduction in the risk of death or myocardial infarction was 43% at 1 week and 22% at 6 months.[8] The drug is indicated for medical stabilization as well as during coronary angiography and coronary angioplasty when indicated. Positive results were also observed with eptifibatide in the PURSUIT trial with a significant risk reduction in the incidence of death and myocardial infarction of 8%.[9] These GPIIb/IIIa antagonists are now under review for approval for indication in acute coronary syndromes. Their use will result in a significant improvement in prognosis.

F *Heparin as Adjunctive Therapy to Thrombolysis*

The indication of heparin as adjunctive therapy to thrombolysis requires special consideration. The GUSTO trial tested four reperfusion strategies: 1) accelerated t-PA with a bolus and infusion of intravenous heparin for at least 48 hours, 2) streptokinase plus IV heparin as with t-PA, 3) streptokinase plus heparin 12,500 U subcutaneously (SQ) commencing 4 hours after streptokinase and repeated every 12 hours for 7 days, and 4) a combination of low dose t-PA and streptokinase plus IV heparin.[10] The best strategy in the trial was accelerated t-PA with heparin; in the absence of a trial with t-PA without heparin, the combination has been universally adopted. A post hoc analysis of the data has shown that the optimal risk benefit ratio of heparin was obtained with aPTT values in the range of 50 to 70 seconds. Prolongation beyond 90 seconds substantially increases the risk of intracranial bleeding. A bolus of 5000 U is administered followed by an infusion at a rate of 1000 U per hour titrated after 12 hours to the aPTT. Lower doses should be considered in older patients and in women who weigh less than 50 kg. Heparin is also administered with reteplase.

G *Heparin with Streptokinase*

The indication for heparin with streptokinase is less clear. Streptokinase is more fibrinogenolytic than t-PA and has a more prolonged biologic activity. The GISSI-2 and ISIS-3 trials evaluated doses of 12,500 U SQ every 12 hours initiated 12 and 4 hours, respectively, after thrombolysis with t-PA or with streptokinase.[11,12] The two studies showed an excess of major bleeding with heparin of 0.44% and 0.27%, respectively, with no excess intracranial hemorrhage in GISSI-2 and an excess of 0.16% in ISIS-3. The former study showed no benefit of heparin with t-PA but some evidence of reduced mortality with streptokinase. The latter showed a modest reduction of reinfarction and mortality with heparin. In GUSTO-1, SQ and IV heparin in conjunction with streptokinase showed similar results.[10] Considering the trials together, no overall important gains of heparin are apparent when administered with streptokinase. Its use remains the physician's choice. Heparin is, however, clearly indicated when a risk of thromboembolic complications is present. Examples are atrial fibrillation and an anterior myocardial infarction with regional wall motion abnormality. Heparin is also indicated in more severe and diffuse left ventricular dysfunction, and in patients at risk of venous thrombosis.

H   *Duration of Heparin Therapy*

The optimal duration for the administration of heparin remains uncertain. It is recommended to administer the drug for 24 to 72 hours following thrombolysis. Most studies that have shown a benefit of heparin in unstable angina and non-Q-wave myocardial infarction have used the drug for more than 72 hours. Reactivation of the disease following the discontinuation of heparin is an important clinical problem.[13] Trials are presently being performed to prevent this rebound. Interventions tested are prolonged administration of subcutaneous low-molecular-weight heparin, the addition of Coumadin to aspirin, and the use of oral inhibitors of the GPIIb/IIIa receptor. In the absence of conclusive data, and considering the cost constraints and the need for a rapid turnover of patients, the best compromise suggested is to administer heparin for 48 hours and stop the medication once the patient has been asymptomatic for a period of 24 hours. A symptom-free period suggests some plaque stabilization. Secondary prevention should have been initiated before the discontinuation of heparin. If Coumadin is used, heparin is stopped once a therapeutic INR in the range of 2.0 to 3.0 is reached.

I   *Secondary Prevention*

Secondary prevention is indicated in all patients who have experienced an acute coronary syndrome. Aspirin is the first choice in the vast majority of patients. Patients intolerant to aspirin should be given ticlopidine or clopidogrel. Clopidogrel is by far a better choice because of a favorable side effect profile. The large CAPRIE trial has shown that clopidogrel was as effective as aspirin for secondary prevention in patients with a previous myocardial infarction, a previous stroke, and in patients with peripheral vascular disease (see Chapter 33).[14] Coumadin is indicated for the prevention of stroke in patients with an anterior myocardial infarction and Q waves. This use is reinforced when the echocardiogram reveals the presence of an intracavitary thrombus. Coumadin is administered for a minimum of 3 months for this indication but can be of benefit in the long term. Coumadin should be administered long term for chronic atrial fibrillation.

Antithrombotic Therapy for Myocardial Infarction

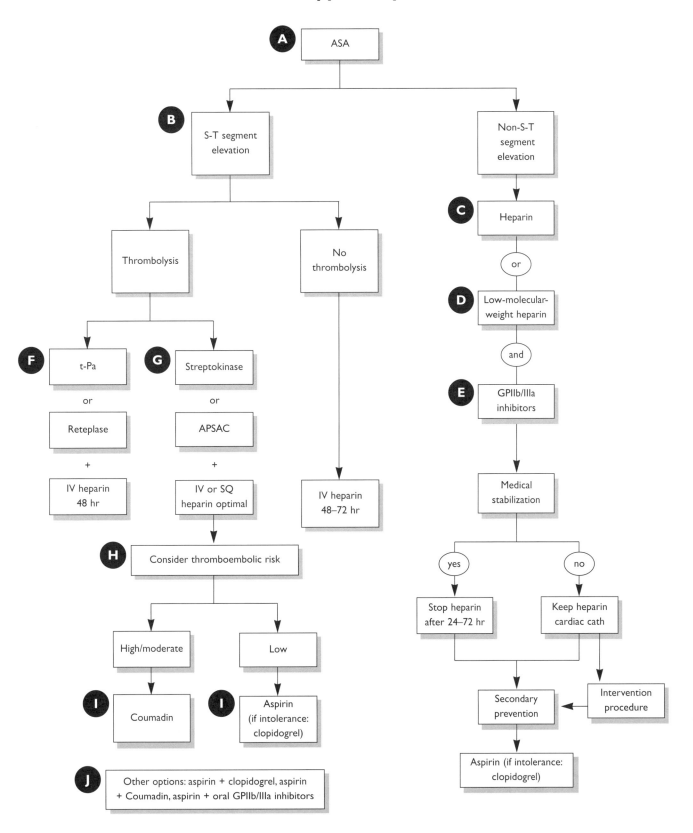

J *Other Therapeutic Options*

Therapeutic options that can be considered for the more unstable patients are the combination of aspirin and clopidogrel, aspirin and Coumadin, or aspirin and an oral GPIIb/IIIa inhibitor. These combined interventions cause a higher risk of bleeding and their efficacy has not yet been documented. The Coumadin Aspirin Reinfarction Study (CARS) failed to show any benefit from the addition of fixed low doses (1 mg or 3 mg per day) of warfarin.[15]

Bibliography

1. The TIMI IIIB Investigators. Effects of tissue plasminogen activator and a comparison of early invasive and conservative strategies in unstable angina and non-Q-wave myocardial infarction. Circulation 1994;89:1545–56.

2. Theroux P, Ouimet H, McCans J, et al. Aspirin, heparin, or both to treat acute unstable angina. N Engl J Med 1988;319:1105–11.

3. The RISC Group. Risk of myocardial infarction and death during treatment with low dose aspirin and intravenous heparin in men with unstable coronary artery disease. Lancet 1990;336:827–30.

4. Oler A, Whooley MA, Oler J, Grady D. Adding heparin to aspirin reduces the incidence of myocardial infarction and death in patients with unstable angina. JAMA 1996;276:811–5.

5. The FRISC Study Group. Low-molecular-weight heparin during instability in coronary artery disease. Lancet 1996;347:561–8.

6. Klein W, Buchwald A, Hillis SE, et al, and for the FRIC Investigators. Comparison of low-molecular-weight heparin with unfractionated heparin acutely and with placebo for 6 weeks in the management of unstable coronary artery disease. Circulation 1997;96:61–8.

7. Cohen M, Demers C, Gurfinkel EP, et al, for the Efficacy and Safety of Subcutaneous Enoxaparin in Non-Q-Wave Coronary Events Study Group. Low molecular weight heparin versus unfractionated heparin for unstable angina and non-Q wave myocardial infarction. N Engl J Med 1997;337:447–52.

8. The PRISM-PLUS Investigators. Specific inhibition of platelet receptor glycoprotein IIb/IIIa with tirofiban in unstable angina and non-Q-wave myocardial infarction. N Engl J Med (in press).

9. The PURSUIT Investigators. A randomized comparison of the platelet glycoprotein IIb/IIIa peptide inhibitor eptifibatide with placebo in patients without persistent S-T-segment elevation acute coronary syndromes. N Engl J Med (in press).

10. The GUSTO Investigators. An international randomized trial comparing four thrombolytic strategies for acute myocardial infarction. N Engl J Med 1993;329:673–82.

11. Gruppo italiano per lo studio della sopravivvenza nell'infarto miocardico. GISSI-2: A factorial randomised trial of alteplase versus streptokinase and heparin versus no heparin among 12 490 patients with acute myocardial infarction. Lancet 1990;336:65–71.

12. ISIS-3 (Third International Study of Infarct Survival) Collaborative Group. ISIS-3: a randomized comparison of streptokinase vs tissue plasminogen activator vs anistreplase and of aspirin plus heparin vs aspirin alone among 41,299 cases of suspected acute myocardial infarction. Lancet 1992;339:754–70.

13. Theroux P, Waters D, Lam J, Juneau M, McCans J. Reactivation of unstable angina after the discontinuation of heparin. N Engl J Med 1992;327:141–5.

14. CAPRIE Steering Committee. A randomized, blinded trial of clopidogrel versus aspirin in patients at risk of ischaemic events. Lancet 1996;348:1329–39.

15. Coumadin Aspirin Reinfarction Study (CARS) Investigators. Randomized double-blind trial of fixed low-dose warfarin with aspirin after myocardial infarction. Lancet 1997;350:389–96.

Additional Reading

U.S. Department of Health and Human Services. Clinical practice guidelines. Unstable angina: diagnosis and management. AHCPR Publication 1994; Report No.:04-0602.

Theroux P, Fuster V. Acute coronary syndromes: unstable angina and non-Q-wave myocardial infarction. Circulation 1998;97:1195–1206.

Chapter 33

ANTITHROMBOTIC THERAPY FOR ANGINA

Pierre Théroux

Angina is a symptom evoked by myocardial ischemia. Myocardial ischemia may be caused by an excess myocardial demand or by decreased blood supply. Inappropriate vasoconstriction of a large coronary artery (i.e., vasospastic or Prinzmetal's variant angina), a disease of the small coronary arteries (i.e., syndrome x) but most often a thrombotic occlusion of an atherosclerotic plaque or a large coronary vessel is at the origin of inadequate supply. Atherosclerosis is a dynamic process. Rapid progression may occur in young plaques rich in cholesterol esters and at the sites of intense inflammation. The inflammation disrupts the endothelium, exposing thrombogenic material that triggers platelet aggregation and intravascular coagulation. Some plaques are more stable and less likely to rupture; when obstructing the lumen diameter by ≥50%, these plaques may create ischemia when myocardial oxygen needs are increased such as during physical stress. Stable and unstable plaques coexist in the same patients. The interactions of platelets, thrombin, and leukocytes in unstable plaque result in release of various active products, including matrix degradation molecules, procoagulant factors and proteins, cytokines, and growth factors that can lead to formation of an obstructive endovascular thrombus, and to accelerated atherosclerosis.

Not surprisingly, therefore, antithrombotic therapy is an important part of the therapeutic armamentarium that can prevent the complications of coronary atherosclerosis, these being myocardial infarction and death. The disease may be at a subclinical stage, yet active; asymptomatic individuals at risk may therefore benefit from therapy.

Acutely or rapidly developing symptoms are usually associated with an active plaque, and stable or slowly developing symptoms with a more stable plaque. The former require aggressive antithrombotic treatment with multiple targets, and the latter prophylactic antithrombotic therapy. Beta blockers, calcium antagonists and nitrates, on the other hand, are useful to decrease myocardial oxygen supply. Calcium antagonists and nitrates also promote coronary vasodilatation.

A *Acute Coronary Syndromes*

The antithrombotic therapy for unstable angina is described in Chapters 31 and 32. Unstable angina is managed as non-Q-wave myocardial infarction.

B *Administration of ASA*

Stable angina patients are administered antiplatelet therapy. Aspirin, at a daily dose of 80 to 325 mg is used, depending on the formulation available. Higher doses are preferably enteric coated. Low doses of aspirin are as effective as higher doses to inhibit thromboxane A_2 generation by platelets and are better tolerated. Although aspirin possesses many physiologic effects, it is believed that its antithrombotic effects are related to inhibition of thromboxane A_2 and thromboxane A_2-induced platelet aggregation. Aspirin has been shown to be effective in the secondary prevention of coronary artery disease in patients with angina and in patients with silent ischemia. Aspirin was also shown to be effective to reduce the risk of a myocardial infarction through primary prevention; the rate of death was, however, unchanged, and a slight excess in intracranial bleeding existed. The absolute benefit increased with advancing age (>50 years) and with the presence of diabetes mellitus, cigarette smoking, and hypertension.[1,2]

C *Administration of Ticlopidine and Clopidogrel*

Many other antiplatelet agents have been evaluated. Dipyridamole is no longer approved as an antiplatelet drug, and sulfinpyrazone has not been associated with reproducible benefit in clinical trials. These agents are not used any more. Thienopyridines, on the other hand, have been shown to be as effective as aspirin, and slightly better in certain circumstances.[3,4] Ticlopidine and clopidogrel are the two thienopyridines approved for clinical use. These agents exert their benefit by inhibiting adenosine diphosphate-induced platelet aggregation. Ticlopidine possesses an unfavorable side effect profile and can cause severe leukopenia and thombocytopenia. Leukocytes and platelet counts should be closely monitored, especially during the first few months. It is currently used in certain patients with stroke and in combination with aspirin for a period of 3 to 4 weeks following intracoronary stent deployment. Clopidogrel was recently approved following the results of the Clopidogrel versus Aspirin in Patients at Risk of Ischaemic Events (CAPRIE) trial.[4] In this trial, a total of 19,185 patients were randomized to aspirin 325 mg/day, or clopidogrel 75 mg/day. The population was composed of subgroups of patients with atherosclerotic vascular disease manifested as recent ischemic stroke, recent myocardial infarction, or symptomatic peripheral disease. Follow-up extended for 3 years. The annual risk of ischemic stroke, myocardial infarction, or vascular death was reduced by 8.7% in favor of clopidogrel from 5.83 to 5.32% (p = .043). The relative risk was reduced by 23.8% (p = .0028) in patients enrolled because of peripheral vascular disease and by 7.3% in patients enrolled because of stroke but was increased by 5.03% (p = .66) in patients enrolled following myocardial infarction (Figure 33.1). Overall, these results can be interpreted as at least equivalent to aspirin, with doubt persisting about patients with coronary artery disease. The low incidence of side effects of clopidogrel in the CAPRIE trial made its use more compelling in patients intolerant to aspirin. Rash and diarrhea were slightly more frequent than with aspirin in the CAPRIE trial but upper gastrointestinal symptoms, gastrointestinal hemorrhage, and abnormal liver function were slightly less frequent. Ticlopidine requires many days before reaching full antiplatelet effects, and is less appropriate for the management of acute situations. Clopidogrel effects are present more rapidly.

Promising new antiplatelet therapies currently investigated are the combination of aspirin and clopidogrel, and oral inhibitors of the GPIIb/IIIa receptor.

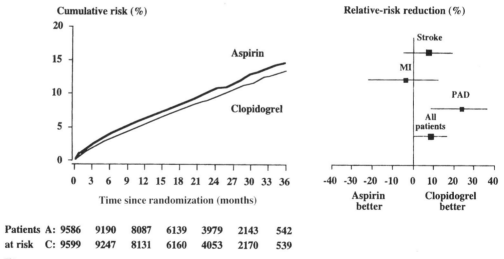

Figure 33.1 Results of the CAPRIE trial. (*Right*) Survival curves in the patients randomized to aspirin and to clopidogrel; (*left*) results in the various predefined subsets. Reproduced with permission of the author and editor; from CAPRIE Steering Committee. A randomized, blinded, trial of clopidogrel versus aspirin in patients at risk of ischaemic events. Lancet 1996;348:1329–39.

Antithrombotic Therapy for Angina

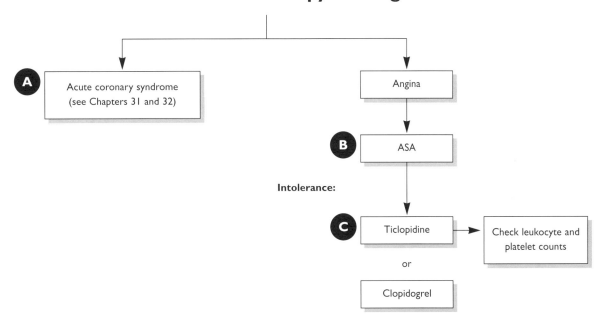

Bibliography

1. The Steering Committee of the Physician' Health Study Research Group. Final report on the aspirin component of the ongoing Physicians' Health Study. N Engl J Med 1989;321:129–35.
2. Manson JE, Stampfer J, Colditz GA, et al. A prospective study of aspirin use and primary prevention in cardiovascular disease in women. JAMA 1991;266:521–7.
3. Hass WK, Easton JD, Adams HP Jr, et al. A randomized trial comparing ticlopidine hydrochloride with aspirin for the prevention of stroke in high-risk patients. N Engl J Med 1989;321:501–7.
4. CAPRIE Steering Committee. A randomized, blinded, trial of clopidogrel versus aspirin in patients at risk of ischaemic events. Lancet 1996;348:1329–39.

Additional Reading

Antiplatelet Trialists' Collaboration. Collaborative overview of randomized trials of antiplatelet therapy—I: Prevention of death, myocardial infarction, and stroke by prolonged antiplatelet therapy in various categories of patients. Br Med J 1994;308:81–106.

Cairns JA, Lewis HD Jr, Meade TW, Sutton GC, Theroux P. Antithrombotic agents in coronary artery disease. Chest 1995;108:380S–400S.

Chapter 34

Patient Selection for Coronary Revascularization, Percutaneous Transluminal Coronary Angioplasty, and Coronary Stenting in Stable Angina Patients

Douglas A Holder

A Severe Angina and/or Severe Ischemia

It is becoming increasingly clear that factors which influence the molecular biology of the atherosclerotic plaque and restore normal endothelial function are most important in contributing to a positive outcome for patients with established coronary artery disease (CAD). Thus, an aggressive approach to lipid lowering and control of modifiable risk factors in all patients, whether or not they undergo a revascularization procedure, is the cornerstone of current therapy.

In spite of optimal medical therapy, including risk factor modification, there are patients who are unacceptably limited in their day-to-day activities by the symptoms of angina pectoris. The majority of these patients have severe, fixed, coronary artery stenoses. In addition, there are other patients who may be less symptomatic but on noninvasive testing show ischemia of large segments of myocardium and/or an inability to exercise beyond 3 minutes on the treadmill, according to the Bruce protocol. Such patients have a poor prognosis and, along with the very symptomatic, should undergo coronary angiography and left ventriculography to determine the extent of coronary artery disease and the degree of left ventricular (LV) dysfunction.

The decision about the most appropriate revascularization method should take into account the following:

1. the exact nature of the coronary stenoses i.e.,

   a) the angiographic appearance of the plaque (smooth, ulcerated, thrombus)

b) the estimated diameter of the stenosis

c) the diameter of the coronary vessel in millimeters

d) the relationship of the stenosis to branch points

e) the amount of myocardium potentially at risk

f) the presence or absence of collateral flow and whether or not the vessel in question is the source or the recipient of the collaterals;

2. the ventricular function;

3. the comorbidity of the patient;

4. the wishes of the patient and family after being informed of the possible risks and benefits.

Generally speaking, the greater the extent of CAD, and the poorer the LV function, the more likely is the patient to benefit from aortocoronary bypass surgery (ACBG),[1,2] providing the nature of the disease, and the health of the patient, allow a successful operation to be done.

B *Coronary Angiography*

The first consideration on viewing the coronary angiogram is whether or not the left main coronary artery has a 50% or greater stenosis and how many other vessels have coronary stenosis ≥70%. Left main coronary stenosis remains a relative contraindication to percutaneous transluminal coronary angioplasty (PTCA) unless it is "protected" by a prior functioning bypass graft to the left anterior descending (LAD) and/or the circumflex coronary artery systems. Furthermore, early randomized controlled trials (RCTs) of medical compared to surgical treatment,[1,2] demonstrated a survival benefit in patients with left main disease who underwent operation. Thus, this subset of patients, approximately 9% of those undergoing angiography, should be selected for surgical management.

The next considerations are whether the patient has single-vessel stenosis of ≥70% (SVD) responsible for morbidity, or more than one major coronary artery stenosed (MVD), the nature of the stenosis itself, as well as the caliber of the runoff vessels.

Table 34.1 lists the characteristics of the coronary stenosis that the interventional cardiologist assesses in deciding suitability for PTCA. The surgeon, of course, looks for an arterial calibre ≥1.5 mm, with the planned anastomotic site accessible (i.e., not intramyocardial) and the downstream vessel free of obstruction.

In addition, the interventional cardiologist must always consider the worst-case scenario when considering a target vessel. For example, if a patient has two-vessel disease with a totally obstructed LAD which is *not* dilatable, and a severely stenotic RCA which is potentially dilatable but is a source of collaterals to the LAD system,the worst-case scenario is total occlusion of the RCA at PTCA with immediate loss of function of the inferior wall and the anterior wall, with probable cardiogenic shock. The prudent course here is to consider ACBG the preferred treatment. There may be occasional circumstances where age, comorbidity, lack of conduit, etc., may make ACBG impossible and the physician and patient may agree to proceed with the PTCA option. However, all are aware of the increased risk, and strategies such as adjunctive intra-aortic balloon counter-pulsation or use of a perfusion balloon for dilatation may be used to minimize the risk of extensive ischemia.

In deciding among the options of ongoing medical treatment, PTCA, or ACBG[3] it should be remembered that ACBG has been shown to confer greater survival benefit compared to medical therapy in patients with left main disease, triple-vessel disease, and some of the subsets of patients with double-vessel disease in whom one of the vessels is the LAD and the stenosis is proximal to the first septal perforator.[4] This is particularly so when there is depression of left ventricular function. No such survival benefit has been shown for PTCA. Thus, when the disease is severe enough to make prognosis a consideration, the choice should almost always

Table 34.1 Coronary Stenosis characteristics and PTCA Selection

Type A (high success >85%; low risk)

Discrete (<10 mm length)
Concentric
Accessible
Non-angulated segment <45%
Not ostial
No major branch

Type B (moderate success 60 to 85%; moderate risk)

Tubular (10 to 20 mm length)
Eccentric
Moderate angulation >45° <90°
Calcification
Total occlusion <3 mo
Ostial
Bifurcation – double wire

Type C (low success x–60%; high risk)

Long >20 mm
Total occlusion >3 mo
Very tortuous
Unable to protect side branches
Angulated >90°
Degenerated vein grafts—friable lesions

be for surgery. Furthermore, symptomatic relief of angina is predictably excellent with surgical revascularization of any patient who is anatomically suitable. Thus it is safe to say that there is no situation in which PTCA has been shown to be superior to ACBG in relieving angina or improving prognosis. However, PTCA is usually chosen where the outcome of symptom relief is potentially as good as ACBG even though the procedure may have to be repeated, since the immediate morbidity and mortality of PTCA is less than with ACBG.

Percutaneous transluminal coronary angioplasty has been compared to medical treatment in patients with single-vessel disease.[5] Angina frequency and treadmill performance were the 6 month endpoints. Patients who were randomized to PTCA had a statistically significant reduction in angina frequency and an increase in exercise capacity. As one would expect, they also underwent more procedures (both PTCA and ACBG) because of restenosis than did those randomized to continue medical treatment.

Recent trials comparing PTCA to ACBG[6,7] in highly selected patients with anatomy suitable for either technique, have shown no difference at 5-year follow-up in new MI, or mortality. However, PTCA patients have undergone many more procedures than ACBG patients and symptomatic relief has been better with surgery. The costs of therapy at 5 years have been virtually equal.[8]

Thus, in MVD where either therapy is possible, and the patient and physician are willing to accept the inevitability of restenosis in a proportion of patients, PTCA can be done with an equivalent benefit to ACBG. In most patients, restenosis does not occur and for them the benefit is striking and the morbidity low. Every patient hopes he/she will have such an outcome. Thus, PTCA is often done as an initial approach in many patients with the option of ACBG later if restenosis is problematic.

In the BARI trial,[6] comparing PTCA to ACBG, the subset of patients with diabetes mellitus had a better outcome with ACBG than PTCA, largely because of a higher restenosis rate in the diabetic patients. Other trials with similar design but fewer patients randomized did not report such a relationship. Nevertheless, in a patient with multivessel disease where the distribution and nature of the coronary disease lends itself to treatment with either strategy, the presence of diabetes makes angioplasty less attractive.

The rapid development of improved coronary stent designs and the consistent benefits noted in RCTs[9,10] have led to adjunctive stenting in the majority of patients undergoing PTCA. An expert panel has recently reported on the current indications for coronary stenting in the province of Ontario.[11] These recommendations are summarized in Table 34.2.

Whereas initial experience with coronary stents was associated with a disappointing frequency of failure to deploy the stent, or thrombosis of the stent in the first week in 8 to 12% of patients, current stent designs and techniques of deployment with associated antiplatelet therapy have greatly minimized these problems.

Currently, all patients are pretreated with ASA and ticlopidine. A standard heparin bolus to achieve an activated clotting time (ACT) 300 to 350 s is used during the procedure and great care is taken with the selection of the stent, positioning in the coronary artery, and deployment pressures to try to achieve an excellent angiographic result. If the procedure becomes complicated with acute closure as a result of possible thrombosis, adjunctive use of abciximab can be very helpful in preventing myocardial infarction or the need to undergo immediate ACBG.[12]

In summary, detailed assessment of the coronary angiogram will determine the extent of CAD. If technical factors do not rule out PTCA or ACBG, then either treatment option remains. Left main, triple-vessel, and double-vessel disease patients in whom LV function is depressed will benefit prognostically as well as symptomatically if operated upon.

Patients with single- or double-vessel disease and normal left ventricular function who are not diabetic, will benefit equally from PTCA or ACBG over 5 years of follow-up, although more patients who have PTCA will undergo additional PTCA

Table 34.2   Coronary Stent Use

Coronary stent use supported by RCT
1. Favourable anatomy and vessel ≥2.5 mm in diameter 2. Proximal LAD stenosis 3. Restenotic lesions after prior PTCA 4. Saphenous vein grafts
Coronary stent use supported by nonrandomized cohort study
1. Acute or threatened closure
Coronary stent use: conditional on extreme need
1. Protected left main stenosis if inoperable 2. Chronic total occlusion 3. Survival dependant vessel
Coronary stent use not recommended
1. Aorto-ostial lesions 2. Long diffuse disease 3. Calcified or tortuous vessels 4. Left main stenosis

Management of Stable Angina Patients

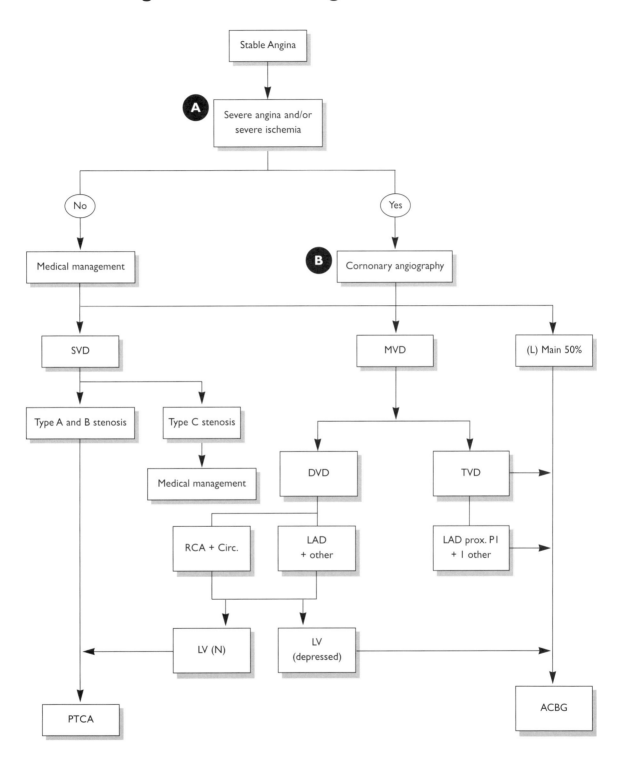

procedures or ACBG compared to those initially operated upon during this interval. Coronary stenting promises to improve the outcome of the PTCA patient by virtue of a reduction in clinical restenosis.

Bibliography

1. Alderman EL, Bourassa M, Cohen LSE. Ten year follow-up of survival and myocardial infarction in the randomized coronary artery surgery study. Circulation 1990;82:1629.

2. European Coronary Surgery Study Group. Long term results of prospective randomized study of coronary artery bypass surgery in stable angina pectoris. Lancet 1982;ii:1173.

3. Rihal CS, Yusuf S. Chronic coronary artery disease: drugs, angioplasty or surgery? BMJ 1996; 312:265–6.

4. Yusuf S, Zuker D, Peduzzi P, et al. Effect of coronary artery bypass graft surgery on survival: overview of 10-year results from randomized trials by the Coronary Artery Bypass Graft Surgery Trialists Collaboration. Lancet 1994;344:563–70.

5. Parisi AF, Folland ED, Hartigan P, for the Veterans Affairs ACME Investigators. A comparison of angioplasty with medical therapy in the treatment of single vessel coronary artery disease. N Engl J Med 1992;326:10.

6. The Bypass Angioplasty Revascularization Investigation (BARI) Investigators. Comparison of coronary bypass surgery with angioplasty in patients with multivessel disease. N Engl J Med 1996;335:217–25.

7. King SB III, Lembo NJ, Weintraub WS, et al. A randomized trial comparing coronary angioplasty with coronary bypass surgery. N Engl J Med 1994;331:1044–50.

8. Hlatky MA, Rogers WJ, Johnstone I, et al. Medical care costs and quality of life after randomization to coronary angioplasty or coronary bypass surgery. N Engl J Med 1997;336:92–9.

9. Serruys PW, de Jagere P, Kiemeneij F, et al. A comparison of balloon-expandable-stent implantation with balloon angioplasty in patients with coronary artery disease. Benestent Study Group. N Engl J Med 1994;331:489–95.

10. Fischman DL, Leon MB, Bain DS, et al. A randomized comparison of coronary stent placement and balloon angioplasty in the treatment of coronary artery disease. Stent Restenosis Study Investigators. N Engl J Med 1994;331:496–501.

11. Cardiac Care Network of Ontario Expert Panel on Intracoronary Stents. Public policy and coronary stenting. Report of an expert panel to the Cardiac Care Network of Ontario. Can J Cardiol 1997;13:731–46.

12. The EPILOG Investigators. Platelet glycoprotein IIb/IIIa receptor blockade and low-dose heparin during percutaneous coronary revascularization. N Engl J Med 1997;336:1689–96.

ANTITHROMBOTIC THERAPY IN PATIENTS UNDERGOING CORONARY ARTERY BYPASS SURGERY

Negin Liaghati-Nasseri

Stephen Edward Fremes

The effects of antiplatelet and anticoagulant therapy on postoperative saphenous vein graft patency have been studied in a number of randomized clinical trials. The results obtained from meta-analyses of the aggregated data demonstrate that either aspirin or warfarin are associated with an approximately 40% odds reduction of saphenous vein graft occlusion within the first year after surgery.[1–3] The addition of dipyridamole to aspirin provides no additional benefit over aspirin alone.[2]

In addition to the data outlined above, the decision tree was created according to the following assumptions: (1) Administration of antiplatelet drugs is preferable to anticoagulation when the two treatment strategies are equally efficacious. (2) Aspirin represents the current standard of care.[4] (3) There is no convincing evidence to support the coadministration of antiplatelet and anticoagulant treatment for this patient population.[2] (4) Patients will also receive deep vein thrombosis (DVT) prophylaxis consisting of 5000 units of unfractionated heparin subcutaneously every 12 hours starting on the first postoperative day. 5) All patients have had coronary artery bypass using cardiopulmonary bypass as opposed to "off-pump" or "MID-CAB" surgery. It should also be recognized that the roles of two potentially useful classes of drugs, low-molecular-weight heparins and glycoprotein IIbIIIa receptor antagonists, have not been evaluated in this clinical situation.

A Bleeding Assessment 6 Hours Post ICU Arrival

Delayed administration of antithrombotic medication (>24 to 48 hours postoperatively) is ineffective. Most positive studies have initiated therapy within 6 hours of surgery. The greatest relative risk reduction was noted in a study in which aspirin was administered 1 hour postoperatively.[5] Preoperative treatment provided no additional benefit when antithrombotic therapy was initiated early postoperatively.[2] Furthermore, preoperative aspirin is associated with increased bleeding.[6] In our institution, we consider excessive bleeding in the early postoperative phase to be of immediate concern, and withhold antithrombotic medication until hemostasis, as determined by chest tube loss, has been achieved. Threshold values either greater than or less than 400 mL in the previous 6 hours may be more relevant for other cardiac surgical centers. Additional information such as the hourly rate of bleeding, the hematocrit of the chest tube fluid, the presence or absence of clots in the chest drainage, etc., may influence the individual clinician's decision to prescribe or withhold antithrombotic drugs in the immediate postoperative period.

B Failure of Hemostasis

Identification and correction of persistent coagulopathy should be considered (as well as the need for surgical re-exploration) should the chest tube losses in the previous 6 hours exceed 400 mL.

C Bleeding Assessment 12 Hours Post ICU Arrival

Patients in whom hemostasis has been achieved should have antithrombotic therapy initiated immediately; however, in patients in whom persistent bleeding remains a concern, therapy should be delayed until postoperative day 1.

D Antithrombotic Drugs

Prior to the initiation of antithrombotic therapy, it is important to determine whether there is a history of aspirin allergy or intolerance, usually upper gastrointestinal bleeding associated with aspirin.

E Indication for Anticoagulation, Aspirin Tolerant

If the patient has an indication for postoperative anticoagulation (and no contraindication) intravenous unfractionated heparin 500 IU/hour should be started initially. "Therapeutic" anticoagulation (>1000 U/hour) with heparin should wait until postoperative day 2 to minimize the risk of postoperative bleeding/tamponade. Warfarin should be given on postoperative day 2 and be titrated to a therapeutic INR (2.5 to 3.5 for mechanical heart valves, otherwise 2.0 to 3.0).

Aspirin 325 mg PO daily should be instituted should warfarin be discontinued in the future. [Note that aspirin 325 mg daily, until the INR is therapeutic, could be substituted for intravenous heparin in the early postoperative period if there is no perceived clinical need for intravenous heparin and/or early therapeutic levels of anticoagulation.]

F *Ticlopidine Sensitivity*

After aspirin, ticlopidine is likely the most commonly prescribed antiplatelet drug in atherosclerotic patients. Ticlopidine has been shown to reduce saphenous vein graft occlusion[7] and is suitable for patients in whom aspirin is contraindicated.

G *Aspirin*

Aspirin 325 mg daily should be prescribed indefinitely. According to results obtained from the aggregated trial data,[2] high doses of aspirin ($\geq$975 mg/daily) are less effective (nonoverlapping confidence intervals) than 325 mg daily. The treatment effect of low-dose aspirin (<150 mg/day) was intermediate to that of 325 mg and high-dose therapy but not significantly different from either dose.

While saphenous vein graft patency is enhanced with aspirin administration, a reduction in clinical events with aspirin has not be conclusively demonstrated in this patient population.[2,3] However, secondary prevention data from other atherosclerotic populations clearly support the use of prolonged aspirin therapy.[8]

H *Indication for Anticoagulation, Aspirin Intolerant, Ticlopidine Tolerant*

If the patient has an indication for postoperative anticoagulation, and no contraindication, intravenous unfractionated heparin 500 IU/hour and warfarin should be administered as described in section E. Ticlopidine 250 mg PO b.i.d. with neutrophil and platelet monitoring can be started should warfarin be discontinued in the future. (Ticlopidine 250 mg PO b.i.d., until the INR is therapeutic, could be substituted for intravenous heparin in the early postoperative period, if there is no perceived clinical need for intravenous heparin and/or early therapeutic levels in anticoagulation.)

I *Other Antithrombotics*

For patients with a contraindication to both aspirin and ticlopidine, other antiplatelet drugs should be considered. The role of clopidogrel with respect to graft patency has not been assessed, although hard clinical events are reduced to a greater extent with clopidogrel than aspirin in atherosclerotic patients.[9] Other antiplatelet drugs maybe of benefit but have not been tested as extensively as aspirin.[1,3,10] Alternatively, long-term anticoagulation could be used in place of antiplatelet drugs.

J *Ticlopidine*

Ticlopidine 250 mg PO b.i.d. with neutrophil and platelet surveillance should be administered indefinitely.

Administration of Postoperative Antithrombotic Therapy

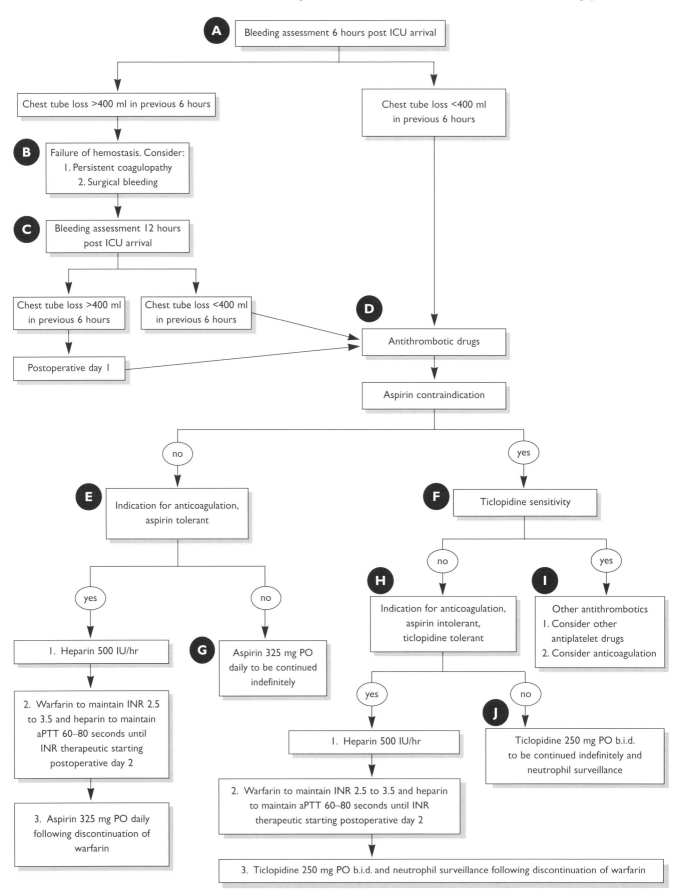

Bibliography

1. Henderson WG, Moritz T, Goldman S, Copeland J, Mortiz TE, Harker LA. Antiplatelet or anticoagulant therapy after coronary artery bypass surgery. A meta-analysis of clinical trials. Ann Intern Med 1989;111:743–50.

2. Fremes SE, Levinton C, Naylor CD, Chen E, Christakis GT, Goldman BS. Optimal antithrombotic therapy following aortocoronary bypass: a meta-analysis. Eur J Cardiothorac Surg 1993;7:169–80.

3. Antiplatelet Trialists' Collaboration. Collaborative overview of randomised trials of antiplatelet therapy II: Maintenance of vascular graft or arterial patency by antiplatelet therapy. BMJ 1994;308:81–106.

4. Hennekens CH, Dyken ML, Fuster V. Aspirin as a therapeutic agent in cardiovascular disease. A statement for healthcare professionals from the American Heart Association. Circulation 1997;96:2751–3.

5. Gavaghan TP, Gebski V, Baron DW. Immediate postoperative aspirin improves vein graft patency early and late after coronary artery bypass graft surgery. Circulation 1991;83:1526–33.

6. Goldman S, Copeland J, Mortiz T, et al. Starting aspirin therapy after operation. Effects on early graft patency. Circulation 1991;84:520–6.

7. Limet R, David JL, Magotteaux P, Larock MP, Rigo P. Prevention of aorto-coronary bypass graft occlusion. J Thorac Cardiovasc Surg 1987;94:773–83.

8. Antiplatelet Trialists' Collaboration. Collaborative overview of randomised trials of antiplatelet therapy I: Prevention of death, myocardial infarction, and stroke by prolonged antiplatelet therapy in various categories of patients. BMJ 1994;308:81–106.

9. CAPRIE Steering Committee. A randomised, blinded, trial of clopidogrel versus aspirin in patients at risk of ischmemic events (CAPRIE). Lancet 1996;348:1329–39.

10. Baur HR, VanTassel RA, Pierach CA, Gobel FL. Effects of sulfinpyrazone on early graft closure after myocardial revascularization. Am J Cardiol 1982;49:420–4.

Chapter 36

Antithrombotic Therapy in Patients Undergoing Catheter-Based Revascularization

Eric A Cohen

The therapeutic objectives for a patient undergoing coronary angioplasty depend on the nature of the clinical presentation. For the patient with stable angina, the objective is to obtain symptom relief and/or reduce the requirement for antianginal medication. For the patient with unstable angina, prevention of myocardial infarction is also a goal of treatment. For the patient with acute myocardial infarction, direct (or primary) angioplasty used as an alternative to thrombolysis has the aim of limiting infarct size and reducing mortality. The major limitations of coronary angioplasty are acute or subacute vessel closure in the initial hours to days following the procedure and late renarrowing (restenosis) at the same site during the first 6 months following the procedure. While antithrombotic agents have had limited, if any, impact on late restenosis, they play a major role in the prevention of acute and subacute vessel closure, in which platelet-thrombus interaction with the injured vessel wall is fundamental. As a general guideline, the intensity of antiplatelet and antithrombotic therapy used is related to the perceived risk of acute or subacute vessel closure. This, in turn, is related to the presenting clinical syndrome and the morphology of the target lesion (more unstable presentations and more complex lesions, each being associated with a higher risk of acute closure). The accompanying flow chart and text outline an approach to antithrombotic therapy according to clinical presentation and lesion morphology in patients undergoing coronary angioplasty.

A *Elective Angioplasty*

An elective angioplasty procedure is generally done for stable angina or stable manifestations of myocardial ischemia on provocative testing. These patients are usually admitted from home for the procedure. The target lesion tends to be a chronic plaque which produces effort-related symptoms by virtue of a stenosis which becomes flow limiting in the presence of increased oxygen demand. The fibrous cap overlying the plaque is intact, and there is no significant thrombotic component. Consequently, the risk of acute thrombotic complications tends to be low.

B Urgent Angioplasty

In this context, "urgent" usually refers to a procedure done on a hospital inpatient who is felt to be too unstable (or potentially unstable) to be discharged home prior to the procedure. Such patients, who have been admitted to hospital with unstable angina or acute myocardial infarction (MI), are almost always treated with aspirin already, and many are also receiving heparin at the time of referral for angioplasty. Depending on the circumstances there may be virtually no delay between referral and intervention, or there may be several days' lead time. The time available has implications for the antithrombotic strategy chosen.

C Emergency Angioplasty

Angioplasty done on an emergency basis as primary therapy for acute MI, cardiogenic shock, or acute vessel closure complicating an earlier angioplasty procedure is associated with a high thrombotic burden. In addition, there may be significant hemodynamic instability, which increases the risk of subsequent vessel closure. Intra-aortic balloon counterpulsation (balloon pump) may be used. Apart from aspirin there is no role for any presently available oral antithrombotic agent.

D Aspirin

Aspirin has been proven to reduce ischemic complications (non-Q-wave MI) associated with coronary angioplasty[1] and should be used routinely in the periprocedural period unless actively contraindicated. Because of the broad indications for and use of aspirin in patients with vascular disease, the majority of patients considered for angioplasty are already on aspirin and will remain on it indefinitely following the procedure.

E Stent Placement

There are a number of anatomic features of the target vessel which influence its suitability for stent placement although with the evolution of stent design the majority of lesions are now amenable to stent placement. Factors which tend to decrease the suitability for stent placement include small vessel size (less than 2.5 mm diameter), excessive angulation of the lesion, and tortuosity of the proximal portion of the vessel (through which the unexpanded stent must pass to reach the target lesion). This is particularly important in the presence of significant calcification of the vessel which reduces its flexibility.

F *Ticlopidine and Aspirin*

Ticlopidine is an antiplatelet agent which inhibits adenosine diphosphate (ADP)-mediated platelet activation. In recent years, it has been used, usually in conjunction with aspirin for the prevention of subacute thrombosis following stent placement. The superiority of the aspirin-and-ticlopidine combination over the older poststent regimen of Coumadin and aspirin has been demonstrated in at least two randomized trials.[2,3] The pharmacodynamics of ticlopidine suggest that its full effect does not occur for 3 to 5 days following initiation of therapy; for this reason ticlopidine should be initiated in stent-eligible patients in advance of the procedure, where feasible. Although the combination of aspirin and ticlopidine is superior to aspirin alone, it is not known if aspirin adds to the efficacy of ticlopidine.

G *Patient and Lesion Characteristics*

Various patient and lesion characteristics predict a higher-than-average risk of acute vessel closure (and subsequent ischemic complications) following coronary angioplasty. Patients may be high risk by virtue of an unstable clinical presentation (acute or recent MI or unstable angina with ongoing symptoms and dynamic electrocardiographic [ECG] changes) or, in the setting of a less acute clinical syndrome, the presence of multiple or severe adverse lesion characteristics. Such adverse features include excessive lesion length, eccentricity, calcification or angulation, vessel tortuosity, involvement of a side branch, presence of an established thrombus or of a chronic total occlusion, or location in a degenerated saphenous vein graft. In general, the presence of an obvious angiographic thrombus, even in the absence of other high-risk lesion morphologic or clinical features, would be considered an indication for the administration of abciximab.

H *Glycoprotein IIb/IIIa Blockade: Abciximab and Other Agents*

Abciximab is a fragment of a human-murine chimeric antibody directed against the glycoprotein IIb/IIIa platelet surface receptor.[4] Virtually all known platelet agonists induce, through a variety of pathways, a conformational change in this receptor, which in turn results in the exposure of its fibrinogen binding site. Blocking this receptor prevents binding of dimeric fibrinogen molecules to platelets, thereby profoundly inhibiting platelet aggregation (which is primarily mediated by fibrinogen cross-linking) regardless of the activating stimulus. Abciximab was the first commercially available agent of this class; a number of other agents are at varying stages of development. Three large randomized trials of abciximab in patients undergoing coronary angioplasty[5–7] have established that it can significantly reduce acute ischemic complications associated with the procedure.

The EPIC (Evaluation of c7E3 for Prevention of Ischemic Complications) trial[5] demonstrated that in high-risk angioplasty patients, abciximab given as a bolus (0.25 mg per kg given 10 minutes before the start of the procedure) followed by an infusion (10 µg per minute for 12 hours) in addition to conventional periprocedural heparin and aspirin reduced the composite endpoint of death, MI, or the need for bailout stent or urgent repeat intervention by 35% at 30 days as compared to heparin and aspirin alone. However, there was a significant increase in bleeding complications, mainly at the vascular access site, in abciximab-treated patients. In a subsequent trial,[6] low- and moderate-risk patients were included, the abciximab infusion was adjusted for patient weight (0.125 µg per kg per minute), and weight-adjusted standard (100 U per kg bolus) and low-dose (70 U per kg bolus) periprocedural heparin regimens were evaluated using specific targets for activated clotting time (ACT). In addition, early removal of vascular access sheaths was strongly recommended. All patients received aspirin. This important trial was halted early due to the efficacy of abciximab (with either heparin regimen) as compared with placebo—a 59% reduction in the 30-day composite endpoint of death, MI, or urgent repeat intervention, which was achieved without any increase in bleeding complications in the abciximab-treated patients. The CAPTURE (c7E3 Fab Anti-Platelet Therapy in Unstable Refractory Angina) trial[7] demonstrated that abciximab (0.25 mg per kg bolus followed by 10 µg per minute infusion) was effective in reducing ischemic endpoints when administered to patients with refractory unstable angina and known coronary anatomy for 18 to 24 hours in advance of the angioplasty procedure. Interestingly, some benefit was evident even prior to the intervention suggesting that the drug was effective in "passivating" the unstable culprit plaque.

Other glycoprotein IIb/IIIa antagonists including tirofiban[8] and eptafibatide (integrelin)[9] have also been found, in large randomized trials, to be effective in reducing ischemic complications of coronary angioplasty. At present, there are no studies comparing the relative efficacy of different glycoprotein IIb/IIIa antagonists.

▌ *High-Risk Unstable Angina*

Refractory or high-risk unstable angina in this context refers to the occurrence, despite treatment with intravenous heparin and nitroglycerin, of at least one episode of ischemic symptoms at rest with associated ECG changes within the preceding 48 hours or at least two such episodes within 24 hours regardless of current treatment.

J Abciximab for Acute MI

Abciximab is indicated as an adjunct in primary angioplasty for acute MI (i.e., without antecedent thrombolytic therapy). Evidence of its efficacy was first noted in a small subgroup of the EPIC trial[5] and more recently demonstrated in a larger randomized trial.[10] Because the efficacy of the low-dose, weight-adjusted heparin dosing regimen (i.e., 70 U per kg bolus) has not been fully evaluated in patients with acute MI, we currently use the standard-dose regimen (i.e., 100 U per kg bolus) in patients undergoing primary angioplasty for acute MI.

K Rescue Angioplasty for Acute MI

When angioplasty is performed on an emergency basis for failure of thrombolytic therapy in the setting of acute MI (rescue angioplasty), the potential bleeding risk is increased regardless of the choice of periprocedural antithrombotic therapy. In addition to the thrombolytic agent, such patients will also have received aspirin and often heparin before arriving at the catheterization laboratory. Although limited data (based on a small subset of patients in the EPIC trial[5]) regarding the role of adjunctive glycoprotein IIb/IIIa blockade in this situation suggests marked benefit of abciximab, its safety has not been established. Until such time, therefore, the risk-benefit tradeoff for each individual patient must be carefully evaluated. Factors such as advanced age, elevated systolic blood pressure, or prior stroke are associated with an increased risk of bleeding, especially intracranial hemorrhage, and are relative contraindications to the use of adjunctive glycoprotein IIb/IIIa blockade while a more pressing clinical need for reperfusion (as manifested by established or impending hemodynamic compromise) would tend to favour its use.

L Heparin Administration

For patients not on a heparin infusion at the start of the procedure, the recommended heparin bolus dose is 100 U per kg if abciximab is not being used, and 70 U per kg if abciximab is being used. Although practices with regard to heparin administration vary between institutions, we do not generally run an infusion during the procedure. If an infusion is already running when the patient arrives at the catheterization laboratory, it is discontinued, ACT is determined, and the subsequent heparin bolus dose is determined from Table 36.1. During the procedure, ACT should be checked every 30 to 60 minutes and additional bolus doses of heparin given according to Table 36.2.

Table 36.1   Heparin Administration Prior to Beginning Intervention

Heparin Infusion Running?	Low-Dose Heparin (with Abciximab)	Standard-Dose Heparin (without Abciximab)
No	70 U/kg	100 U/kg
Yes—obtain baseline ACT		
ACT <150	70 U/kg	100 U/kg
ACT 150–199	50 U/kg	75 U/kg
ACT 200–299	—	50 U/kg

M Optimal Angiographic Result and Stent Use

An optimal angiographic result implies minimal residual stenosis (less than 25% stenosis for a balloon dilation and less than 10% stenosis for a stent implant), the absence of intraluminal filling defects, and normal flow in the vessel. Furthermore, following stent implantation, there should be no residual dissection proximal or distal to the stent(s). Major side branches within or adjacent to the lesion should be patent. In some situations, intravascular ultrasound rather than contrast angiography is used to assess the adequacy of the final result.

Stent use may be planned at the outset of the procedure (primary stenting) or may be predicated by a suboptimal result following balloon angioplasty (provisional stenting). Bailout stenting refers to the use of one or more stents to reverse acute or threatened closure (impaired or absent flow with signs of ischemia) occurring during the procedure. Abciximab may also be used with or without stents in a bailout manner, in response to the development of angiographic complications or the presence of a suboptimal result. However, the efficacy of abciximab and other glycoprotein IIb/IIIa antagonists used in a bailout manner has not been established.

N Risk of Subacute Stent Thrombosis

Despite an optimal angiographic result, the risk of subacute stent thrombosis may be increased in smaller vessels (i.e., less than 2.5 mm), when multiple stents are used, or when the stent use was for a bailout indication. In such situations, additional antithrombotic measures may be warranted.

Table 36.2   Heparin Administration during Intervention

	Low-Dose Heparin (with Abciximab)	Standard-Dose Heparin (without Abciximab)
ACT <200	20 U/kg	50 U/kg
ACT 200–275	—	50 U/kg
ACT 275–299	—	25 U/kg

Management of Patients Undergoing Catheter-Based Revascularization

A Elective procedure

B Urgent procedure
Unstable angina

C Emergent procedure
Acute MI
• direct
• rescue
Cardiogenic shock

D ASA 325 mg OD
(if not already on)

E Vessel and lesion
potentially amenable
to coronary stent?

no → **G** High risk lesion
morphology?

yes →

F Ticlopidine
250 mg b.i.d.

yes

G High risk lesion
morphology?

yes →

no →

I Refractory unstable
angina or high risk
unstable angina?

yes →

no →

H Abciximab bolus
(0.25 mg/kg) plus infusion
(0.125 µg/kg/min)

J Thrombolytic agent
administered prior to
emergency angioplasty?

yes →

no →

K Evaluate risk-benefit
tradeoff with respect to
bleeding and clinical need;
consider use of
Abciximab

Bleeding risk low
and/or
clinical need high

Bleeding risk
high and/or
clinical need low

Commencement of
coronary angioplasty
procedure

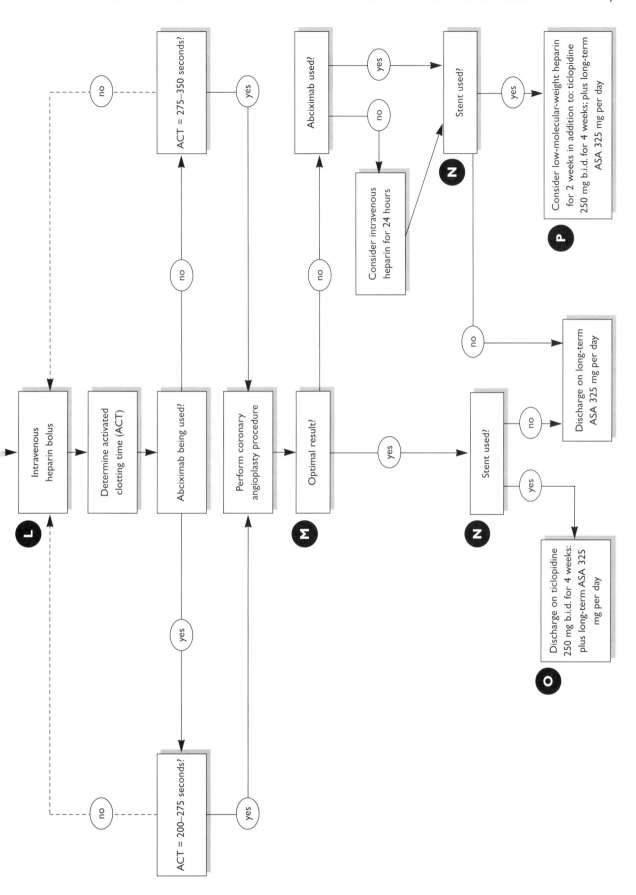

O *Ticlopidine Therapy*

The optimal duration of ticlopidine therapy is not known. Most regimens have employed a 4- to 6-week course although as little as 2 weeks following angioplasty may be equally effective. When using ticlopidine, it is recommended that the white blood cell count be monitored every 2 weeks because of the potential for neutropenia. Other rare but serious side effects include a serum-sickness-type reaction and thrombotic thrombocytopenic purpura.[11] Ticlopidine is also associated with a variety of minor side effects, the most common being gastrointestinal upset and skin rash. Clopidegrel is a newer, chemically similar drug with an improved side-effect profile. It may replace ticlopidine for prevention of stent thrombosis although, to date, studies evaluating this indication have not been completed.

P *Addition of LMWH*

The addition of therapeutic-dose low-molecular-weight heparin (e.g., 100 antifactor Xa U per kg SQ twice daily) to ticlopidine and aspirin may help prevent stent thrombosis in patients at increased risk. A large randomized trial addressing this question is ongoing.

Bibliography

1. Schwartz L, Bourassa MG, Lesperance J, et al. Aspirin and dipyridamole in the prevention of restenosis after percutaneous transluminal coronary angioplasty. N Engl J Med 1988;318:1714–9.

2. Schomig A, Neumann FJ, Kastrati A, et al. A randomized comparison of antiplatelet and anticoagulant therapy after the placement of coronary-artery stents [comments]. N Engl J Med 1996;334:1084–9.

3. Leon MB, Baim DS, Gordon P, et al. Clinical and angiographic results from the Stent Anticoagulation Regimen Study (STARS) [abstract]. Circulation 1996;94 (Suppl I):I685.

4. Coller BS. Platelet GPIIb/IIIa antagonists: the first anti-integrin receptor therapeutics. J Clin Invest 1997;100(11 Suppl):S57–60.

5. The EPIC Investigators. Use of monoclonal antibody directed against the platelet glycoprotein IIb/IIIa receptor in high risk coronary angioplasty. N Engl J Med 1994; 330:956–61.

6. EPILOG Investigators. Effect of the platelet glycoprotein IIb/IIIa receptor inhibitor abciximab with lower heparin dosages on ischemic complications of percutaneous coronary revascularization. N Engl J Med 1997;336:1689–96.

7. The CAPTURE Investigators. Randomized placebo-controlled trial of abciximab before and during coronary intervention in refractory unstable angina: the CAPTURE study. Lancet 1997;349:1429–35.

8. The RESTORE Investigators. Effects of platelets glycoprotein IIb/IIIa blockade with tirofiban on adverse cardiac effects in patients with unstable angina or acute myocardial infarction undergoing coronary angioplasty. Circulation 1997;96:1445–53.

9. The IMPACT-II Investigators. Randomized placebo-controlled trial of effect of eptifibatide on complications of percutaneous coronary intervention: IMPACT-II. Lancet 1997;349:1422–28.

10. Brener SJ, Barr LA, Burchenal JEB, et al, on behalf of the RAPPORT Investigators. A randomized, placebo-controlled trial of platelet glycoprotein IIb/IIIa blockade with primary angioplasty for acute myocardial infarction. Circulation, in press, 1998.

11. Bennett CL, Weinberg PD, Rozenberg-Ben-Dror K, Yarnold PR, Kwaan HC, Green D. Thrombotic thrombocytopenic purpura associated with ticlopidine. A review of 60 cases. Ann Intern Med 1998;128:541–4.

Chapter 37

Investigation of Acute Cerebral Ischemia

Robert J Duke

Stroke remains the third leading cause of death in North America, and the leading cause of acquired neurological disability. Stroke survivors have a high risk of future stroke as well as vascular events, in general. An efficient yet thorough investigation of stroke patients identifies the cause in most individuals, allows appropriate management of the acute stroke situation, and suggests strategies for secondary stroke prevention. The algorithm outlines an approach to the investigation of the patient presenting with a probable stroke, emphasizing the importance of bedside clinical evaluation as well as selection of appropriate investigations.

A *History and Physical Examination*
The neurological examination allows one to determine whether an organic lesion of the brain is present. Recognition of certain stroke syndromes, such as the lateral medullary syndrome or lacunar syndromes listed in Table 37.1, may allow inferences about the underlying mechanisms of stroke (Table 37.2). More often, it is a careful analysis of the temporal profile that provides information regarding probable stroke mechanisms; for example, cerebral emboli generally manifest abruptly while a more gradual evolution might suggest thrombosis or hemorrhage. Antecedent transient ischemic attacks (TIAs) would weigh against a cerebral hemorrhage and in favor of thromboembolism from a proximal arterial source. Multifocal TIAs could point to a cardiac source.

Past history, with special attention to risk factors for stroke (Table 37.3), and age of the patient (see Table 37.4), will serve to increase the probability of the presence of certain conditions and reduce the probability of others.

B *"Mimics" of Stroke*
Approximately 10% of patients presenting with possible stroke are found to have other causes for their condition. These "mimics" of stroke are generally identified

Table 37.1   Lacunar Syndromes

Pure motor stroke	Dysarthria—clumsy hand syndrome
Pure sensory stroke	Ataxic hemiparesis

by careful history and physical or, less frequently, by CT scan (see Table 37.5). Conversely, some stroke patients present with problems not initially recognized as being due to focal brain disease—e.g., the patient with dysphasia or apraxia is misinterpreted as having a global confusional state or dementia. This can also occur in patients with cortical blindness who may not express concerns about their vision.

C   *Imaging and Other Diagnostic Procedures*

Computed tomography (CT) scan remains the preferred initial imaging investigation for stroke. An unenhanced CT scan serves to effectively exclude intracranial hemorrhage. A magnetic resonance imaging scan can provide more detailed anatomic definition of a cerebral infarct but in the acute situation, it is less likely to accommodate a restless or intubated patient, is less likely to be available, and is more expensive. More rarely, a lumbar puncture may be necessary to definitively exclude a small subarachnoid hemorrhage in the patient who presents with likely symptoms, such as sudden new headache. The timing of a CT scan will be determined not only by availability but also by the purpose of the scan. Highest priority for immediate scanning includes stroke patients with a history or signs of significant head trauma; patients with progressive neurological deterioration, especially involving a deteriorating level of consciousness; and patients with a hyperacute stroke who are being considered for thrombolytic therapy. A somewhat lower priority can be justified for clinically stable candidates for anticoagulation. A repeat or delayed scan at 1 week may be more helpful when the objective of scanning is to determine the anatomical location and extent of cerebral infarction.

Table 37.2   Diagnostic Subtypes of Stroke*

	Percent
Large vessel atherosclerosis	10
Lacunar	19
Other identified (migraine, vasculitis, etc.)	3
Cardioembolic	14
Infarct of undetermined cause	28
Hemorrhage: intracerebral	13
subarachnoid	13

*based on 1805 cases in the NINCDS Stroke Data Bank[1]

Table 37.3   Risk Factors for Stroke

Age	Smoking	Hyperlipidemia
Hypertension	Diabetes	Oral contraceptives
Heart disease	Heavy alcohol consumption	Family history
Atrial fibrillation	Obesity	

D *Findings on CT Scan*

The majority of patients with acute stroke will have a normal CT scan in the first 6 hours. A small number may show early signs of infarction, including loss of gray/white matter differentiation (especially in the insular ribbon and basal ganglia) and subtle brain swelling causing effacement of sulci or ventricular compression. A hyperdense middle cerebral artery sign strongly suggests thrombotic or embolic occlusion of this vessel. The presence of a clear-cut infarct or lacuna evident on a very early CT scan should suggest either pre-existing pathology not directly related to the present stroke or, if it fits precisely with the patient's neurological deficit, it may be an indication that the stroke occurred earlier than initially recognized. Cortical infarcts within multiple arterial territories might relate to extensive craniovascular disease or, alternatively, could suggest a cardiac source for the emboli. Hemorrhagic infarction is more likely in embolic stroke or in cortical venous thrombosis. Lacunar infarcts are often "silent."

E *Causes of Ischemic Brain Infarction*

Determining the underlying etiology and pathophysiology of a patient's stroke is best carried out by considering the three fundamental causes of ischemic brain infarction: disease of blood vessels, disease of the heart, and blood disorders. It is

Table 37.4   Cause of Ischemic Stroke in Younger Patients (expressed as percent)[2,3]

	Childhood	16–30 Years	31–45 Years
Undetermined	27	14	28
Cardioembolism	21	23	23
Arterial dissection	5	16	23
Migraine	–	20	12
Arteritis	–	7	3
Large artery atherosclerosis	–	2	7
Hypertensive small artery disease	–	–	3
Fibromuscular hyperplasia	–	4	1
Pregnancy-associated	–	4	–
Venous thrombosis	25	5	<1
Mitochondrial cytopathy	2	–	–
Dehydration, infection	20	–	–

Table 37.5   Mimics of Stroke

Other focal brain lesions	
Postictal palsy	Migraine
Trauma (e.g., subdural hematoma)	Multiple sclerosis
Brain tumor	
Metabolic encephalopathy	
Hypoglycemia	Drugs
Focal peripheral neurological lesions	
Bell's palsy	Peroneal nerve palsy
Radial nerve palsy	
Simulated neurological deficit	

important to pursue all three avenues of investigation to avoid the error of accepting one risk factor such as migraine or nonstenosing plaque of the internal carotid artery as the cause of the stroke, when another factor such as patent foramen ovale or anticardiolipin antibody goes undetected.

F Basic Investigations of Stroke Patients

Noninvasive and readily available investigations constitute the basic investigations in the majority of stroke patients. In terms of blood vessel disease, it is important to consider not only atherosclerosis and hypertension but less common varieties of vascular disease such as arterial dissection, fibromuscular hyperplasia, and vasculitis. Standard transthoracic echocardiography with a "bubble test" will suffice to identify most, but not all, patients with a cardiac source of the emboli, and is more rational than screening all patients with transesophageal echocardiography.[4] The importance of routine blood tests should never be underestimated in serving to identify the occasional patient whose stroke is due to polycythemia, thrombocytosis, leukemia, etc.

G Cardiac Investigations

Life-threatening arrythmia is rarely present in conscious stroke patients but atrial fibrillation, which can reflect associated cardiovascular disease and which may represent the source of the patient's stroke, can be identified with Holter monitoring. Transesophageal echocardiography is more sensitive than transthoracic examination in identifying potential cardiac sources of embolism in the majority of patients presenting with unexplained stroke. It is especially sensitive in identifying patent foramen ovale, atrial septal aneurysm, and ulcerated plaques in the ascending aorta but its impact on treatment is less certain. For example, better definition of an embolic source in a stroke patient with atrial fibrillation is not likely to alter the decision to anticoagulate the patient. Transesophageal echocardiography should be reserved for use in patients who would be anticoagulated if a potential source of embolism were identified.

H   Imaging of Intra- and Extracranial Disease

Angiography remains the gold standard for imaging both intracranial and extracranial disease but it is not without risk. Magnetic resonance angiography (MRA), which does not involve injection of contrast, can be helpful in identifying extracranial disease, such as carotid bifurcation atherosclerosis, and carotid dissection. It is also useful for imaging intracranial disease, including that involving the cerebral veins and venous sinuses. The resolution of MRA is somewhat poorer than traditional arteriography, so for suspected CNS vasculitis, arteriography is still essential. Carotid duplex imaging is a useful screening tool for detecting significant atherosclerotic narrowing of the common and internal carotid arteries[5] but it can miss disease beyond the proximal internal carotid artery, such as fibromuscular hyperplasia, dissection, and tandem atherosclerotic lesions. Cervical CT, following administration of contrast, can be useful in the diagnosis of dissection of carotid or vertebral arteries by showing on transverse section the true and false lumen as a "bull's eye" phenomenon.

I   Systemic Investigations

Patients with protein C and protein S deficiency are at higher risk of further thrombotic events as are those with activated protein C resistance or persistently present antiphospholipid antibodies (lupus anticoagulant and anticardiolipin antibody). Such screening tests should be considered in young patients with stroke, even in those with an identified cofactor.

J   Stroke of Undetermined Origin

Although a substantial minority of documented cerebral infarctions remain cryptogenic, it is important to consider rare causes of stroke such as MELAS syndrome (mitochondrial myopathy, encephalopathy, lactic acidosis, and stroke-like episodes) and to consider repeating neuroimaging investigations. The risk of recurrent stroke in patients with stroke of undetermined etiology is lower than in those with identified specific causes.

Acute Focal Neurological Deficit

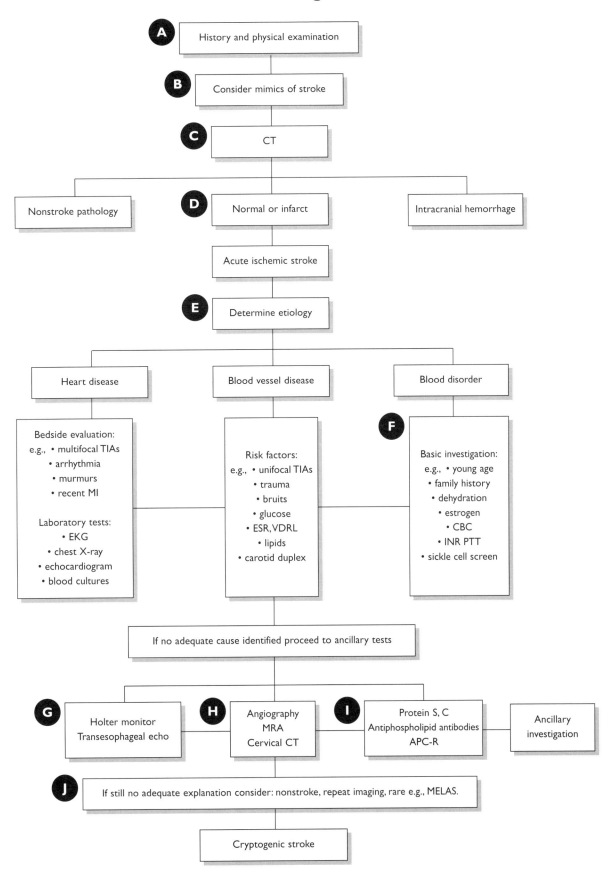

Bibliography

1. Sacco RL, Ellenberg JH, Mohr JP, Tatemichi TK, Hier DB, Price JR, Wolf PA. Infarcts of undetermined cause: the NINCDS stroke data bank. Ann Neurol 1989;25:382–90.
2. Bogousslavsky J, Pierre P. Ischemic stroke in patients under age 45. Neurol Clin 1992;10:113–24.
3. deVeber GA. Canadian pediatric ischemic stroke registry (abstract). Can J Neurol Sci 1995; 22(S1):S24.
4. Cabanes L, Mas JL, Cohen MD, et al. Atrial septal aneurysm and patent foramen ovale as risk factors for cryptogenic stroke in patients less than 55 years of age: a study using transesophageal echocardiography. Stroke 1993;24:1865–74.
5. Blakeley DD, Oddone EZ, Hasselblad V, Simel DL, Matchar DB. Noninvasive carotid artery testing: a meta-analytic review. Ann Intern Med 1995;122:360–7.

Additional Reading

Adams RD, Victor M, Ropper AH. Principles of neurology. New York: McGraw-Hill, 1997.
Caplan LR. Stroke: a clinical approach. Boston: Butterworth-Heinemann, 1993.

Chapter 38

ANTITHROMBOTIC THERAPY IN PATIENTS WITH CEREBROVASCULAR DISEASE

Robert J Duke

The two strongest predictors of future stroke are the occurrence of a previous stroke, or a transient ischemic attack (TIA). A variety of antithrombotic agents have been used for primary and secondary stroke prevention, and are also used to reduce the risk of stroke complications such as deep vein thrombosis (DVT) and pulmonary embolism. Thrombolysis with tissue plasminogen activator (t-PA) appears to be effective in selected patients with very early ischemic stroke. While recent studies allow some firm recommendations for the use of antithrombotic agents, there are a number of persisting uncertainties that await the results of definitive clinical trials (Table 38.1).

A *Asymptomatic Patients*

Although aspirin appears effective in the primary prevention of ischemic heart disease, any reduction in the risk of ischemic stroke appears to be almost neutralized by an increase in the risk of hemorrhagic stroke. Individuals with asymptomatic carotid artery stenosis may benefit from antiplatelet therapy but this has not been proven.

B *Patients with TIAs*

Although most TIAs are embolic and reflect atherosclerosis of the extracranial blood vessels, it is important to consider alternative explanations, particularly those which require more specific or different therapy, such as cardioembolism. Migraine can mimic TIA at any age and tends to be quite benign, so is generally not treated with antiplatelet agents.

C *Patients with Acute Stroke*

Despite an increased incidence of symptomatic intracerebral hemorrhage, treatment with intravenous t-PA within 3 hours of onset of ischemic stroke has been shown to improve clinical outcome at 3 months. The optimal dose for the treatment of stroke appears to be significantly less than that for acute myocardial infarction. Thrombolysis for ischemic stroke should be considered only when the time of the stroke can be ascertained with confidence and treatment can begin within 3 hours of stroke onset, when the patient has no contraindication to thrombolytic agents (such as a patient already on warfarin, or with uncontrolled hypertension, or who has had recent surgery), and after a CT scan has excluded hemorrhage or early changes of very large infarction. Streptokinase appears more likely to cause hemorrhage and is not recommended.

D Patients with Cardioembolic TIAs

Warfarin is established as the agent of choice in most patients who have had a TIA or stroke and who have a well-defined cardiac source for potential recurrent emboli. The safety of anticoagulation in bacterial endocarditis remains uncertain but it is no longer considered an absolute contraindication. Some less definite potential cardiac sources of emboli such as mitral valve prolapse may not justify treatment with warfarin, since the likelihood of recurrent stroke appears to be quite low. Recent studies have shown the combination of aspirin plus warfarin to be safe and effective for patients with mechanical heart valves, and it is increasingly used in patients experiencing cerebral ischemic events while on warfarin alone.

Table 38.1   Generally Accepted Indications for Antithrombotic Agents in Cerebrovascular Disease

Antiplatelet Agents

1. Primary stroke prevention in high-risk patients—e.g., carotid stenosis or TIA
2. Secondary stroke prevention in stroke survivors

Heparin

1. Stroke prevention in patients with clearly defined cardioembolic source
2. Prevention of DVT and pulmonary embolism in stroke patients with paresis and confined to bed (subcutaneous 5000U q12h or low molecular weight)
3. Arterial dissection
4. Cerebral venous thrombosis
5. Crescendo TIAs
6. Deteriorating stroke, "stroke-in-evolution"

Warfarin

1. Primary stroke prevention in rheumatic heart disease, atrial fibrillation, and mechanical heart valves
2. Antiphospholipid antibody syndrome
3. Stroke prevention postmyocardial infarction
4. Failure of antiplatelet agents

E *Noncardiac Emboli*

Transient ischemic attack patients and stroke survivors without a cardiac source for emboli have significant risk of further stroke and other ischemic events, including sudden death. Aspirin, ticlopidine, and more recently clopidogrel have all been shown to be effective in this group of patients. A recent meta-analysis involving over 100,000 patients in 145 trials included platelet inhibitors of all types and reported that the overall odds-reduction for vascular events was 25%. Specifically, among patients with previous minor strokes or TIAs, the odds-reduction was 22% for vascular events and 23% for nonfatal strokes. Aspirin is generally the drug of first choice for patients with cerebral ischemia but the optimal dose remains uncertain. Doses ranging from 30 mg per day to 1300 mg per day have been advocated, and, at the present time, enteric-coated aspirin at a dose of 325 or 650 mg per day seems reasonable. If poorly tolerated, the dose can be lowered. If the patient suffers recurrent TIA or stroke, or if there is a contraindication to aspirin, ticlopidine at a dose of 250 mg twice daily is an effective alternative.

F *Antiplatelet "Failures"*

Therapy combining two antiplatelet agents may be helpful in selected patients who continue to have thromboembolic events. While heparin is often used in a patient with "crescendo" TIAs, this has not been proven effective in preventing stroke.

G *The Deteriorating Stroke*

After arrival in hospital, many stroke patients will deteriorate with either a gradual or step-wise progression to increasing disability or death. An increase in the neurological deficit may be due to one or a combination of several mechanisms including propagation of an intra-arterial thrombus, re-embolization from a cardiac or proximal arterial source, delayed cerebral hemorrhage, cerebral edema, and systemic factors such as hypotension, hyponatremia, and sedation. Although administration of heparin has never been shown to be effective in the prevention of such deterioration, it is often used in patients with progressing or fluctuating stroke after alterative causes for the patient's symptoms have been excluded.

H *Embolic Stroke*

In presumed embolic stroke, anticoagulants are administered to reduce the likelihood of further emboli. However, anticoagulants increase the likelihood of symptomatic intracerebral hemorrhage, especially when given to patients with massive neurological deficits (perhaps reflecting the volume of infarcted brain), in those with uncontrolled hypertension and in the elderly. Many embolic strokes undergo

Patient with Cerebrovascular Disease

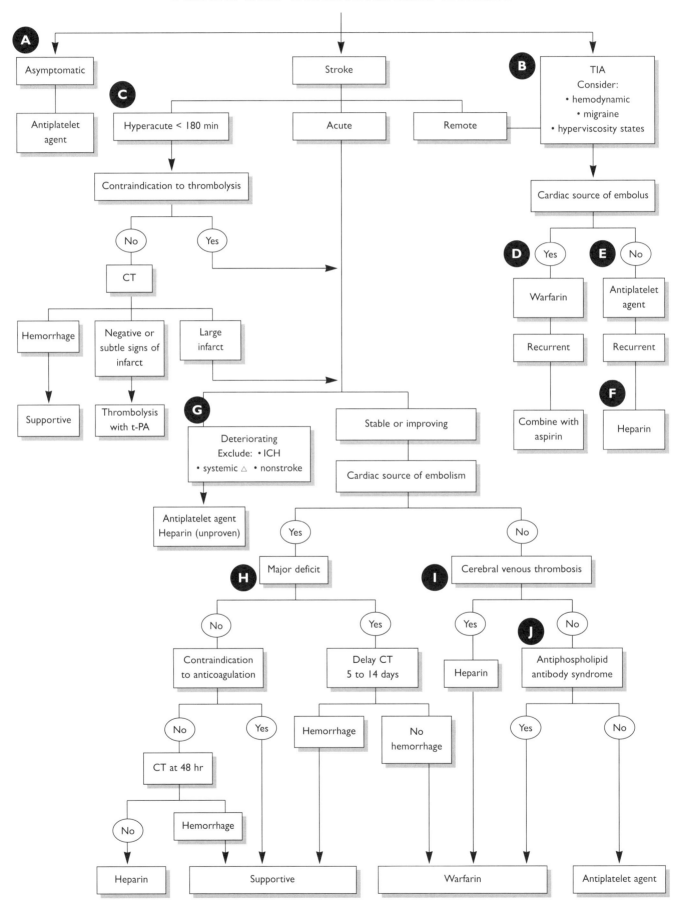

asymptomatic hemorrhagic transformation, even in the absence of anticoagulant therapy. The risk of recurrent embolism is approximately 1% per day. A prudent policy is to carry out a noncontrast CT scan 48 hours after stroke onset and, if negative for hemorrhage, to treat with intravenous heparin without a loading bolus. Delayed scanning and anticoagulation is recommended for patients with more profound neurological deficits.

I *Antithrombotic Therapy in Cerebral Venous Thrombosis*

For the role of antithrombotic therapy in cerebral venous thrombosis, see Chapter 24.

J *Systemic Disease and Recurrent Thrombosis*

Antiphospholipid antibody syndrome is defined by the presence of an antiphospholipid antibody (anticardiolipin antibody or lupus anticoagulant) and recurrent clinical events such as arterial or venous thromboses, or fetal loss. The risk of recurrent thrombosis in such patients has been reported to be high, and long-term anticoagulation therapy in which the INR is maintained at or above 3 has been recommended in these patients.

Additional Reading

Adams RD, Victor M, Ropper AH. Principles of neurology. New York: McGraw-Hill, 1997.

Antiplatelet Trialists' Collaboration. Collaborative overview of randomized trials of antiplatelet therapy—I: prevention of death, myocardial infarction and stroke by prolonged antiplatelet therapy in various categories of patients. BMJ 1994;308:91–106.

Barnett HJM, Eliasziw M, Meldrum H. Drugs and surgery in the prevention of ischemic stroke. N Engl J Med 1995;332:238–48.

Caplan LR. Stroke: a clinical approach. Boston: Butterworth-Heinemann, 1993.

CAPRIE Steering Committee. A randomised, blinded trial of clopidogrel versus aspirin in patients at risk of ischemic events (CAPRIE). Lancet 1996;348:1329–36.

Cote R, Battista RN, Abramowicz M, et al., and the Asymptomatic Cervical Bruit Study Group. Lack of effect of aspirin in asymptomatic patients with carotid bruits and substantial carotid narrowing. Ann Intern Med 1995;123:649–55.

Duke RJ, Bloch RF, Turpie AGG, Trebilcock R, Bayer N. Intravenous heparin for the prevention of stroke progression in acute partial stable stroke: a randomized controlled trial. Ann Intern Med 1986;105:825–8.

Khamashta M, Cuadrado MJ, Mujic F, Taub NA, Huut BJ, Hughes GRV. The management of thrombosis in the antiphospholipid-antibody syndrome. N Engl J Med 1995;332:993–7.

The National Institute of Neurological Disorders and Stroke rt-PA Stroke Study Group. Tissue plasminogen activator for acute ischemic stroke. N Engl J Med 1995;333:1582–7.

Turpie AGG, Gent M, Cote R, Levine MN, Ginsberg JS. A low-molecular weight heparinoid compared with unfractionated heparin in the prevention of deep vein thrombosis in patients with acute stroke. Ann Intern Med 1992;117:353–7.

Chapter 39

Patient Selection for Carotid Endarterectomy

Robert J Duke

Patient selection for carotid endarterectomy involves identification of patients most likely to benefit from surgery as well as those patients in whom the risk of the procedure is likely to exceed the benefit. In recent years, large clinical trials have yielded confident results for certain groups of patients while for other patients, optimal management remains uncertain. The two algorithms in this chapter are based on the stratification of patients according to whether or not symptoms are present.

CAROTID ENDARTERECTOMY FOR SYMPTOMATIC DISEASE

A *Symptoms of Carotid Artery Disease*

The first task in *symptomatic* patients is to decide whether the symptomatology is consistent with carotid territory origin. Symptoms characteristic of the carotid territory include ipsilateral monocular visual symptoms, and contralateral hemispheral symptoms, including sensory/motor deficits in the face and/or limbs, and aphasia. Certain symptoms such as aphasia or transient monocular visual loss are essentially pathognomonic of carotid artery distribution; others such as unilateral sensory or motor deficits or dysarthria may relate to carotid or posterior circulation territory. It is reasonable to assume that such symptoms may relate to the carotid territory, and investigations should be pursued in this direction. Other symptoms such as diplopia are inconsistent with carotid territory symptomatology. More nonspecific symptoms such as lightheadedness, syncope, or bilateral facial or limb numbness may occasionally relate to bilateral high-grade carotid stenosis or occlusion. A collateral history from family members is often helpful in supplementing even the most detailed history taken from patients.

B *Comorbidity and the Risk of Surgery*

Before proceeding further, it is useful to identify patients who have either coexistent disease, which makes carotid endarterectomy highly risky, or who have such a poor prognosis that they are unlikely to reap the benefits of endarterectomy. Such patients are those with congestive heart failure, dementia or advanced malignancy, and the extremely elderly.

C *Angioplasty and Perioperative Stroke*

Angioplasty, with or without stent, is occasionally used in symptomatic patients considered too frail to undergo surgical endarterectomy although the scant data available does not suggest that the associated perioperative stroke rates are lower than those of the surgical procedure.

D *Degree of Stenosis and the Risk of Stroke*

In both symptomatic and asymptomatic individuals, the risk of stroke rises as the degree of stenosis increases. Carotid arteriography has been the gold standard for determining the degree of stenosis and has the advantage of being able to evaluate the presence of disease proximal and distal to the carotid bifurcation and to most readily identify other conditions such as fibromuscular hyperplasia or carotid dissection. The main disadvantage is its associated morbidity, including stroke, and death. See Figure 39.1 which explains how to measure carotid stenosis. Ultrasound is a useful, safe screening tool for identifying disease at the carotid bifurcation but correlation with arteriography is only moderate and, therefore, only in rare instances should carotid endarterectomy be recommended on the basis of this information alone. Magnetic resonance angiography (MRA) represents a significant advance, having no appreciable risk and allowing imaging of more proximal and distal vasculature but again correlation with standard arteriography is incomplete.

E *Mild Stenosis and Surgical Risk*

The immediate risk of surgery outweighs any potential long-term benefit in symptomatic patients with mild stenosis (0 to 25% reduction in luminal diameter).

F *Moderate Stenosis and Risk/Benefit Assessment*

The role of carotid endarterectomy in symptomatic patients with *moderate* degrees of stenosis (30 to 69%) remains uncertain. The European Carotid Surgery Trials' Collaborative Group concluded that endarterectomy is not indicated for most, or possibly all, patients with moderate symptomatic stenosis.[1] The results of NASCET's moderate stenosis group will be known shortly. In the interim, symptomatic patients with moderate disease should usually be managed medically although it is reasonable to recommend endarterectomy for patients who have stenosis towards the high end of the scale of moderate stenosis, or if there are associated factors that might confer higher risk of stroke, such as plaque ulceration, contralateral occlusion, or the presence of multiple medical risk factors.

G *Severe Stenosis and the Risk of Subsequent Stroke*

It is the group of patients with severe (70 to 90%) stenosis who derive the most benefit from carotid endarterectomy. NASCET data revealed that a cumulative risk of any ipsilateral stroke at 2 years was 26% in medical patients and 9% in surgical patients.[2] Subsequent analysis of the data reveals that benefit was greater for patients with hemispheral symptoms as opposed to retinal symptoms; patients with ulcerated plaque, especially with very high degrees of stenosis, in comparison to nonulcerative plaques;[3] or in the presence of contralateral carotid artery occlusion. In TIA patients, the presence of infarction on CT scan conferred no higher risk of subsequent stroke.

H *Chronic Occlusion and the Risk of Stroke*

Endarterectomy for chronic occlusion is associated with an unacceptably high risk of stroke, probably due to intracranial embolization. Endarterectomy for acute occlusions (within 6 hours) in patients with moderate deficits has occasionally been reported to be associated with clinical improvement but is not of proven value, in general.

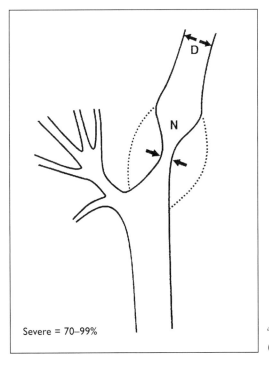

Severe = 70–99%

Figure 39.1   How to measure carotid stenosis (Adapted from Fox[4])

I   *Complication Rates and Risk/Benefit Assessment*

The theoretical benefit of carotid endarterectomy can be undermined in part or in total by high complication rates. In NASCET, the 30-day perioperative complication rate for stroke or death was 5.8% and for disabling stroke or death was 2.1%. Complication rates substantially higher than these can result in greater harm than benefit.

J   *Medical Management*

Optimal medical management, which must be extended to those who have had carotid endarterectomy as well as those who have not, includes antithrombotic therapy (see Chapter 38), risk factor modification, and education, including instruction about recognizing and reporting further TIA or stroke symptoms.

TIA or Stroke

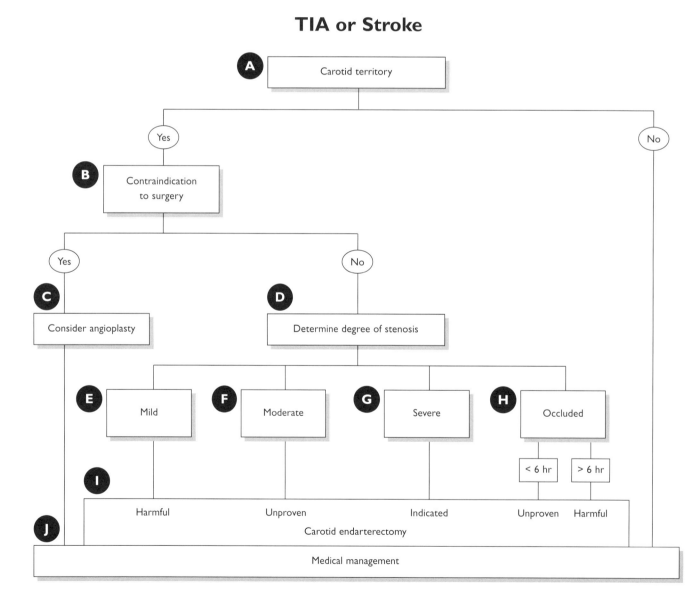

CAROTID ENDARTERECTOMY FOR ASYMPTOMATIC DISEASE

Patients in this category are generally referred after an audible cervical bruit has been detected, or because of ultrasound evidence of carotid bifurcation atherosclerosis. The following algorithm will assist in appropriate investigation of such patients, but it is important to recognize that there is considerable controversy in this area.

A *Symptomatic versus Asymptomatic Disease*

Be aware that a substantial number of patients referred for asymptomatic bruits or stenosis will admit to relevant symptoms when questioned carefully. Identification of such patients is important since asymptomatic carotid artery disease is more benign than symptomatic disease. Such symptomatic patients should be investigated according to the algorithm on page 246.

B *Patient Selection*

Before proceeding with further investigations, it is reasonable to identify for medical treatment those patients who are either too frail to undergo surgery or have such a poor prognosis that they are unlikely to survive long enough to reap the benefit of endarterectomy. Only patients with a life expectancy of more than 5 years should be considered surgical candidates for asymptomatic carotid disease, regardless of severity.

C *Degree of Stenosis and the Risk of Stroke*

The risk of stroke rises as the degree of stenosis increases. The Asymptomatic Carotid Endarterectomy Study[5] showed that patients with >60% stenosis had an estimated 5-year risk of 11% for ipsilateral stroke or death (6.0% for major ipsilateral stroke), or a stroke rate of just over 2% per annum. However, higher stroke rates occur in asymptomatic individuals with very high degrees of stenosis identified by ultrasound or angiography.[6] In determining the severity of stenosis, duplex ultrasound is an acceptable screening tool, allowing medical management for patients with mild or moderate degrees of stenosis. Those identified by ultrasound as having high-grade stenosis and who are being considered for carotid endarterectomy should have angiography to define the degree of stenosis and the associated risk of stroke. Ultrasound has a "false-positive" rate of 8 to 15%.

D *High-Grade Stenosis and the Risk of Stroke*

Patients with asymptomatic high-grade carotid stenosis who are being considered for coronary artery bypass grafting (CABG) often present special concerns. However, the perioperative stroke rate in patients with asymptomatic high-grade carotid stenosis undergoing CABG is surprisingly low, even when the stenosis is bilateral.[7] The added morbidity associated with endarterectomy rarely justifies "prophylactic" endarterectomy in this group of patients. It should be noted that the scales are tipped in the opposite direction for patients with symptomatic high-grade carotid stenosis who need CABG. In this latter group of patients, where there is clear indication for both carotid endarterectomy and CABG, the clinical dilemma relates to staging of the procedures. Since the most serious cerebral complication of CABG in such patients is stroke, a combined procedure under one anesthetic is favored, when feasible.

E *Moderate Stenosis and the Risk of Stroke*

The ACAS Study demonstrated that patients with asymptomatic carotid artery stenosis of ≥ 60%, whose general health makes them good candidates for elective surgery, will have a reduced 5-year risk of ipsilateral stroke if carotid endarterectomy can be performed and a perioperative morbidity and mortality of 3% or less. However, the absolute risk reduction is small, approximately 1% per annum, reducing the stroke rate from 2% per year to 1% per year. It has been calculated that 67 patients would have to undergo surgery to prevent one stroke in the first 5 years of follow-up, and 17 patients would need an operation to prevent a single major stroke within 5 years. Since patients with very high grade stenosis have a substantially higher risk of stroke, these are the patients most likely to benefit from endarterectomy. It is likely that patients with multiple risk factors, ulcerated plaques, progressive stenosis on sequential ultrasounds, and possibly those with clinically "silent" strokes or retinal emboli are at highest risk for stroke, and it is this group of patients that should be targeted for endarterectomy.

A prerequisite for recommendation of endarterectomy in asymptomatic individuals is having access to a surgeon who has a proven record of very low perioperative morbidity and mortality. Another important factor to be considered is the patient's philosophy and temperament. It should be remembered that a perioperative stroke next week is worse than the same stroke occurring 3 years hence. Patients differ in their willingness to accept an immediate and dangerous procedure to decrease the future risk of death or chronic disability due to stroke, and many patients will have strong opinions on these matters. Many, though not all, patients with asymptomatic stenosis will have warning transient ischemic attacks, and in lower-risk patients, a wait-and-see approach remains a reasonable therapeutic option.[8]

F *The Role of Patient Education in Risk Reduction*

In addition to the standard medical management (see Chapter 38), asymptomatic carotid stenosis patients should be educated to recognize TIAs or stroke symptoms and to seek medical attention should they occur. It is important that this education be individualized to minimize needless anxiety.

Asymptomatic Carotid Stenosis

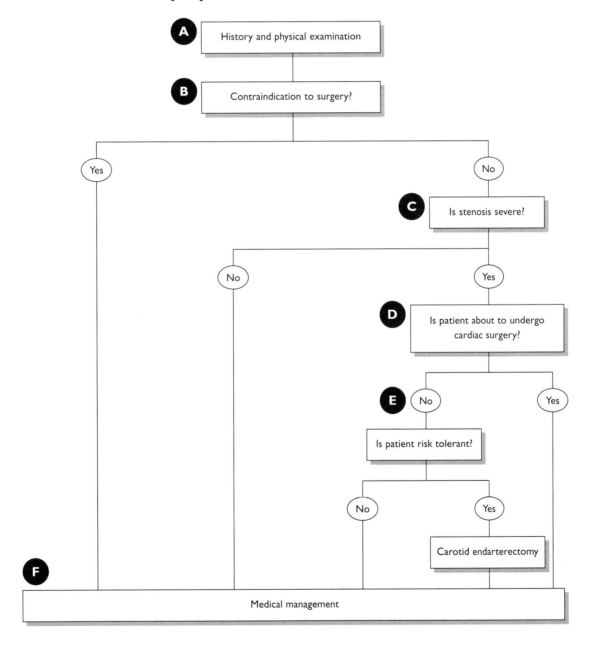

Bibliography

1. European Carotid Surgery Trialists' Collaborative Group. Endarterectomy for moderate symptomatic carotid stenosis: interim results from the MRC European carotid surgery trial. Lancet 1996;347:1591–3.

2. North American Symptomatic Carotid Endarterectomy Trial Collaborators. Beneficial effect of carotid endarterectomy in symptomatic patients with high-grade carotid stenosis. N Engl J Med 1991;325:445–53.

3. Eliasziw M, Streifler JY, Fox AJ, Hachinski VC, Ferguson GG, Barnett HJM. Significance of plaque ulceration in symptomatic patients with high-grade carotid stenosis. Stroke 1994; 25:304–8.

4. Fox AJ. How to measure carotid stenosis. Radiology 1993;186:316–8.

5. Executive committee of the asymptomatic carotid atherosclerosis study. Endarterectomy for asymptomatic carotid stenosis. JAMA 1995;273:1421–8.

6. Chambers BR, Norris JW. Outcome in patients with asymptomatic neck bruits. N Engl J Med 1986;315:860–4.

7. Gerraty RP, Gates PC, Doyle JC. Carotid stenosis and perioperative stroke risk in symptomatic and asymptomatic patients undergoing vascular or coronary surgery. Stroke 1993; 24:1115–8.

8. Sarasin FP, Bounameaux H, Bogousslavsky J. Asymptomatic severe carotid stenosis: immediate surgery or watchful waiting? A decision analysis. Neurology 1995;45:2147–53.

Additional Reading

Barnett HJM, Eliasziw M, Meldrum HE. Drugs and surgery in the prevention of ischemic stroke. N Engl J Med 1995;332:238–48.

Chapter 40

Diagnosis of Acute Ischemic Limb

Ryan T Hagino

G Patrick Clagett

Patients who present with acute lower extremity ischemia have a significant risk for limb loss and death. The progression from ischemia to irreversible cellular damage, membrane failure, and cell death is rapid in untreated limbs, occurring within 4 to 6 hours. Even with aggressive intervention, the rate of limb loss ranges from 5 to 40%.[1–6] Mortality ranges from 7.1 to 25%.[1–5] Proven methods of restoring circulation to the limb exist; however, their effectiveness depends on timely and appropriate application. An acute ischemic limb can be easily recognized; the signs and symptoms are classic and unmistakable. More difficult is determining the etiology of the ischemia, which may alter the application of further diagnostic tests and/or the method of restoring blood flow.[3,4] Much has been written about distinguishing an embolism from in-situ thrombosis based on history and physical examination alone.[1,7,8] Modern series document that this is difficult[1–4,7,8] and that distinguishing between an embolic and a thrombotic cause may ultimately require surgical exploration. A more difficult and perhaps more important task for the clinician comes after the diagnosis is made. The ability to distinguish between limbs in which revascularization would salvage the extremity and those in which ischemia has progressed beyond the hope of preserving a functional limb is necessary to achieve acceptable outcomes.

A History and Physical Examination

The history and physical examination are the most important tools for diagnosing acute limb ischemia. Patients who present with acute lower extremity ischemia are often elderly and have significant comorbid medical disease. Particular attention should be directed at cardiac history. Atrial fibrillation, when untreated or inadequately treated with oral anticoagulant therapy, can produce macroemboli. Retrospective studies suggest that the fibrillating left atrium is the most common source of peripheral emboli.[1,8] In addition, myocardial infarction, especially within the first 2 weeks, can also be a source of embolism.[1] The high mortality associated with acute limb ischemia is more a result of cardiac comorbidities than of complications directly related to the ischemic limb.[3,5,6] Over 50% of patients have New York Heart Association Class III or IV cardiac function or are classified as Goldman cardiac risk index of III or IV.[7,9] Careful attention should also be directed toward the central nervous system, the gastrointestinal tract, and kidneys, which may also be directly affected by macroemboli.

The classic "six ps" of acute limb ischemia are pain, paresthesias, pallor, paralysis, pulselessness, and poikylothermia. The presence of all "ps" is not essential in establishing a diagnosis. Pain is the most frequent and first symptom. The time of onset, the character of the pain and the presence of pre-existing symptoms of chronic ischemia, all yield important clues in determining the etiology of the ischemia. Pain of sudden onset (patients are often able to recall the exact time of onset) often suggests an embolic arterial occlusion. Ill-defined, gradual onset of pain over several days may suggest acute worsening of a chronic problem. A history of pre-existing intermittent claudication in the affected limb suggests thrombosis superimposed upon a chronic stenosis. A history of prior arterial surgery or bypass in the affected extremity strongly suggests thrombotic failure of the reconstruction. An attempt should be made at distinguishing between an embolic cause and a thrombotic cause for ischemia. Such a distinction helps in choosing the most appropriate therapy. However, such a distinction based on history and physical exam alone should be made with the understanding that the clinician will be wrong in a significant number of cases.[3]

Ischemia involving nerves results in varying degrees of paresthesias and motor dysfunction. The smaller caliber sensory nerves are more susceptible to ischemia. As a result, pain, paresthesias, and loss of proprioception are present early in the ischemic process. As the ischemia persists, gross sensation is lost, followed by a loss of motor function. The rapidity of this progression is dependent upon the degree of ischemia. Paralysis of the affected limb is a grave sign, and is due to motor neural dysfunction combined with muscle death and compartment swelling. In the severely ischemic limb, the loss of motor function is a precursor to irreversible tissue loss.[10]

B *Pulse Examination*

The pulse examination must be carefully performed and documented. Intuitively, limbs affected by acute arterial obstruction will have no palpable pulse distal to the level of occlusion. The pulse just proximal to or at the level of occlusion is often exaggerated and expansile. Emboli lodge at branch points along the arterial tree; the most common site of occlusion is the bifurcation of the femoral arteries.[7,8] Thrombosis develops at locations typically involved with athero-occlusive lesions, such as the distal superficial femoral artery. In addition, arterial aneurysms may thrombose. The presence or absence of a palpable pulse in a given location may add information vital in planning appropriate therapy or operative approach.

Equally important is the pulse examination of the contralateral, asymptomatic limb. Reduced or absent pulses in the contralateral, asymptomatic limb suggests pre-existing athero-occlusive disease in the lower limb, implying a thrombotic cause of ischemia. In addition, the presence of a popliteal aneurysm in the limb opposite to the ischemic extremity suggests a diagnosis of a thrombosed ipsilateral popliteal aneurysm.

C *Differential Diagnosis*

The presence of a palpable pedal pulse essentially rules out arterial occlusion of the major axial arteries of the lower extremity. Digital or forefoot ischemia accompanied by palpable pedal pulses suggests involvement of the small vessels of the foot or the digital arteries. The differential diagnosis includes atheroemboli (microemboli), vasospastic disease, or collagen vascular diseases. The risk of major tissue loss in these patients remains high but the diagnostic workup can proceed at a more leisurely pace.

D *Use of Doppler Ultrasound*

The continuous wave Doppler ultrasound detects frequency shift produced by moving erythrocytes insonated with sound waves. Sound waves of a particular wave length are produced at a frequency of 3 to 10 mHz by a piezoelectric crystal in the Doppler probe. The resulting Doppler shift caused by sound reflected by moving blood is translated as sound. This instrument is invaluable in the diagnosis and treatment of acute limb ischemia and is readily available in most hospitals. The utility of Doppler ultrasound lies in its ability to detect blood flow in vessels that may not have a palpable pulse. Blood flow detected distal to an occlusion is a reflection of flow through collaterals, or flow through a nonocclusive lesion. The character of the sound produced suggests the velocity of the moving red blood cells as well as the nature of the flow. Sluggish blood flow distal to an arterial occlusion translates into a slow, monophasic Doppler signal. When arteries proximal to occlusions are insonated, a distinctive "thump" can be heard; the lack of arterial outflow effectively stops any diastolic blood flow, sharply truncating the sound on continuous wave Doppler. The presence or absence of Doppler flow in both arteries and veins in the affected limb are important factors in stratifying the degree of ischemia and predicting the outcome of intervention.

The pedal arterial pressures are obtained by measuring the systolic blood pressure in the foot using a continuous wave Doppler. The appropriate-sized cuff is placed two fingerbreadths above the malleolus. Pressures are measured in both dorsalis pedis and posterior tibial arteries. The higher of the two values is used. The pedal pressure can be a useful means of quantifying distal arterial perfusion and can be used to stratify the degree of ischemia. It is important to remember that these values may be falsely elevated in patients with diabetes and significant medial calcinosis of the tibial vessels.

The ankle-brachial index (ABI) is an effective means of quantifying the degree of arterial insufficiency in an ischemic limb. The ABI is determined by dividing the highest pedal arterial pressure obtained by Doppler with the highest brachial arterial pressure obtained by Doppler. Normal limbs have ABIs of >1.0. Patients with moderate arterial insufficiency associated with intermittent claudication have ABIs between 0.5 and 0.9. Limbs with severe arterial insufficiency typically show ABIs of < 0.5. The absence of Doppler flow in an ischemic limb is a poor prognostic indicator.

E   *Acute Leg Ischemia*

Aortic dissection may produce lower limb ischemia if the dissection extends into the aortic bifurcation. Massive iliofemoral deep venous thrombosis may produce acute ischemia by severely impeding venous outflow to the lower limb, eventually compromising arterial inflow. Both aortic dissection and phlegmasia cerulea dolens should be considered as possible causes of acute leg ischemia.[4] These diagnoses may drastically alter diagnostic and therapeutic strategies.

F   *Gradations of Acute Lower Extremity Ischemia*

The Ad Hoc Committee on Reporting Standards for the Society of Vascular Surgery of the North American Chapter of the International Society for Cardiovascular Surgery has developed three gradations of acute lower extremity ischemia: viable, threatened viability, and irreversible.[1] The criteria are summarized in Table 40.1. As some of the criteria are subjective, overlap may exist among categories. Temporal criteria are deliberately excluded. The degree of ischemia and outcome of treatment in an ischemic limb is related more to the location of the occlusion and the presence of collateral circulation, than to the duration of symptoms. Such criteria are useful in predicting those patients who will respond to revascularization as well as providing a standardized method of comparing patients. The criteria allow a lucid, realistic approach to determining which patients should undergo further, more invasive procedures in an attempt to salvage a limb (see Chapter 41).

Diagnosis of Acute Ischemic Limb

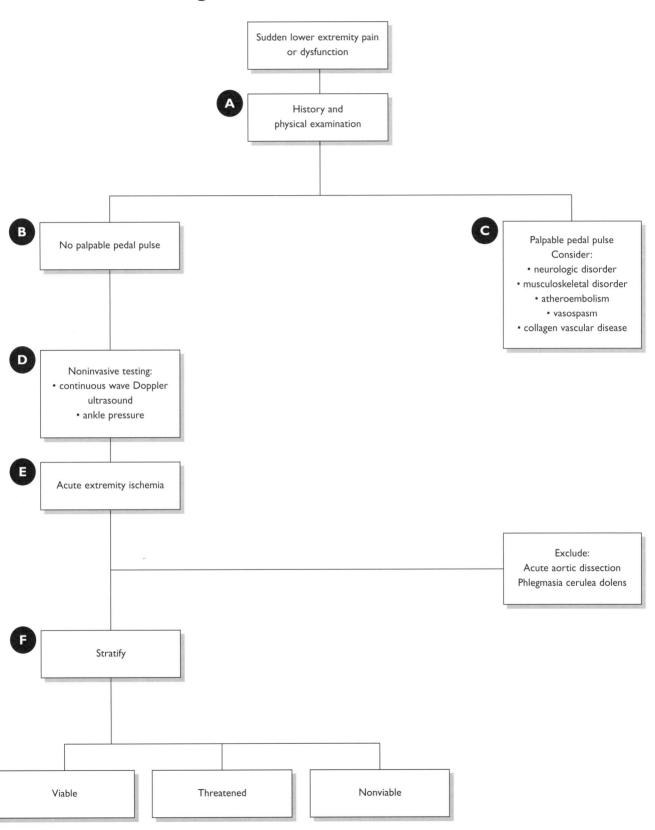

Table 40.1   SVS/ISCVS Clinical Categories of Acute Limb Ischemia[10]

Category	Description	Capillary Refill	Motor	Sensory	Doppler Signals	
					Arterial	Venous
Viable	Not immediately threatened	Intact	No deficit	No deficit	Audible (AP > 30 mm Hg)	Audible
Threatened	Salvageable with prompt treatment	Slow	Mild/partial deficit	Mild/incomplete deficit	Inaudible	Audible
Irreversible	Major tissue loss or amputation regardless of treatment	Absent (marbling)	Profound deficit/ paralysis	Profound deficit/ anesthetic	Inaudible	Inaudible

AP = ankle pressure

Data from Ad Hoc Committee on Reporting Standards, Society for Vascular Surgery/North American Chapter, International Society for Cardiovascular Surgery. Suggested standards for reports dealing with lower extremity ischemia. J Vasc Surg 1986;4:80–94.

Bibliography

1. Baxter-Smith D, Ashton F, Slaney G. Peripheral arterial embolism: a 20-year review. J Cardiovasc Surg (Torino) 1988;29:453–7.

2. Blaisdell FW, Steele M, Allen RE. Management of acute lower extremity arterial ischemia due to embolism and thrombosis. Surgery 1978;84:822–34.

3. Cambria RP, Abbott WM. Acute arterial thrombosis of the lower extremity: its natural history contrasted with arterial embolism. Arch Surg 1984;119:784–7.

4. Dale WA. Differential management of acute peripheral arterial ischemia. J Vasc Surg 1984; 1:269–78.

5. Tawes RL, Harris EJ, Brown WH, et al. Arterial embolism: a 20-year perspective. Arch Surg 1985;120:595–9.

6. Yeager RA, Moneta GL, Taylor LM, Hamre DW, McConnell DB, Porter JM. Surgical management of severe acute lower extremity ischemia. J Vasc Surg 1992;15:385–93.

7. Dregelid EB, Stangeland LB, Eide GE, Trippestad A. Characteristics of patients operated on because of suspected arterial embolism: a multivariate analysis. Surgery 1988;104:530–6.

8. Elliott JP, Hageman JH, Szilagyi E, Ramakishnan V, Bravo JJ, Smith RF. Arterial embolization: problems of source, multiplicity, recurrence, and delayed treatment. Surgery 1980;88:833–44.

9. Ouriel K, Shortell CK, DeWeese JA, et al. A comparison of thrombolytic therapy with operative revascularization in the initial treatment of acute peripheral arterial ischemia. J Vasc Surg 1994;19:1021–30.

10. Ad Hoc Committee on Reporting Standards, Society of Vascular Surgery/North American Chapter, International Society for Cardiovascular Surgery. Suggested standards for reports dealing with lower extremity ischemia. J Vasc Surg 1986;4:80–94.

Chapter 41

MANAGEMENT OF ACUTE ISCHEMIC LIMB

Ryan T Hagino

G Patrick Clagett

The severity of acute limb ischemia is determined mainly by the location of the arterial lesion, the collateral circulation, and the ischemia time.[1–5] Despite the advent of new treatment modalities and improvements in perioperative care, the rates of mortality and limb loss remain surprisingly high, with estimates of 33% and 25%, respectively.[2–11] Outcomes are heavily influenced by comorbid factors such as low cardiac output, recent myocardial infarction and patient's age.[3,5,6,8,11] Although early and aggressive surgical intervention is associated with the most favorable limb salvage, this is achieved at the cost of increased patient mortality.[3,5] Therefore, the clinician must weigh the usefulness of all treatments with full understanding that each treatment option is associated with major shortcomings.

A *Rapid Administration of Heparin*

Once the diagnosis of acute lower limb ischemia has been made (see Chapter 40), the first and foremost step is the rapid administration of heparin. Bolus heparin (150 IU/kg) is given to ensure adequate, rapid, and complete systemic anticoagulation. This bolus, accompanied by continuous heparin infusion (18 IU/kg/hr), is essential in preventing the progression of thrombus formation. The activated partial thromboplastin time (aPTT) should be used to monitor heparin therapy; the target intensity of anticoagulation should be an aPTT of 1.5 to 2.5 times control. Continued propagation of thrombus may lead to occlusion of vital collaterals, obliterating any reserve an ischemic limb may have had left.[3,4,7]

B *Is the Limb Viable, Threatened, or Nonviable?*

Limb viability may not fall clearly into one category.[1] Careful evaluation of all aspects of a particular patient is mandatory; pre-existing medical conditions and functional status should be considered when stratifying a patient.

C *Consider Nonoperative Therapy*

Blaisdell et al. were first to suggest that initial nonoperative treatment in selected patients with high-dose heparin offered the lowest overall mortality with acute limb ischemia.[3] This observation has since been corroborated by other investigators.[5] However, initial nonoperative therapy does not imply that later surgical intervention will not be necessary. For instance, initial nonoperative heparin therapy may be advisable in patients with viable extremities and thrombosed arterial reconstructions or nonreconstructable arterial anatomy prior to surgery. The change from emergency intervention to "urgent" intervention allows careful planning of these complex operative procedures.[7] Unfortunately, initial nonoperative therapy is not without significant shortcomings. Nonoperative therapy is clearly associated with higher rates of limb loss.[3–5] Failure of "conservative" treatment necessitating early operative intervention or amputation occurs in 16 to 72% of cases.[2–7,11] Its application should be limited to those patients with clearly viable extremities, or those with threatened limbs who are considered too frail from associated comorbid conditions to undergo early intervention.

D *Consider Primary Amputation*

Nonviable extremities should be amputated at the most distal level where successful healing can be anticipated. Little is gained by revascularizing a nonfunctional, insensate extremity with severe, permanent neurologic damage. In such a patient, primary amputation is in the patient's best interest.

E *Angiography*

In cases of thrombotic occlusion, and selected cases of peripheral embolism, emergent arteriography is performed. Such patients often have underlying intrinsic arterial pathology or failed bypass grafts. As a result, local thromboembolectomy is often inadequate treatment. Angiography will delineate arterial anatomy, allowing assessment of target vessels for arterial reconstruction and, if appropriate, provide access for thrombolytic therapy.

F *Thromboembolectomy*

In cases of suspected iatrogenic or embolic occlusion, the site of arterial occlusion is focal and predictable. When treating threatened limbs with suspected embolic or iatrogenic occlusion, the delay in obtaining a confirmatory angiogram can be avoided, and prompt surgical thromboembolectomy should be performed. Using local anesthesia, an arterial cut-down can be performed in most cases, and the embolus or focal thrombus can be extracted using well-described techniques.[6,7]

Antegrade and retrograde embolectomy using a balloon-embolectomy catheter device allows rapid restoration of blood flow to the limb. Backbleeding from distal vessels, although encouraging, is a poor predictor of adequate embolectomy.[7] Qualitative success can only be defined by restoration of a palpable pedal pulse and by an on-table angiogram.

G *Arterial Reconstruction*

The goal of any arterial reconstruction is to provide unobstructed blood flow from an unaffected inflow source to an appropriate outflow vessel, thus restoring perfusion to the ischemic region. Bypass procedures are ideally suited for native arterial thrombosis of stenotic lesions and thrombosed aneurysms. Thrombectomy of a failed arterial reconstruction must often be coupled with surgical correction of the anatomic cause of graft failure or placement of a new bypass graft. An occluded aortofemoral graft limb will usually require revision of the distal anastomosis, or profundaplasty. Infrainguinal bypasses may fail because of intrinsic midgraft lesions, anastomotic stenoses, or progression of distal disease. Durable results can be achieved using these reconstructive techniques.[11] However, long-term survival in this group is disappointingly low with mortality rates of 50% after 3 years.[6,11]

H *Thrombolysis*

Catheter-directed, intra-arterial thrombolysis is an attractive therapy for acute lower extremity ischemia. Because of the high mortality associated with emergent operative intervention, and the low rate of limb salvage associated with nonoperative therapy, thrombolytic therapy may offer a compromise between the extremes of therapy. The less invasive approach of percutaneous arterial access and direct application of lytic therapy appears attractive in high-risk patients provided that effective and rapid clot lysis can be achieved. Several randomized prospective studies[8–10] comparing initial surgical treatment with thrombolytic therapy for acute arterial occlusions have been published. These studies demonstrated comparable rates of limb salvage and mortality with initial thrombolytic therapy and initial arterial reconstruction. Several important points should be remembered when thrombolysis is considered in an ischemic limb: 1) Technical failures and incomplete thrombolysis occurred in 28 to 40% of attempts.[8–10] 2) Adequate and complete thrombolysis required an average of 22 to 36.6 hours.[8–10] The time to reperfusion averaged 7.6 (range 1 to 35) hours, in one study.[8] Therefore, thrombolytic therapy should be initiated only if delay in reperfusion would not result in a nonviable extremity. Severely ischemic limbs should be treated with prompt surgery. 3) In the majority of patients, complete thrombolysis will uncover anatomic lesions that may have initiated the thrombotic process. Further invasive intervention such as balloon angioplasty, patch angioplasty, or arterial bypass surgery is often required to maintain patency. Thrombolytic therapy alone was a durable treatment of ischemia in only 20 to 33% of patients.[8–10] It would seem from these studies that major advantage of intra-arterial thrombolysis is the ability to reduce the complexity of additional surgical procedures without compromising limb salvage or survival. Ongoing prospective trials may ultimately show a clear advantage in late outcome of one technique over another; however, currently such data is lacking.

Realizing the lack of absolute consensus regarding the optimal protocol for intra-arterial thrombolytic therapy, our recommendations for such treatment clearly reflect institutional biases. However, we generally conform to the recommendations of McNamara and associates whose protocol for catheter-directed intra-arterial thrombolysis has been widely adopted.[12] Briefly, following initial transthrombus passage of a guidewire and infusion catheter, a starting dose of high-dose (4000 IU/min) urokinase is initiated. Serial advancement of the catheter into any remaining thrombosed segments is performed every 1 to 2 hours until antegrade flow is re-established. The catheter is then pulled back proximally, and the dose is reduced to 1000 IU/min and continued for 8 to 12 hours. Infusion is continued until complete thrombolysis has occurred, or complications or ischemia preclude continued thrombolytic therapy. Our rates of technical failure, complications, and time to reperfusion parallel those reported earlier.

I Intraoperative Angiogram

Intraoperative angiography is invaluable in assessing the qualitative technical results of both embolectomy and arterial reconstruction. The presence of a residual thrombus or arterial spasm may alter further treatment strategies.

J Residual Thrombus Removal

Complete removal of residual thrombus in the distal arterial circulation should be actively pursued. Although frustrating, repeat thromboembolectomy should be performed if durable results are to be expected. However, repeated balloon catheter extraction attempts can be associated with considerable intimal trauma. Others have turned to intraoperative, intra-arterial thrombolysis.[13] The typical technique involves selective catheter placement through a proximal arteriotomy and direct infusion of 250,000 IU of urokinase over a 20- to 30-minute period. Investigators with considerable experience with this technique have not shown significant systemic effects and have achieved successful, localized thrombolysis.[14]

Management of Acute Ischemic Limb

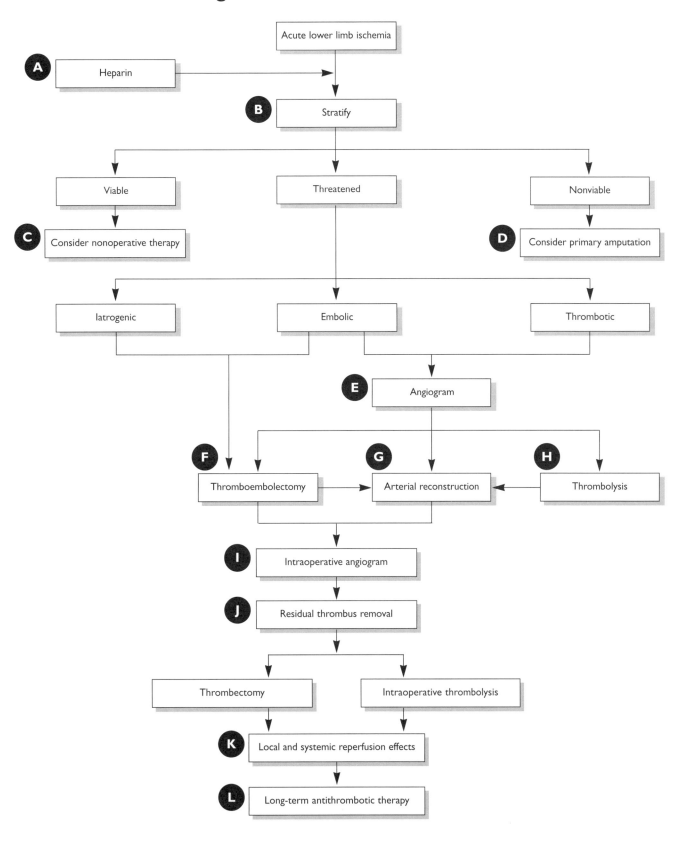

K *Local and Systemic Reperfusion Effects*

After restoration of arterial blood flow, significant local and systemic problems may arise related to reperfusion injury.[3,4,11] Local muscle swelling within the inelastic fascial compartments of the limb may result in a compartment syndrome. Prompt incision of these fascial layers will effectively release the pressure within the compartments, preventing further neurologic damage and muscle death. Systemic effects related to metabolic acidosis, hyperkalemia, release of myoglobin, complement activation, and cytokine release can lead to remote organ injury. The morbidity associated with this reperfusion syndrome can be considerable.[3] Prevention of these effects may be achieved by rapid intervention, thus minimizing the effects of prolonged ischemia. In patients with severe, prolonged ischemia, prophylactic mannitol can be administered, and steps taken to alkalinize the urine in order to protect the kidneys from deposition of myoglobin pigments. Proactive measures including invasive hemodynamic monitoring, aggressive fluid replacement, frequent blood gas and electrolyte studies, and testing of the urine for myoglobin are recommended.

L *Long-Term Antithrombotic Therapy*

Recurrent embolism occurs in 10 to 28% of cases.[2,4] Events may be multiple and involve carotid, visceral, or renal circulation. Aggressive diagnostic work-up and treatment of the source of emboli is mandatory. For the most part, chronic warfarin anticoagulation has been used with good results. Less convincing data are available regarding chronic antithrombotic therapy for arterial reconstructions performed for acute limb ischemia. In general, we adhere to the recommendations proposed by the American College of Chest Physicians regarding the use of antithrombotic therapy in peripheral arterial occlusive disease.[15] They recommend oral anticoagulation with warfarin following treatment for acute thrombosis or embolism, antiplatelet therapy for infrainguinal bypass patients to reduce the incidence of stroke and myocardial infarction, and no routine administration of warfarin in patients following infrainguinal bypass. Exceptions may include patients with grafts in low-flow, high-resistance systems with small caliber conduits.

Bibliography

1. Ad Hoc Committee on Reporting Standards, Society for Vascular Surgery/North American Chapter, International Society for Cardiovascular Surgery. Suggested standards for reports dealing with lower extremity ischemia. J Vasc Surg 1986;4:80–94.

2. Baxter-Smith D, Ashton F, Slaney G. Peripheral arterial embolism: a 20-year review. J Cardiovasc Surg 1988;29:453–7.

3. Blaisdell FW, Steele M, Allen RE. Management of acute lower extremity arterial ischemia due to embolism and thrombosis. Surgery 1978;84:822–34.

4. Elliott JP, Hageman JH, Szilagyi DE, Ramakishnan V, Bravo JJ, Smith RF. Arterial embolization: problems of source, multiplicity, recurrence, and delayed treatment. Surgery 1980;88: 833–44.

5. Jivegard L, Bergqvist D, Holm J. When is urgent revascularisation unnecessary for acute lower extremity ischaemia? Eur J Vasc Endovasc Surg 1995;9:448–53.

6. Cambria RP, Abbott WM. Acute arterial thrombosis of the lower extremity: its natural history contrasted with arterial embolism. Arch Surg 1984;119:784–7.

7. Dale WA. Differential management of acute peripheral arterial ischemia. J Vasc Surg 1984; 1:269–78.

8. Ouriel K, Shortell CK, DeWeese JA, et al. A comparison of thrombolytic therapy with operative revascularization in the initial treatment of acute peripheral arterial ischemia. J Vasc Surg 1994;19:1021–30.

9. Ouriel K, Veith FJ, Sasahara AA, for the TOPAS Investigators. Thrombolysis or peripheral arterial surgery: Phase I results. J Vasc Surg 1996;23:64–75.

10. The STILE Investigators. Results of a prospective randomized trial evaluating surgery versus thrombolysis for ischemia of the lower extremity: the STILE trial. Ann Surg 1994;220: 251–68.

11. Yeager RA, Moneta GL, Taylor LM, Hamre DW, McConnell DB, Porter JM. Surgical management of severe acute lower extremity ischemia. J Vasc Surg 1992;15:385–93.

12. McNamara TO, Bomberger RA, Merchant RF. Intra-arterial urokinase as the initial therapy for acutely ischemic lower limbs. Circulation 1991;83(Suppl I):106–19.

13. Comerota AJ, White JV. Intraoperative, intra-arterial thrombolytic therapy as an adjunct to revascularization in patients with residual and distal arterial thrombous. Semin Vasc Surg 1992;5:110–7.

14. Comerota AJ, Rao AK, Throm RC, et al. A prospective, randomized, blinded placebo-controlled trial of intraoperative intra-arterial urokinase infusion during lower extremity revascularization: Regional and systemic effects. Ann Surg 1993;218:534–43.

15. Clagett GP, Krupski WC. Antithrombotic therapy in peripheral arterial occlusive disease. Chest 1995;108(Suppl):431S–43S.

Additional Reading

Brewster DC, Chin AK, Hermann GD, Fogarty TJ. Arterial thromboembolism. In: Rutherford RB, ed. Vascular Surgery. 4th ed. Philadelphia: W.B. Saunders Company, 1995.

Chapter 42

Diagnosis and Management of Peripheral Vascular Disease

Shannon M Bates

Jeffrey I Weitz

Vascular occlusive disease of the lower extremities commonly occurs in people as they age. Some 5% of men and 2.5% of women 50 years or older have symptoms of intermittent claudication.[1] When sensitive noninvasive tests are used to make the diagnosis of arterial insufficiency in either symptomatic or asymptomatic individuals, the prevalence is at least threefold higher.[2] Atherosclerosis is the most common cause of peripheral vascular disease. In symptomatic individuals, the prognosis for the affected limb is relatively good since after 5 to 10 years, more than 70% of patients report either no change or improvement of their symptoms, 20 to 30% have disease progression requiring intervention, and <10% require amputation.[3] However, patients with symptomatic lower extremity arterial disease have an increased risk of stroke, myocardial infarction, and cardiovascular death than are asymptomatic age-matched patients.[4] Seventy-five percent of patients with lower extremity arterial disease will die of a coronary or cerebrovascular event.[4] The life expectancy of patients with claudication has been estimated to be approximately 10 years less than individuals of the same age without symptoms.[1] Peripheral vascular disease should, therefore, be viewed as a marker of generalized atherosclerosis and an indicator of an increased risk of premature death.

Risk factors for atherosclerotic disease of the lower extremities include increasing age, male gender, tobacco use, hypertension, hyperlipidemia, diabetes mellitus, and impaired glucose tolerance.[1,4]

A Clinical Assessment of Nonlimb-Threatening Peripheral Vascular Disease

Patients with nonlimb-threatening peripheral vascular disease may be asymptomatic or may present with impotence or intermittent claudication. Claudication, the pain of muscle ischemia, has been described as a sensation of fatigue, dull aching, or cramping felt in the leg muscles that is induced by a fixed degree of exercise and completely relieved by 5 to 10 minutes of rest. In patients with peripheral vascular disease, the location of the ischemic pain is determined by the site of obstruction. Pain in the buttocks and thighs suggests aortoiliac disease while calf muscle pain implies femoral or popliteal artery disease. Aortoiliac disease in men produces the so-called Leriche syndrome, in which there is claudication of the hip, thigh, and buttock muscles, impotence, and diminished or absent femoral pulses.

Physical signs of peripheral arterial insufficiency may include hair loss on the toes and dorsum of the foot, thickening of the toenails, coolness of the skin to touch, and extreme pallor of the forefoot with elevation and rubor with dependency. The presence of a pulse deficit or a bruit at the site of vessel narrowing can help determine the distal level of disease involvement.

B Clinical Assessment of Limb-Threatening Peripheral Vascular Disease

Patients with critical leg ischemia can present with rest pain, ulcers, or gangrene.[2] In addition to the usual signs of arterial insufficiency, patients with advanced peripheral arterial disease may develop subcutaneous tissue atrophy, painful ulcers, or gangrene.

C Differential Diagnosis

Musculoskeletal disease, venous insufficiency, neurospinal compression, and acute arterial occlusions can also produce lower extremity pain. Patients with musculoskeletal disease or venous insufficiency may complain of pain produced by exercise and relieved by rest, their exercise tolerance is variable, and relief with rest can be delayed for several hours or days. In patients with venous claudication, elevation of the affected limb often results in pain relief whereas in those with arterial insufficiency, elevation may exacerbate symptoms. Accompanying signs of chronic venous insufficiency such as venous ulcers, hemosiderin pigmentation, varicosities, and lower extremity edema are common. Symptoms of neurospinal compression due to osteophytic narrowing of the lumbar neurospinal canal are exacerbated by increasing lumbar lordosis. Therefore, standing, as well as walking, causes lower extremity pain, which is not relieved until the patient straightens the lumbar spine by sitting or lying down. The discomfort of neurological claudication usually follows a dermatomal distribution, and there may be abnormal neurologic signs on physical examination. Sudden onset of severe, constant leg pain accompanied by pallor, parasthesias, diminished or absent pulses, or paralysis raises the possibility of acute arterial occlusion.

D *Laboratory Assessment of Peripheral Vascular Disease*

As arterial narrowing progresses, systolic blood pressure distal to the affected site decreases. The severity of occlusive disease is reflected by the extent to which pressure falls. The sensitivity of pressure measurements can be heightened by using exercise to decrease resistance distal to the lesion and, thereby, accentuate the pressure drop.[2]

The ankle-brachial index (ABI) can be used to establish the diagnosis and severity of peripheral vascular disease. The ABI is derived by dividing the highest ankle pressure (posterior tibial or dorsalis pedis pressure) by the brachial pressure. The pressure at the ankle is normally slightly greater than the brachial pressure. An ABI <0.95 is indicative of occlusive disease. There is an inverse correlation between the ABI and disease severity.[2] Serial measurements of the ABI can be used to follow up patients with chronic peripheral vascular disease or to monitor the success of vascular surgery.

The ABI may have limited utility in patients with diabetes mellitus and chronic renal failure as calcification of the arterial media may render the arteries incompressible. Because medial calcification does not extend into the digital arteries, toe systolic pressure can be used to assess perfusion in this setting. The toe systolic pressure index (TSPI) can be derived by dividing the toe pressure by the brachial pressure. Normally, the TSPI is greater than 0.60.[5]

Segmental pressures of the leg can be used to localize the diseased arterial segment. Standard pneumatic cuffs are placed at the level of the upper thigh, lower thigh, calf, and ankle, and the pressures are measured. Differences in pressure greater than 30 mm Hg between segmental levels are suggestive of significant arterial obstruction.[2]

Continuous wave Doppler can be used to assess arterial flow velocity patterns in the lower extremities. The normal pattern at rest is triphasic: forward flow, reverse flow, and late forward flow. With pressure- and flow-reducing lesions proximal to the recording site, a reduction in peak systolic velocity distal to the lesion, loss of reverse flow, turbulence distal to the lesion, or an increase in peak systolic velocity at the site of the lesion may be seen.[2] Continuous wave Doppler retains its utility in diabetic patients with noncompressible arteries.

Contrast angiography remains the reference method for assessing the cause and severity of peripheral vascular disease. It is seldom required for management decisions in patients with peripheral vascular disease but it is necessary if reconstructive surgery is planned.

E *Treatment*

The goals of treatment should be (1) to relieve ischemic symptoms and arrest disease progression, and (2) to prevent associated cardiovascular complications. To achieve the first, both conservative measures such as exercise, risk factor modification, and pharmacotherapy, and surgical treatments such as percutaneous transluminal angioplasty, endarterectomy, vascular reconstruction, and amputation are used. Currently, the best treatment for the prevention of cardiovascular complications from diffuse atherosclerosis is aspirin.[6] Ticlopidine is a reasonable alternative for those intolerant of aspirin.[7]

As the risk of progressive leg ischemia is low in patients without limb-threatening ischemia or disabling claudication,[3] conservative therapy should be attempted first. Patients with disabling claudication that interferes with their work or lifestyle, or limb-threatening ischemia manifesting as rest pain, nonhealing ulcers, infection, or gangrene may be candidates for more aggressive intervention in addition to conservative therapy.

F *Management of Risk Factors*

Risk factor management may prevent the cardiovascular complications associated with widespread atherosclerosis and reduce the risk of progressive lower extremity vascular occlusion. Smoking cessation can improve maximal walking distance in patients with intermittent claudication.[8] While there is no evidence that treatment of hyperlipidemia with 3-hydroxy-3-methylglutaryl-coenzyme A (HMG-CoA) reductase inhibitors alters the course of peripheral vascular disease, it is reasonable to use these agents as they may reduce cardiovascular mortality.[9,10] Improved glycemic control may reduce the risk of peripheral vascular and cardiovascular events in insulin-dependent diabetics.[11]

G *Physical Training*

Exercise therapy is the cornerstone of conservative treatment for peripheral vascular disease. There is some evidence that it is the most consistently effective treatment for intermittent claudication.[12] The mechanism accounting for documented improvements in pain-free and maximal walking distances is unknown. Simple walking regimens, dynamic leg exercises, and individualized treadmill exercise performed three to four times per week for several months have all been used. Longer training periods are more successful than shorter ones. Regularity is more important than intensity. Unstable angina pectoris, severe chronic obstructive pulmonary disease, symptomatic congestive heart failure, and manifestations of severe limb ischemia requiring vascular reconstruction may, however, preclude participation in exercise training.[2]

H *Antithrombotic Therapy*

Aspirin, alone or in combination with dipyridamole, has been shown to slow progression of established peripheral arterial disease as assessed by serial angiography[13] and to reduce the need for arterial reconstruction when used for primary prevention in men.[14] While these data suggest that platelet inhibitors may slow the progression of peripheral vascular disease, no trial has shown that their use improves limb prognosis. Therefore, the best reason for aspirin therapy in patients with peripheral vascular disease remains the prevention of death and morbidity from cerebrovascular disease and myocardial infarction. Aspirin in doses of 75 to 325 mg daily is at least as effective as higher doses, and lower doses are associated with fewer side effects and complications.[6]

Small randomized trials have suggested that ticlopidine may relieve symptoms, increase walking distances, and improve ABIs.[2] Also, a meta-analysis of these trials has demonstrated a significant decrease in both fatal and nonfatal cardiovascular events in patients with intermittent claudication receiving ticlopidine compared to those receiving placebo therapy.[7] Ticlopidine is, therefore, a reasonable alternative for patients who are intolerant of aspirin.[2,7]

I *Other Agents*

While many drugs have been evaluated, few, if any, have shown convincing clinical benefit. Pentoxifylline has been reported to improve abnormal erythrocyte deformability, reduce blood viscosity, and decrease platelet reactivity and plasma hypercoagulability in patients with peripheral vascular disease.[2] However, overall, there are no good data to support claims of its effectiveness.[12] Vasodilators, EDTA chelation, fish oil supplementation, naftidrofuryl, suloctidil, ketanserin, and nifedipine have all been found ineffective in the treatment of intermittent claudication.[2]

J *Percutaneous Transluminal Angioplasty*

Percutaneous transluminal angioplasty (PTA) is appropriate only when arterial disease is restricted to a vessel segment <10 cm in length and a skilled vascular interventionist is available.[2] Limited data are available comparing the outcome of patients with lower extremity peripheral vascular disease who are treated surgically with those treated with PTA. Success rates for PTA appear to be operator dependent.[2]

Diagnosis and Management of Peripheral Vascular Disease

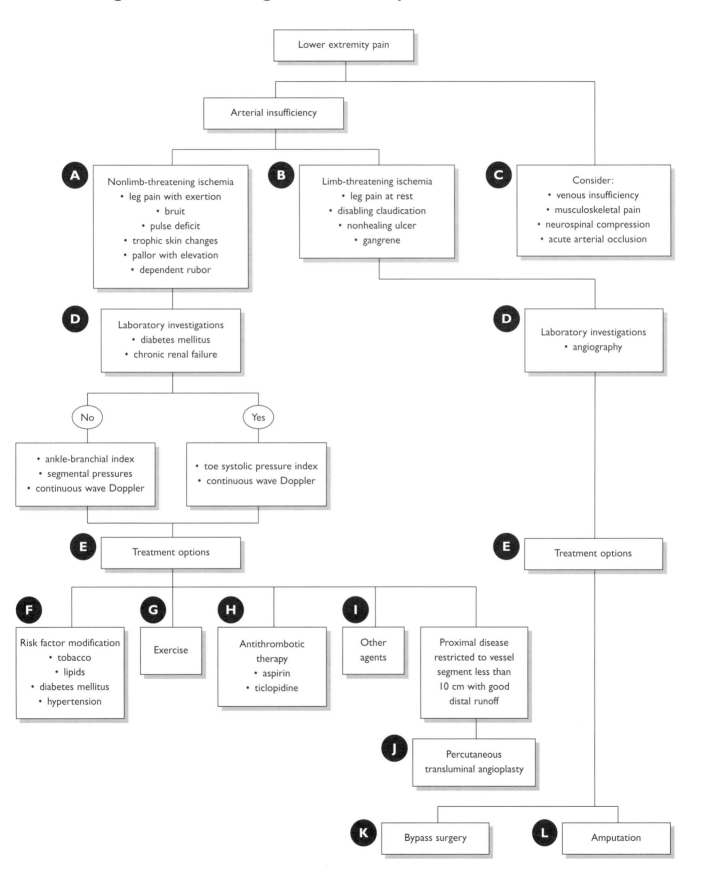

While sometimes used in patients with critical leg ischemia, the failure rate appears high when performed in patients with limb-threatening disease. Stenotic rather than occlusive disease, a proximal rather than distal lesion, and good distal run-off predict a more favorable outcome. The role of stents in primary PTA is not clear but stent placement may be reasonable in the presence of a complex lesion or when dissection occurs.[2] In the absence of contraindications, patients undergoing PTA should receive lifelong aspirin therapy to reduce cardiovascular morbidity and mortality.

K *Lower Extremity Bypass Surgery*

Surgical intervention is able to provide durable salvage of limbs threatened by ischemia in 85 to 90% of cases with aggressive reoperation for recurrent symptoms or lesions necessary in 10 to 15% of patients. Surgical mortality is less than 5%. The choice of surgical procedure and material depends on the level of arterial disease. Conventional treatment for proximal occlusive disease has been aortofemoral bypass with the size of the vessels involved determining the use of prosthetic bypass material. There is no convincing evidence that any one currently available prosthesis is superior to others for aortofemoral bypass. When performed by individuals skilled in the procedure, endarterectomy is as successful as bypass for proximal occlusive disease.[2]

The conduit of choice for infrainguinal bypass is the intact great saphenous vein.[2] There appears to be no difference in the results obtained with in situ and reversed techniques nor has the overall superiority of one synthetic graft material for infrainguinal bypass been clearly established.[2] All bypass patients without contraindications should receive lifelong aspirin therapy to reduce the incidence of myocardial infarction and stroke.

L *Amputation*

Primary amputation appears to hold no advantages over revascularization in terms of operative risk[15] or overall cost (when the expense of the prosthesis and rehabilitation is included).[16] Therefore, only in permanently nonambulatory patients is it the treatment of choice for critical limb ischemia.

Bibliography

1. Dormandy J. Peripheral vascular disease. Med North Am 1994;17:353–60.
2. Weitz JI, Byrne J, Clagett GP, et al. Diagnosis and treatment of chronic arterial insufficiency of the lower extremities: a critical review. Circulation 1996;94:3026–49.

3. Imparato AM, Kim GE, Davidson T, Crowley JG. Intermittent claudication: its natural course. Surgery 1975;78:795–9.

4. Kannel WB, McGee DL. Update on some epidemiologic features of intermittent claudication: the Framingham Study. J Am Geriatr Soc 1985;33:13–8.

5. Orchard TJ, Strandness DE Jr. Assessment of peripheral vascular disease in diabetes: report and recommendations of an international workshop sponsored by the American Diabetes Association and the American Heart Association, September 18–20, 1992, New Orleans, Louisiana. Circulation 1993;88:819–28.

6. Antiplatelet Trialists' Collaboration. Collaborative overview of randomized trials of antiplatelet therapy, I: prevention of death, myocardial infarction, and stroke by prolonged antiplatelet therapy in various categories of patients. BMJ 1994;308:81–106.

7. Boissel JP, Peyrieux JC, Destors JM. Is it possible to reduce the risk of cardiovascular events in subjects suffering from intermittent claudication of the lower limbs? Thromb Haemost 1989;62:681–5.

8. Quick CRG, Cotton LT. The measured effect of stopping smoking on intermittent claudication. Br J Surg 1982;69(Suppl):S24–S26.

9. Randomized trial of cholesterol lowering in 4444 patients with coronary heart disease: the Scandinavian Simvastatin Survival Study (4S). Lancet 1994;344:1383–9.

10. Shepherd J, Cobbe SM, Ford I, et al. Prevention of coronary heart disease with pravastatin in men with hypercholesterolemia: West of Scotland Coronary Prevention Study Group. N Engl J Med 1995;333:1301–7.

11. The Diabetes Control and Complications Trial Research Group. The effect of intensive treatment of diabetes on the development and progression of long-term complications in insulin-dependent diabetes mellitus. N Engl J Med 1993;329:977–86.

12. Radack K, Wyderski RJ. Conservative management of intermittent claudication. Ann Intern Med 1990;113:135–46.

13. Hess H, Mietaschk A, Deichsel G. Drug-induced inhibition of platelet function delays progression of peripheral occlusive arterial disease: a prospective double-blind arteriographically controlled trial. Lancet 1985;1:415–9.

14. Goldhaber SZ, Manson JE, Stampfer MJ, et al. Low-dose aspirin and subsequent peripheral arterial surgery in the Physicians' Health Study. Lancet 1992;340:143–5.

15. Ouriel K, Fiore WM, Geary JE. Limb-threatening ischemia in the medically compromised patient: amputation or revascularization? Surgery 1988;104:667–72.

16. Veith FJ, Gupta SK, Samson RH, et al. Progress in limb salvage by reconstructive arterial surgery combined with new or improved adjunctive procedures. Ann Surg 1981;194:386–401.

Chapter 43

Management of Patients with Atrial Fibrillation

Michael D Ezekowitz

Patients with atrial fibrillation have a five times greater risk of stroke than comparably aged patients in sinus rhythm. The absolute risk of stroke, however, varies from being very low in patients with lone atrial fibrillation, i.e., patients with atrial fibrillation without structural heart disease, to being very high in patients with risk factors such as age > 65 with a history of hypertension, diabetes mellitus, previous TIA, or poor ventricular function.

A Evaluation of Clinical Status

The first step in evaluating a patient with atrial fibrillation is to determine whether the patient is symptomatic, i.e., either hemodynamically compromised or ischemic. If the patient is unstable and cannot be restored to a compensated state, either with rate control or other measures directed at heart failure or ischemia, immediate cardioversion is indicated. Cardioversion, under these circumstances, should be performed with the patient heparinized. If the patient is a candidate for long-term Coumadin therapy, it should also be initiated. Intravenous heparin is discontinued when the anticoagulant effect of Coumadin produces an INR range of 2.0 to 3.0.

Patients who are stable (i.e., minimally symptomatic or asymptomatic) offer a window for more rigorous evaluation. First, it is important to evaluate the patient for a reversible cause of the atrial fibrillation; these are found in Table 43.1. Any reversible cause should be eliminated. At the same time, it is advisable to institute pharmacologic measures for rate control. The drugs that are currently used are digoxin, beta-blockers (both short- and long-acting), and the calcium antagonists, verapamil and diltiazem.

Table 43.1   Conditions Associated with Atrial Fibrillation

Cardiac	Systemic
Cardiac surgery	Age
Cardiomyopathy	Alcohol
Congenital heart disease	Cerebrovascular disease
Hypertension	Chronic pulmonary disease
Ischemic heart disease	Electrocution
Lipomatous hypertrophy	Electrolyte abnormalities
Pericarditis	Fever
Pre-excitation syndromes	Hypothermia
Tachycardia-bradycardia syndrome	Hypovolemia
Tumors	Pregnancy
Valvular heart disease	Sudden emotional change
Ventricular hypertrophy	Swallowing
Ventricular pacing	Trauma

B *Rate Control and Prophylaxis against Stroke versus Cardioversion*

Once a reversible cause has been eliminated and rate control has been achieved, the decision for cardioversion rests on the premise that a patient in sinus rhythm is hemodynamically better off than a patient in atrial fibrillation. As well, if cardioversion can be maintained permanently, then the risk of systemic embolization reverts back to the risk in a patient with sinus rhythm.

Cardioversion can be achieved using either of two strategies. The first requires 4 weeks of anticoagulation at an INR of 2.0 to 3.0 prior to cardioversion. The warfarin is then continued for at least 1 month or until the patient is permanently in sinus rhythm, at which time it can be discontinued.

An alternative method of cardioversion is to perform transesophageal echocardiography to rule out the presence of a left atrial clot. The heparinized patient can be cardioverted immediately, thus saving a second hospitalization. In this circumstance, the patient needs to be maintained on warfarin for at least 4 weeks or until sinus rhythm is maintained permanently. Alternatively, cardioversion is not attempted and the patient is anticoagulated indefinitely.

The basis of this approach is the recognition that cardioversion is not always successful in the long term, despite using the most efficacious drugs. It is estimated that only 50% of patients remain in sinus rhythm 12 to 18 months following successful cardioversion. In addition, it has been demonstrated that patients who can tolerate antithrombotic therapy are protected against thromboembolic disease. Thus, if rate control allows the patient to be clinically stable and hemodynamically uncompromised and nonischemic and the patient is a candidate for anticoagulant therapy, this approach is justified.

C Stratification of Risk for Stroke in Patients with Atrial Fibrillation

The overall risk of developing a stroke in patients with atrial fibrillation is five times the risk of age-matched patients in sinus rhythm. By pooling the data from the placebo groups of the primary prevention trials, it is possible to identify clinical risk factors that, when absent, convey a low risk of stroke and, when present, increase the risk of stroke. If a patient is under the age of 65, has no risk factors (i.e., a history of hypertension, history of diabetes, history of previous TIA, and stroke) and has normal ventricular function by echocardiography, anticoagulant therapy is not indicated because the benefits of a reduction in stroke are outweighed by the risk and inconvenience of treatment. Provided there are no contraindications for anticoagulation therapy, in patients under the age of 65 with one or more of these risk factors or over age 65, anticoagulation with warfarin is indicated. Patients who cannot be anticoagulated should be treated with aspirin at a dose of 325 mg.

D Contraindication to Warfarin Therapy

This includes patients who have an active bleeding diathesis and patients with the contraindications shown in Table 43.2.

E Anticoagulation with Warfarin in Patients with Atrial Fibrillation

If the patient is under the age of 70, initiation of anticoagulation therapy should be with 4 mg of warfarin. If the patient is over the age of 70, the dose should be 3 mg of warfarin. During the initiation phase, an INR should be obtained at 7 days. If the patient is below the therapeutic range, the dose should be increased by 1 mg. If above the range, the dose should be decreased by 1 mg until the patient has a therapeutic INR result. Thereafter, INRs should be obtained every month. Monitoring is

Table 43.2   Contraindications to Anticoagulation Therapy

Chronic alcoholism, psychologically or socially unsuitable	Active peptic ulcer
Advanced liver disease	Planned invasive procedure/surgery
Disseminated malignancy	Platelet count < 50,000
Active bleeding	Poorly controlled hypertension

Approach to Patient with Atrial Fibrillation

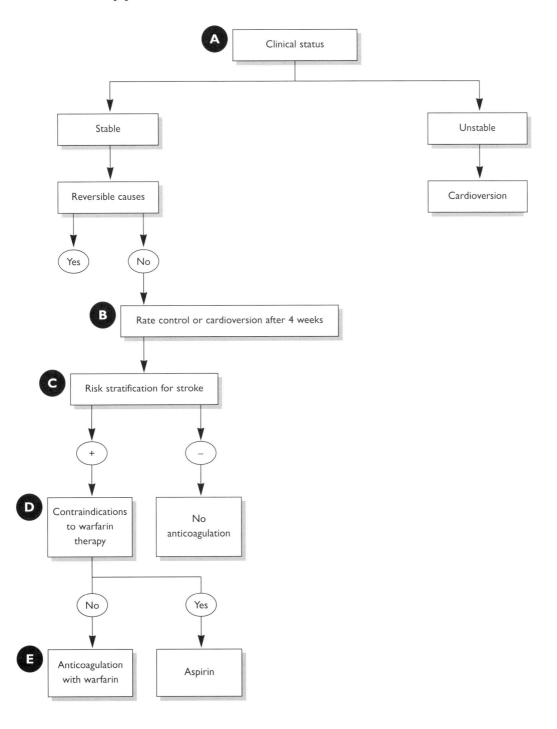

essential. Fixed low-dose warfarin trials have uniformly failed to show the benefit that is seen with dose-adjusted warfarin due to the failure to maintain patients in the therapeutic range.

Additional Reading

Atrial Fibrillation Investigators. Risk factor for stroke and efficacy of antithrombotic therapy in atrial fibrillation; analysis of pooled data from five randomized controlled trials. Arch Intern Med 1994;154:1449–57.

Connolly SJ, Laupacis A, Gent M, et al. Canadian Atrial Fibrillation Anticoagulation (CAFA) Study. J Am Coll Cardiol 1991;18:349–55.

Ezekowitz MD, Bridgers SL, James KE, et al, and SPINAF Investigators. Warfarin in the prevention of stroke asssociated with nonrheumatic atrial fibrillation. N Engl J Med 1992;327:406–12.

Peterson P, et al. Placebo-controlled, randomized trial of warfarin and aspirin for prevention of thromboembolic complications in chronic atrial fibrillation: the Copenhagen AFASAK Study. Lancet 1989;1:175–8.

Stroke Prevention in Atrial Fibrillation Investigators. Adjusted dose warfarin versus low-intensity, fixed-dose warfarin plus aspirin for high-risk patients with atrial fibrillation: stroke prevention in atrial fibrillation III randomized clinical trial. Lancet 1996;348:633–8.

Stroke Prevention in Atrial Fibrillation Investigators. Stroke prevention in atrial fibrillation study; final results. Circulation 1991;84:527–39.

The Boston Area Trial for Atrial Fibrillation Investigators. The effect of low-dose warfarin on the risk of stroke in patients with nonrheumatic atrial fibrillation. N Engl J Med 1990;323:1505.

Chapter 44

Valvular Heart Disease and Heart Valve Replacement

Alexander GG Turpie

NATIVE VALVE DISEASE

Prior to surgical implantation of prosthetic heart valves, native valvular disease, particularly rheumatic mitral valve disease, was associated with a significant risk of systemic embolism, of which stroke was the most frequent clinical manifestation.[1]

A Heart Valve Replacement

Almost all patients with severe valvular heart disease are now treated surgically with heart valve replacement. Thus, for most patients, the requirement for anti-thrombotic therapy is dependent on the thromboembolic risk associated with the valve replacement.

B No Additional Risk Factors

Valvular heart disease in the absence of additional risk factors such as atrial fibrillation or enlargement of the left atrium carries a low risk of systemic embolism, and in general, anticoagulant therapy is not indicated.

C Additional Risk Factors Present

Patients with native valve disease who have additional risk factors for systemic embolism should be considered for anticoagulant therapy. Although there are no randomized trials evaluating antithrombotic therapy in such patients, the American College of Chest Physicians (ACCP) developed recommendations for antithrombotic therapy in patients with valvular heart disease based on extrapolation from other studies involving patients with similar risk factors. These guidelines are largely empiric. A summary of the American College of Chest Physicians recommendations for antithrombotic therapy in valvular heart disease is given in Table 44.1.[1]

Table 44.1   Summary of the ACCP Recommendations for Patients with Native Valvular Disease

Rheumatic Mitral Valvular Disease	
Previous embolism	Oral anticoagulants INR 2.0–3.0
Atrial fibrillation	Oral anticoagulants INR 2.0–3.0
LA diameter >5.5 cm	Oral anticoagulants INR 2.0–3.0
Sinus rhythm and no left atrial enlargement	Anticoagulants optional
Recurrent embolism despite adequate oral anticoagulants (INR >2.0)	Add ASA (160–325 mg/day) or increase INR to 2.5–3.5
Mitral Valve Prolapse	
Uncomplicated	No antithrombotic treatment
Transient cerebral ischemia	ASA 325 mg/day
Systemic embolism, chronic or paroxysmal atrial fibrillation	Oral anticoagulants INR 2.0–3.0
Recurrent TIA despite ASA	Ticlopidine 250 mg or oral anticoagulants INR 2.0–3.0
Mitral Annular Calcification	
Uncomplicated	No antithrombotic treatment
Systemic embolism or atrial fibrillation	Oral anticoagulants INR 2.0–3.0
Aortic Valve Disease	
Sinus rhythm	No oral anticoagulants
Chronic atrial fibrillation or systemic embolism	Oral anticoagulants INR 2.0–3.0
Infective Endocarditis	
Sinus rhythm	No antithrombotic treatment
Mechanical prosthetic valve	Continue oral anticoagulants INR 2.5–3.5
Systemic embolism and native valve thrombus	Uncertain—consider oral anticoagulants if AF or LA

Levine HJ, et al. Chest 1995;108:360S–70S.

D *Heart Valve Replacement*

The development of new materials and improvement in the design of prosthetic valves has greatly improved the success of heart valve replacement surgery. Despite these improvements, however, thromboembolism remains a serious complication in patients after heart valve replacement. Oral anticoagulant therapy has greatly reduced the risk of thromboembolism in patients with mechanical prosthetic valves and in patients with tissue valves, if they have atrial fibrillation or a history of thromboembolism, and is generally recommended for life.

E *Bioprosthetic Heart Valves*

The risk of thromboembolism is less with bioprosthetic valves than with mechanical valves and some authorities suggest that they do not require anticoagulants, particularly if there are no additional risk factors. Although this recommendation remains controversial, most cardiac centers recommend oral anticoagulants for 3 months until the sewing ring is completely endothelialized.[1]

In uncomplicated patients with tissue valves, the highest risk of thromboembolism is in the first 3 months postoperatively but is present indefinitely in patients with atrial fibrillation.[2]

F *No Risk Factors*

Patients with bioprosthetic valves are at low risk of systemic embolism, particularly those with aortic prostheses.

G *ACCP Recommendations*

Anticoagulant therapy is recommended for 3 months (INR 2.0–3.0) in patients with mitral prostheses and is optional in patients with aortic prostheses. However, this latter recommendation is not universally accepted, and many authorities recommend 3 months of treatment for all patients.

H *Risk Factors Present*

Risk factors include atrial fibrillation, atrial thrombus detected at echocardiography, and development of a systemic embolism.

I *ACCP Recommendations*

The current guidelines by the American College of Chest Physicians for antithrombotic therapy for patients with tissue valves are shown in Table 44.2.[2]

J *Mechanical Prosthetic Heart Valves*

Patients with mechanical heart valve prostheses require life-long anticoagulation therapy.

K *Caged-Ball Valves*

In the 1995 guidelines, the American College of Chest Physicians recommended long-term oral anticoagulant therapy for patients with caged-ball valves, with a target International Normalized Ratio (INR) of 3.5 to 4.5.[2]

Table 44.2   Antithrombotic Therapy in Heart Valve Replacement

Bioprosthetic Valves	INR	Duration
Mitral	2.0–3.0	3 months
Aortic	A/C optional, 2.0–3.0	3 months
Atrial fibrillation	2.0–3.0	Long term
Left atrial thrombosis	2.0–3.0	3 month minimum, duration uncertain
Systemic embolism	2.0–3.0	3–12 months, duration uncertain

(Aspirin optional long-term in uncomplicated patients who are not anticoagulated)

Stein, et al. Chest 1995;108:371.

L *Tilting Disk or Bileaflet Valves*

For patients with tilting disk or bileaflet valves, the recommended INR is 2.5 to 3.5.

The recommendations for anticoagulant therapy for patients with mechanical valves by the American College of Chest Physicians are shown in Table 44.3.[2] The recommendations of an INR target of 2.5 to 3.5 is lower than that suggested in a report from Europe that recommended a higher target range of 3.0 to 4.0.[3] However, the European recommendation is based on retrospective data and largely on events that occurred in patients with older caged-ball valve prostheses. Thus, recommendations based on these data are unlikely to be applicable for use in patients with the modern bileaflet and tilting disc valves that are currently in use.

ANTIPLATELET PLUS ANTICOAGULANT THERAPY

A major limitation to the current approach used to treat high-risk patients with prosthetic heart valves is that systemic embolism, which may result in a disabling

Table 44.3   Antithrombotic Therapy in Heart Valve Replacement

Mechanical Valves (Type)	INR
Bileaflet	2.5–3.5
Tilting disc	2.5–3.5
Caged-ball/disc	Consider higher INR
Systemic embolism	2.5–3.5
	Plus aspirin 80 mg/day or dipyridamole 400 mg/day

Stein, et al. Chest 1995;108:371.

stroke, still occurs at a rate of approximately 2 to 3% per year, even with well-controlled anticoagulant therapy.

M *Anticoagulation Therapy*

The addition of platelet inhibitors to oral anticoagulants has been advocated as an approach to improve the treatment for patients with mechanical valves and patients with tissue valves at high risk of systemic embolism.[4,5]

SUMMARY

The demonstration that for most indications for oral anticoagulant therapy, less intense anticoagulation (INR 2.0 to 3.0) is as efficacious as standard intensity anti-coagulation (INR 3.0 to 4.5) but is associated with significantly less bleeding is an important advance.[6] This has greatly improved the safety of long-term oral anti-coagulant therapy and has resulted in its more widespread use in the prevention and treatment of thromboembolism. Thus, an INR of 2.0 to 3.0 is the level of choice in uncomplicated patients with tissue prostheses and in patients with native valvular disease without additional risk factors. However, further evidence is

Management of Valvular Heart Disease

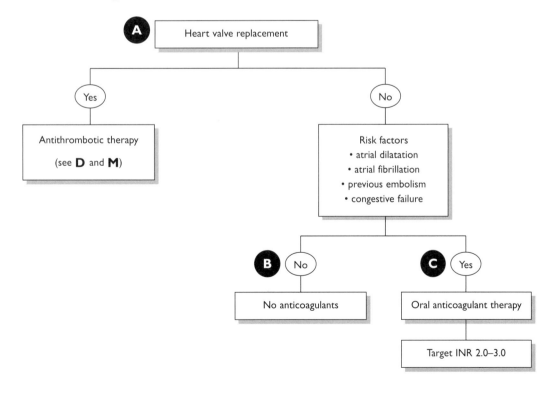

Heart Valve Replacement

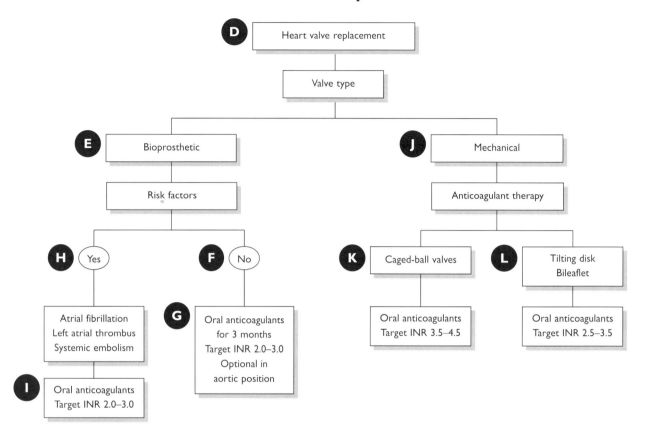

Heart Valve Replacement

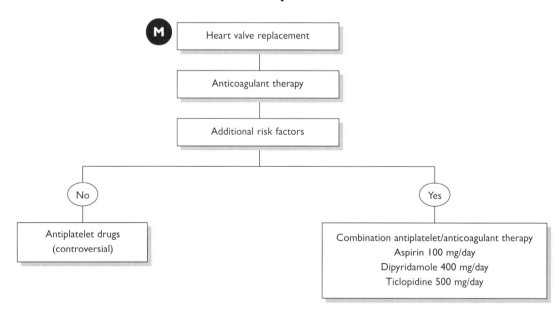

required before this less intense regimen is routinely adopted for patients with mechanical valves and patients with tissue valves at high risk for embolism. In this patient population, the recommended anticoagulant regimen is an INR of 2.0 to 3.0. The addition of low dose aspirin to anticoagulants is more efficacious in the prevention of systemic embolism and vascular death in heart valve replacement patients than anticoagulants alone. However, the risk of bleeding with the use of combination therapy may limit its use, particularly in older patients.

Bibliography

1. Levine HJ, Pauker SG, Eckman MH. Antithrombotic therapy in valvular heart disease. Chest 1995;108:360S–70S.
2. Stein PD, Alpert JS, Copeland JG, et al. Antithrombotic therapy in patients with mechanical and biological prosthetic heart valves. Chest 1995;108:371S–9S.
3. Cannegieter SC, Rosendaal FR, Wintzen AR, et al. Optimal oral anticoagulant therapy in patients with mechanical heart valves. N Engl J Med 1995;333(1):11–7.
4. Turpie AGG, Gent M, Laupacis A, et al. A comparison of aspirin with placebo in patients treated with warfarin after heart-valve replacement. N Engl J Med 1993;329:524–9.
5. Pouleur H, Buyse M. Effects of dipyridamole in combination with anticoagulant therapy on survival and thromboembolic events in patients with prosthetic heart valves. A meta-analysis of the randomized trials. J Thorac Cardiovasc Surg 1995;110:463–6.
6. Hirsh J, Dalen JE, Deykin D, Poller L. Oral anticoagulants: mechanism of action, clinical effectiveness and optimal therapeutic range. Chest 1995;108:231S–46S.

Chapter 45

ANTITHROMBOTIC THERAPY
IN PREGNANT PATIENTS WITH
VALVULAR HEART DISEASE

Agnes YY Lee

Jeffrey S Ginsberg

The optimal antithrombotic therapy for pregnant patients with valvular heart disease remains controversial. Although there is no doubt that patients with mechanical heart valves, or bioprosthetic valves plus atrial fibrillation or a history of thromboembolism, require continuation of their antithrombotic therapy during pregnancy, the choice of anticoagulant regimen (heparin alone, warfarin alone, or a combination of heparin and warfarin) is debated. Due to the lack of reliable data on the efficacy and safety of these regimens, there are no definitive recommendations. There are significant and potentially fatal risks for both the mother and fetus, and the final decision of which antithrombotic regimen is "best" should be made only after counseling the pregnant woman and her family so that an informed decision is based on balancing the risk of thromboembolism in the mother and the risk of potential congenital anomalies for the fetus.

A Prepregnancy Counseling

For women of childbearing age with either a mechanical or a bioprosthetic heart valve, prepregnancy counseling is essential. Although pregnancy is not absolutely contraindicated in these women, the maternal risk is increased, partly due to the cardiovascular changes associated with pregnancy and partly due to potential complications (both thromboembolic and hemorrhagic) from the anticoagulant therapy. Women with New York Heart Association Class III or IV heart disease should be advised to avoid pregnancy because maternal mortality is high and fetal prematurity is increased.[1-3] For patients with bioprostheses who do not require long-term anticoagulation, their tissue valves can deteriorate at an accelerated rate during pregnancy, necessitating replacement in up to 47% of cases.[2,4,5] Although surgical intervention during pregnancy can be performed safely in the mother, fetal mortality with cardiopulmonary bypass is 20%.[3]

Once pregnancy is considered, the woman must be informed of the maternal and fetal risks of pregnancy and anticoagulant therapy. Risks to the mother include increased likelihood of bleeding, thromboembolism despite antithrombotic therapy, and side effects specific to heparin treatment such as osteoporosis and heparin-induced thrombocytopenia. Risks to the fetus include warfarin embryopathy, central nervous system (CNS) anomalies, bleeding, and demise secondary to maternal morbidity[6] (see Chapter 15). The rates of spontaneous abortions and stillbirths are reportedly elevated, likely due to placental hemorrhage but the true incidences and etiology are unknown.

If the woman is not yet pregnant, she has the choice of continuing warfarin until pregnancy is confirmed, or switching to subcutaneous (SQ) heparin. The latter approach avoids warfarin exposure at conception for the fetus but can add months to the total duration of heparin exposure for the mother. This prepregnancy decision partly depends on the antithrombotic regimen the mother plans to use during her pregnancy. If she does not wish to expose the fetus to any warfarin, then she should switch to heparin before conception and carry through the pregnancy with SQ heparin; if she chooses to remain on warfarin throughout her pregnancy, then there is no need for heparinization. The woman who chooses the "combination" approach can conceive while on warfarin, monitor weekly for conception, then switch to SQ heparin as soon as pregnancy is confirmed. This will minimize maternal heparin exposure and avoid fetal warfarin exposure during weeks 6 to 12 of gestation when the risk of warfarin embryopathy is highest.

B *Review Maternal Options*

Once pregnancy is confirmed, the risks and options of antithrombotic therapy should be reviewed with the pregnant woman and her family. If she decides not to carry through with her pregnancy or if her health deteriorates significantly, then a therapeutic abortion should be offered as an option. In general, there are three different regimens for anticoagulation during pregnancy in patients with valvular heart disease: warfarin only, heparin only, or heparin and warfarin. Each is associated with a different degree of risk to the mother and the fetus. In our opinion, there are no right or wrong options, and the physician must be flexible to the needs of the patient and be vigilant in the monitoring of antithrombotic therapy and complications.

Recently, a randomized trial in nonpregnant patients with mechanical or bioprosthetic heart valves and either atrial fibrillation or previous thromboembolic events showed that the addition of low-dose aspirin (80 to 100 mg/d) to warfarin reduced mortality and major systemic embolism without a significant increase in major bleeding.[7] Although there is no comparable data on pregnant patients on a combination of heparin and aspirin, it is reasonable to add low-dose aspirin throughout pregnancy to any of the three anticoagulant regimens because of the high thromboembolic risk in this population. Women with the highest risks are those with previous thromboembolic events and those with older-generation mechanical valves (Starr-Edwards, Björk-Shiley), especially in the mitral position.[3,8,9] Antiplatelet agents alone are not adequate for prophylaxis in this group of patients.

C Warfarin Therapy

The manufacturers of Coumadin state that it is teratogenic and its use is contraindicated in pregnancy. However, advocates of the use of warfarin therapy throughout pregnancy believe the risk of thromboembolic events on heparin outweighs the risk of fetal anomalies from warfarin exposure.[2,9,10] Unfortunately, because prospective data are lacking, it is difficult to confirm or refute this belief. If a mother chooses to continue warfarin therapy throughout pregnancy, a therapeutic International Normalized Ratio (INR) of 2.5 to 3.5 for those with mechanical heart valves has been recommended by the American College of Chest Physicians (ACCP) consensus conference, 1995.[11] This is based on data from nonpregnant patients with mechanical valves. It is not known whether the pregnant patient warrants a higher therapeutic range. Thromboembolism has been reported in pregnant patients receiving oral anticoagulants.[2,9] This is more likely in those with older-generation valves and those with mechanical valves in the mitral position. For women with bioprosthetic valves and chronic atrial fibrillation, a therapeutic INR of 2.0 to 3.0 is likely adequate. Patients must be intensely monitored, with weekly INRs performed, while on warfarin therapy. When a patient fails on warfarin therapy, the choice of anticoagulation depends on the specific circumstances (e.g., subtherapeutic versus therapeutic INR, embolic versus thrombotic event) and the hemodynamic stability of the patient (see section I).

To avoid coagulopathy in the fetus at the time of delivery, we believe that patients on warfarin should be switched to SQ heparin at about 36 weeks of pregnancy (see sections F and G).

D Heparin and Warfarin Therapy

This option aims to minimize the risks of thromboembolic events in the mother and to prevent warfarin embryopathy in the fetus by using warfarin throughout pregnancy, except for weeks 6 to 12 and close to term. Subcutaneous heparin is given during these periods as twice daily injections. Dosing and monitoring of heparin therapy is discussed in section E. At week 13, warfarin is restarted and adjusted to a therapeutic INR of 2.5 to 3.5. Heparin is stopped only after the INR is within the therapeutic range for 2 consecutive days. At week 36, treatment is switched back to heparin to avoid coagulopathy in the fetus at delivery (see sections F and G). Warfarin exposure in this regimen is still associated with a low risk of (<5%), but potentially serious, fetal central nervous system (CNS) abnormalities (see Chapter 15), and thrombosis can occur during the short periods of heparin therapy. Salazar managed 40 pregnancies with 22 live births using this combination approach and reported no cases of warfarin embryopathy in all 16 infants examined by a geneticist, one case of myelomeningocele, and two cases of fatal, massive valve thrombosis in the mother while on SQ heparin. Both of the latter patients had Björk-Shiley valves.[10]

E *Heparin Therapy*

If the mother does not wish to risk any teratogenic effect from warfarin, heparin can be given throughout pregnancy. Recent studies showed that heparin therapy is not associated with any increased fetal morbidity.[12] The initial dose should be 17,500 to 20,000 units every 12 hours, adjusted to prolong the activated partial thromboplastin time (aPTT) to at least twice the control value at 6 hours after injection. Although there is no data to verify this approach, there is evidence that fixed low-dose SQ heparin (5000 units bid or less) and an aPTT ratio of 1.5 times control are inadequate.[10,13] Strict monitoring, by initially checking the aPTT daily until a therapeutic dose is determined, then by checking once weekly, is absolutely essential. Heparin requirement will fluctuate over time and will increase with gestation due to the rise in acute-phase plasma proteins to which heparin binds nonspecifically. Long-term heparin therapy is associated with increased maternal risk of osteoporosis and heparin-induced thrombocytopenia (see Chapter 15). Weekly platelet counts should be done while a patient is receiving heparin therapy.

The major concern for heparin therapy is its efficacy in preventing thromboembolic events. Failure of heparin, given via the SQ or intravenous (IV) route, has been documented in case reports and retrospective studies, sometimes with fatal consequences for the mother and fetus. Although SQ heparin is probably less effective than warfarin, it is uncertain whether heparin failure only occurs when the aPTT is inadequate. When SQ heparin therapy fails, warfarin is a better alternative than IV heparin.[14] Other alternatives depend on the type of complication and the hemodynamic status of the patient (see section I).

Low-molecular-weight heparins (LMWH) have received increasing attention as alternatives to unfractionated heparin for the treatment and prophylaxis of acute venous thrombosis. Although their use in pregnancy is not recommended by the ACCP 1995, these agents have been used safely in pregnant women with acquired or hereditary thrombophilia, or allergies to unfractionated heparin. Their use is especially attractive in pregnancy because LMWHs do not cross the placental barrier and are probably associated with reduced risks of bleeding, thrombocytopenia, and osteoporosis (see Chapter 15). Dulitzki recently reported using enoxaparin in 34 pregnant women for treatment or prophylaxis of venous thrombosis. Nineteen underwent surgical procedures and 9 received epidural anesthesia without excessive bleeding.[15] There are no published reports of LMWH use in pregnant patients with valvular heart disease.

F At Term (Week 36)

Because the fetal liver is immature and produces low concentrations of vitamin-K-dependent clotting factors, it is incapable of rapidly reversing the anticoagulant effect of warfarin.[9] There is a high risk of cerebral hemorrhage with vaginal delivery in a baby who is still anticoagulated.[9,11] Therefore, for all anticoagulant regimens, only heparin should be given starting at week 36. Dosing and monitoring of heparin are discussed in section E.

G Labour and Delivery

At the onset of spontaneous labour at term, SQ heparin should be stopped. The aPTT should be monitored closely because heparin clearance can be delayed and an anticoagulant effect can persist for up to 28 hours after the last injection.[16] If the aPTT is greater than 1.5 times control at the time of delivery, protamine sulfate should be given. If the aPTT is less than 1.5 times control, vaginal delivery and epidural anesthesia are not contraindicated, and a cesarean section should be performed only for obstetrical reasons.

Another way to avoid delivering an anticoagulated fetus is to arrange for an elective induction at term. The mother can be admitted to hospital, and SQ heparin is discontinued 24 hours prior to induction. Intravenous heparin should be started while preparing for induction, then stopped when labour starts. Protamine sulfate should be given if the aPTT is prolonged to greater than 1.5 times control at the time of delivery.

If a mother goes into premature labor (<36 weeks gestation) or is still on warfarin at the onset of labor, vitamin K 10 mg IV should be administered and the baby should probably be delivered by cesarean section because of high risk of traumatic cerebral hemorrhage from vaginal delivery (see section F).

Management of Pregnant Patients with Valvular Heart Disease

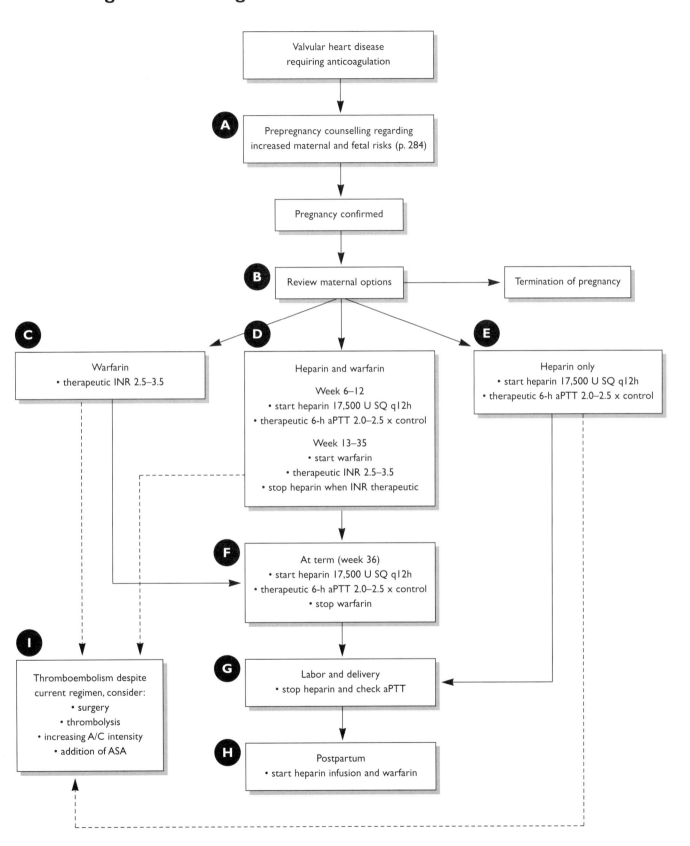

H *Postpartum*

Besides the need for indefinite anticoagulation in these women, the postpartum period is associated with a higher risk of thromboembolism. When hemostasis is achieved after delivery, intravenous heparin can be started. A standard bolus of 5000 units followed by an infusion of 30 to 35,000 units over 24 hours can be initiated within 24 to 48 hours of delivery. The aPTT should be adjusted to at least twice control or within the therapeutic range for the specific reagent used. Warfarin can be started the next day, aiming for a therapeutic INR of 2.5 to 3.5. When the INR is therapeutic for 2 consecutive days, heparin can be stopped. Both heparin and warfarin are safe for the breastfed infant because they are not secreted significantly into breast milk (see Chapter 15).

I *Thromboembolism Despite Anticoagulation*

Despite the most stringent monitoring of anticoagulant therapy, thromboembolic events can still occur during pregnancy. This is an extremely difficult and dangerous situation for both mother and fetus; without intervention, both may die. The optimal treatment for acute valvular thromboembolism in pregnant patients is unknown. There are three alternatives to consider: surgery to remove the valve thrombus and replace the valve, thrombolytic therapy, and/or intensification of anticoagulation. The successes and failures of these options have been the subject of case reports, and there are no criteria or guidelines to identify which is the best option under different circumstances. For valve thrombosis, a cardiovascular surgeon should be consulted to evaluate the potential risks and success of thrombectomy and valve replacement. Thrombolytic therapy has been successfully given without maternal or fetal adverse outcomes.[17,18] If the patient is hemodynamically stable with valve thrombosis, and/or has suffered an embolic event, intensification of the anticoagulation regimen, replacement of SQ heparin with warfarin, or addition of aspirin should be considered.

Bibliography

1. Born D, Martinez EE, Almeida PAM, et al. Pregnancy in patients with prosthetic heart valves: the effects of anticoagulation on mother, fetus, and neonate. Am Heart J 1992;124:413–7.

2. Sbarouni E, Oakley CM. Outcome of pregnancy in women with valve prostheses. Br Heart J 1994;71:196–201.

3. Sullivan HJ. Valvular heart surgery during pregnancy. Surg Clin North Am 1995;75:59–75.

4. Badduke ER, Jamieson RE, Miyashima RT, et al. Pregnancy and childbearing in a population with biological valvular prostheses. J Thorac Cardiovasc Surg 1991;102:179–86.

5. Lee CN, Wu CC, Lin PY, Hsieh FJ, Chen HY. Pregnancy following cardiac prosthetic valve replacement. Obstet Gynecol 1994;83:353–6.

6. Ginsberg JS, Hirsh J, Turner DC, Levine MN, Burrows R. Risks to the fetus of anticoagulant therapy during pregnancy. Thromb Haemost 1989;61:197–203.

7. Turpie AGG, Gent M, Laupacis A, et al. A comparison of aspirin with placebo in patients with treated with warfarin after heart-valve replacement. N Engl J Med 1993;329:524–9.

8. Sareli P, England MJ, Berk MR, et al. Maternal and fetal sequelae of anticoagulation during pregnancy in patients with mechanical heart valve prostheses. Am J Cardiol 1989;63:1462–5.

9. Oakley CM. Anticoagulants in pregnancy. Br Heart J 1995;74:107–11.

10. Salazar E, Izaguirre R, Verdejo J, Mutchinick O. Failure of adjusted doses of subcutaneous heparin to prevent thromboembolic phenomena in pregnant patients with mechanical cardiac valve prostheses. J Am Coll Cardiol 1996;27:1698–703.

11. Ginsberg JS, Hirsh J. Use of antithrombotic agents during pregnancy. Chest 1995;108(Suppl): 305S–11S.

12. Ginsberg JS, Kowalchuk G, Hirsh J, Brill-Edwards P, Burrow R. Heparin therapy during pregnancy: risks to the fetus and mother. Arch Intern Med 1989;149:2233–6.

13. Iturbe-Alessio I, Del Carmen Fonseca M, Mutchinik O, Santos MA, Zajarias A, Salazar E. Risks of anticoagulant therapy in pregnant women with artificial heart valves. N Engl J Med 1986;315:1390–3.

14. Golby AJ, Bush EC, DeRook FA, Albers GW. Failure of high-dose heparin to prevent recurrent cardioembolic strokes in a pregnant patient with a mechanical heart valve. Neurology 1992;42:2204–6.

15. Dulitzki M, Pauzner R, Langevitz P, Pras M, Many A, Schiff E. Low-molecular-weight heparin during pregnancy and delivery: preliminary experience with 41 pregnancies. Obstet Gynecol 1996;87:380–3.

16. Anderson DR, Ginsberg JS, Burrows R, Brill-Edwards P. Subcutaneous heparin therapy during pregnancy: a need for concern at the time of delivery. Thromb Haemost 1991;65:248–50.

17. Ramamurthy S, Talwar KK, Saxena A, Juneja R, Takkar D. Prosthetic mitral valve thrombosis in pregnancy successfully treated with streptokinase. Am Heart J 1994;127:446–7.

18. Turrentine MA, Braems G, Ramirez MM. Use of thrombolytics for the treatment of thromboembolic disease during pregnancy. Obstet Gynecol 1995;50:534–41.

Chapter 46

Antithrombotic Therapy in Patients with Left Ventricular Systolic Dysfunction

Eric Grubman

Evan Loh

Left ventricular systolic contractile dysfunction is the most common underlying cause of congestive heart failure (CHF). Reduced cardiac contractility is associated with an initially compensatory process, which results in hypertrophy, increased wall stress, and ventricular remodeling. The pathophysiologic causes of systolic dysfunction are varied, and are outlined in Table 46.1. Less commonly, CHF occurs secondary to diastolic dysfunction, which is characterized by normal left ventricular chamber dimensions, preserved systolic contractile function, and markedly reduced ventricular compliance. A decision-making algorithm for the use of antithrombotic therapy in patients with CHF secondary to left ventricular systolic dysfunction is the focus of this chapter.

Systolic Dysfunction and the Risk of Stroke

Systolic contractile dysfunction with left ventricular enlargement is associated with increased intracavitary stasis and decreased shear forces.[1] These factors predispose to left ventricular mural thrombus formation, which in turn, increases the risk of peripheral embolization. Thrombus formation in the right atrium or ventricle will most commonly embolize to the lungs, resulting in a pulmonary embolus. In contrast, thrombus formation in either the left atrium or ventricle may embolize to the systemic circulation, with a wide variety of possible consequences, including myocardial infarction, limb ischemia, and stroke.

The incidence of stroke in the presence of left ventricular systolic dysfunction depends upon many factors, including severity of left ventricular dysfunction, idiopathic versus ischemic etiology of the cardiomyopathy, temporal proximity to an acute myocardial infarction, the presence of symptomatic congestive heart failure,

Table 46.1   Common Causes of Congestive Heart Failure

Causes of Systolic Dysfunction	Causes of Diastolic Dysfunction
Alcohol-induced heart disease	Constrictive cardiomyopathy
Arrhythmias	Idiopathic hypertrophic subaortic stenosis (IHSS)
Beriberi	Restrictive cardiomyopathy
Idiopathic dilated cardiomyopathy	Hemochromatosis
Infective endocarditis	
Ischemic heart disease	
Hyperthyroidism	
Myocarditis	
Valvular heart disease	

atrial fibrillation, and visualizable left ventricular thrombus.[1–3] Despite the potentially devastating sequelae of an embolic event, the potentially protective effect of systemic anticoagulation continues to be debated.

The absence of a consensus recommendation for systemic anticoagulation in patients with left ventricular systolic dysfunction reflects the lack of prospective data defining a threshold reduction in left ventricular ejection fraction (LVEF) at which stroke risk exceeds the hemorrhagic risk associated with long-term systemic anticoagulation. Therapeutic strategies have also been clouded by studies suggesting a lack of benefit with systemic anticoagulation therapy or antiplatelet therapy with aspirin[4] in patients with congestive heart failure. Unfortunately, these studies have failed to include LVEF as a variable, and have used a combined endpoint of venous thromboembolic and arterial stroke events. Venous thromboembolic events (e.g., deep venous thrombosis and pulmonary embolism) may represent a disparate pathophysiologic mechanism, which may be alleviated by alternative therapies, which include 1) early mobilization; 2) use of subcutaneous heparin; and 3) venous compression stockings during the hospitalization admissions for congestive heart failure (see Chapter 3).

The goal of this chapter is to identify those patients at greatest risk for systemic embolic events, and to provide an algorithm that defines the role of antithrombotic therapy in these patients.

A *Signs and Symptoms of Patients with Heart Failure*

The clinical symptoms of patients with CHF represent the manifestation of the body's compensatory response to inadequate cardiac output by producing excessive levels of aldosterone, ADH, and renin. The kidneys act to retain fluid in an attempt to improve forward stroke volume (Frank-Starling mechanism). The clinical signs and symptoms of CHF reflect both the severity and chronicity of the heart failure syndrome. Patients with symptomatic CHF in the presence of left ventricular enlargement and decreased systolic function appear to have a significantly increased risk of stroke.

Acute impairment of left ventricular systolic function, such as that seen with acute myocardial ischemia, will result in a sudden increase in left heart filling pressures, followed by transudation of fluid into the alveoli of the lungs. Pulmonary rales will be evident on auscultation, initially in the dependent portions of the lung (bases). Insidious fluid retention with resultant weight gain is often the first sign of chronic CHF. Chronic elevations in left ventricular filling pressures will lead to progressive swelling of the lower extremities, evidence of jugular venous distention, abdominal fullness, liver engorgement, and right upper quadrant pain. Despite increases in total body volume, the absence of pulmonary rales on examination is commonly seen in patients with chronic CHF.

Volume overload secondary to left ventricular dysfunction with increased transudation of fluid into the alveoli impairs oxygen delivery to hemoglobin in the lungs. This increase in total lung water results in complaints of dyspnea on exertion, orthopnea, and paroxysmal nocturnal dyspnea. As lung water continues to increase, dyspnea may be present even with minimal physical activity or at rest. Chronic congestive heart failure is also associated with volume overload in the tissues that deliver blood to the right ventricle. This results in peripheral edema, which begins in the lowest and most gravity-dependent portion of the body, the feet and lower extremities. As the volume overload syndrome worsens, edema may extend upward through the legs, and eventually involve the abdomen and chest. Abdominal edema may give rise to hepatic congestion, which will result in right upper quadrant fullness and pain, with anorexia, nausea, and vomiting.

B   *Cardiac Echocardiography*

Echocardiography is perhaps the single most valuable diagnostic tool in the evaluation of patients with CHF. Two-dimensional echocardiography will provide important information about the presence of wall motion abnormalities, valvular disease, an accurate assessment of left ventricular systolic function, and the presence or absence of atrial or ventricular mural thrombi. Doppler echocardiography can enhance these data with information about the severity of valvular abnormalities and the presence or absence of diastolic dysfunction.

C   *Left Ventricular Systolic Dysfunction following Myocardial Infarction*

We used the Survival and Ventricular Enlargement (SAVE) trial[5] to evaluate post-myocardial infarction patients with LVEF ≤ 40% and no overt congestive heart failure, to determine 1) the cumulative and longitudinal risk of stroke; 2) the relationship of stroke to the extent of left ventricular dysfunction; and 3) the effect of systemic anticoagulation and antiplatelet therapy on stroke risk .

In the early, postmyocardial infarction phase of the SAVE trial prior to randomization to captopril or placebo (mean, 11 days post MI), we found a small risk of early stroke (0.5%). However, in contrast to previous reports, which suggested that the risk of stroke no longer increases after the first 3 months following myocardial infarction,[6] we reported a progressive stroke risk, which continued for the duration of the follow-up period of the SAVE trial (42 ± 10 months). Further, we demonstrated that the magnitude of reduction in LVEF, as a marker of left ventricular systolic dysfunction, was an independent predictor of stroke risk in patients following myocardial infarction. There was an 18% increase in stroke risk for every 5% reduction in LVEF over the duration of the study period. The postmyocardial infarction patients with LVEF ≤ 28% had the greatest stroke risk. These observations were true irrespective of the location of the infarction or whether the myocardial infarction was a Q-wave or non-Q-wave myocardial infarction. We observed an overall 81% reduction in total stroke risk in patients treated with systemic anticoagulation therapy and a 56% reduction in total stroke risk in patients treated with aspirin. These effects were observed with patients with an ejection fraction ≤ 28% and also those with an ejection fraction between 29% and 40%. Therefore, patients with left ventricular systolic dysfunction following myocardial infarction (LVEF ≤ 40%) should be strongly considered for systemic antithrombotic therapy.

The SAVE trial was designed specifically to include only patients without signs and symptoms of heart failure. Therefore, it appears that symptomatic heart failure may not be a major risk factor for stroke in this patient population. Despite observing that increasing age was an independent risk factor for increased stroke risk, recommendations for initiation of anticoagulant therapy in elderly patients with significant hemorrhagic potential should be balanced by the risk profile for increased bleeding tendencies (i.e., age, history of previous intracranial hemorrhage, recent trauma, history of bleeding dyscrasias, or unstable gait). We found that 96% of the strokes were ischemic in origin and that patients treated with systemic anticoagulation therapy did not appear to have an increased rate of hemorrhagic stroke. Nevertheless, if patients do possess absolute contraindications to systemic anticoagulation therapy, aspirin appears to be a reasonable therapeutic alternative.

D *Left Ventricular Systolic Dysfunction without Previous Myocardial Infarction*

The role of anticoagulation in patients whose systolic dysfunction is not due to myocardial ischemia is less well defined. Postmortem studies have revealed that up to 60% of patients with global systolic dysfunction as a result of a dilated cardiomyopathy had evidence of embolic events.[7] The majority of these embolic events were pulmonary emboli; however, stroke occurred in a significant number as well. In one retrospective study, the risk of stroke in patients with dilated cardiomyopathy appears to be decreased with the use of warfarin.[8] Further, in patients with dilated cardiomyopathies, the presence of left ventricular thrombus on echocardiographic evaluation, is felt to present a significant risk of distal embolization.[1] These patients should be strongly considered for long-term systemic antithrombotic therapy, although specific data concerning the optimal duration of therapy in these patients is lacking. In summary, in patients with dilated cardiomyopathy and reduced left ventricular ejection fraction (at least ≤ 40%) without absolute contraindications to systemic anticoagulant therapy, warfarin therapy should be strongly considered.

E *Duration of Anticoagulation Therapy*

Longitudinal and prospective data defining the incidence of stroke in patients with left ventricular dysfunction following myocardial infarction were unavailable prior to the SAVE stroke study. In contrast to previously reported literature and the current recommendations for anticoagulant therapy, we observed that a stroke risk continued to be present in each year of follow-up. Anticoagulant and/or antiplatelet therapy was beneficial over the entire duration of follow-up (mean follow-up = 42 months). These beneficial effects of anticoagulant therapy were also observed in each LVEF tercile, including patients with the least impairment in ventricular function (LVEF 35 to 40%). Therefore, at this time, it appears that therapy with warfarin should be continued indefinitely in patients with LVEF ≤ 40% following myocardial infarction.

F *Unanswered Questions*

Several questions regarding anticoagulation therapy in patients with left ventricular dysfunction remain unanswered. The first question is whether the current observations from the SAVE trial are applicable to patients with nonischemic systolic dysfunction or to patients with diastolic dysfunction. The second question is whether these recommendations apply to other syndromes associated with a clinical heart failure presentation, such as aortic or mitral insufficiency. The third question is whether to anticoagulate patients with other known risk factors for stroke such as atrial fibrillation. As stroke risk is known to be increased in patients with atrial fibrillation and preserved left ventricular systolic function,[9] clinical intuition guides our recommendations to more strongly favor systemic anticoagulation in these individuals who also have significant reductions in LVEF. The final important question

Left Ventricular Systolic Dysfunction

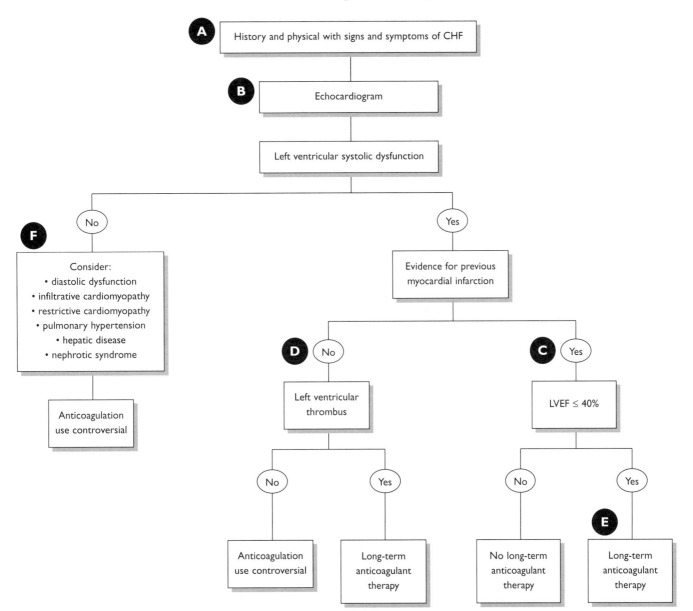

to resolve is at what INR range should these at-risk individuals be anticoagulated? A recent analysis of the ASPECT trial[10] suggested that the stroke rate fell at INR values of ≥ 2.0 while hemorrhagic complications (major CVA or hemorrhage requiring hospitalization or leading to death) rose precipitously at INR values ≥ 4.0. In postmyocardial infarction patients with left ventricular dysfunction, chronic therapy with warfarin to reduce the risk of ischemic cerebral stroke, carefully monitored to INR values between 2.0 and 4.0, should be the goal.

Recommendations

Patients with left ventricular dysfunction (LVEF ≤ 40%) secondary to ischemic heart disease regardless of the presence or absence of symptoms of CHF should be strongly considered for therapy with systemic anticoagulation. The INR range, at this time, should be between 2.0 and 4.0. In the absence of other absolute contraindications to systemic anticoagulation, patients with idiopathic cardiomyopathy and valvular heart dysfunction with severe left ventricular systolic dysfunction should be considered for anticoagulation therapy. At this time, in patients in whom warfarin may carry an unacceptable risk of bleeding, aspirin appears to be a reasonable therapeutic alternative.

Bibliography

1. Hirsh J, Fuster V. Guide to anticoagulant therapy. Part 2: oral anticoagulants. Circulation 1994;89:1469–80.

2. The Stroke Prevention in Atrial Fibrillation Investigators. Predictors of thromboembolism: II. echocardiographic features of patients at risk. Ann Intern Med 1992;116:6–12.

3. The Stroke Prevention in Atrial Fibrillation Investigators. Predictors of thromboembolism in atrial fibrillation: I. clinical features of patients at risk. Ann Intern Med 1992;116:1–5.

4. Dunkman WB, Johnson GR, Carson PE, et al. Circulation 1993;87:VI94–VI101.

5. Loh E, St. John Sutton M, Wun CC, et al. Ventricular dysfunction and the risk of stroke after myocardial infarction. N Engl J Med 1997;336:251–7.

6. Keating EC, Gross SA, Schlamowitz RA, et al. Mural thrombi in myocardial infarctions. Prospective evaluation by two-dimensional echocardiography. Am J Med 1983;74:989–95.

7. Roberts WC, Siegel RJ, McManus BM. Idiopathic dilated cardiomyopathy: analysis of 152 necropsy patients. Am J Cardiol 1987;60:1340–55.

8. Fuster V, Gersh BJ, Giuliani ER, et al. The natural history of idiopathic dilated cardiomyopathy. Am J Cardiol 1981;47:525–31.

9. Laupacis A, Albers G, Dalen J, et al. Antithrombotic therapy in atrial fibrillation. Chest 1995;108:352S–9S.

10. Azar AJ, Cannegieter SC, Deckers JW, et al. Optimal intensity of oral anticoagulant therapy after myocardial infarction. J Am Coll Cardiol 1996;27:1349–55.

Chapter 47

INVESTIGATION OF ACUTE RETINAL ISCHEMIA

Robert J Duke

Acute visual failure is a medical emergency and most often represents an ocular stroke. Even when visual loss is transient, prompt attention and investigation are warranted to identify either ocular or systemic causes. The algorithm in this chapter, based on the temporal profile as well as a funduscopic examination, will allow appropriate management of patients with acute visual failure.

A *History and Physical Examination*

A detailed history will usually allow one to determine whether the visual disturbance has been monocular or binocular. Inability to read or see faces properly implies a binocular visual disturbance but patients can mistake hemianopic vision for visual loss in one eye. Knowing the character of the visual loss is often helpful; is it, for example, the scintillations and fortification spectra of migraine that evolve over minutes, the abrupt shade or blind-like visual loss of embolic amaurosis fugax, or the iris-like loss of vision with ocular hypoperfusion or presyncope? A focused general physical examination can identify evidence of carotid atherosclerosis, hypertension, hyperlipidemia, and cardiac sources for the emboli.

B *Transient versus Persistent Visual Disturbance*

Patients with acute visual failure are best divided into those with transient visual disturbance and those with persistent visual loss. On physical examination of the patient with persistent visual loss, visual field examination will allow one to determine whether the lesion responsible is monocular (anterior to the optic chiasm) or binocular, which would generally indicate either bilateral ocular pathology or a solitary lesion at or behind the chiasm. The ocular fundus provides a unique opportunity for visual analysis of vessels, hemorrhages, and retinal infarctions (Figures 47.1 to 47.5). When funduscopic examination appears normal but the patient is blind ("the patient sees nothing, and the doctor sees nothing"), retrobulbar ischemia, inflammation, or compression are most likely, and the temporal profile determines the pathologic probabilities. Nonorganic monocular blindness can easily be identified by the persistence of normal pupillary light reflexes.

C   Presence of Scintillations

In the evaluation of a patient reporting transient visual disturbance, it is helpful to determine whether positive phenomena such as scintillations were experienced. Such features are highly characteristic of a migrainous mechanism, even in the absence of headache, particularly when the disturbance evolves gradually over several minutes.

D   Transient Binocular Visual Loss

Transient binocular visual loss can occur as brief obscurations related to papilledema, and are most typically seen in benign intracranial hypertension, and are often

Table 47.1   Funduscopic Findings Associated with Acute Visual Failure

Condition	Arteries	Veins	Disc	Retina	Vision
Central retinal artery occlusion	Narrowed, segmentation of blood column Embolus in 20%	Boxcar segmentation, blood dark	Normal or pale	White opaque, cherry red macula	Sudden blindness (see Figure 47.1)
Branch retinal artery occlusion	Embolic occlusion	Normal	Normal	Focal white retinal infarct	Sectoral defect (see Figures 47.2 and 47.3)
Anterior ischemic optic neuropathy	Normal	Normal	Pale, swollen one or more flame hemorrhages on disc	Normal	Severe loss often altitudinal
Posterior ischemic optic neuropathy	Normal	Normal	Normal early	Normal	Severe loss
Central retinal vein occlusion	Normal	Dilated, tortuous dark	Swollen	"Blood and thunder" blot and dot (deep), flame-shaped (nerve fibre layer)	Variable (see Figure 47.4)
Branch retinal vein occlusion	Often sclerotic	Locally dilated, tortuous	Normal	Focal hemorrhages ± cotton wool spots (infarcts)	Variable (see Figure 47.5)

Table 47.2   Comparison of Three Types of Microemboli in Retinal Arterioles

	Cholesterol	Platelet-Fibrin	Calcific
Colour	Orange-yellow bright metalic gold	Gray-white nonreflective	Gray-white nonreflective
Shape	Irregular, angulated	Long with flat ends	Discrete ovoid
Size	Appear larger than blood column	Same as blood column	Same or larger than blood column
Source	Eroding atheroma in carotid bifurcation	Mural or tail thrombus in carotid	Calcific valve or aorta

triggered by postural change. Transient binocular visual loss can also be a benign condition with presyncope and stretch syncope of adolescence but may also reflect focal transient ischemia of calcarine cortex due to atheroemboli.

E *Transient Monocular Visual Loss*

Transient monocular visual loss is most frequently due to platelet or cholesterol emboli from atherosclerotic plaque in the ipsilateral internal carotid artery. Investigation and management of amaurosis fugax is addressed in sections G to K.

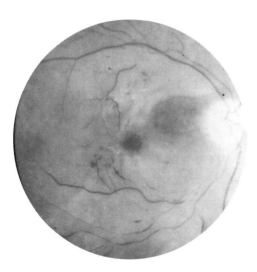

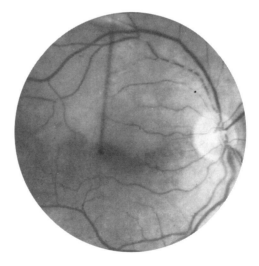

Figure 47.1   Central Retinal Artery Occlusion. This 59-year-old woman awoke following right carotid endarterectomy to note loss of vision in the ipsilateral eye. Note the pale infarcted retina contrasting with the normally perfused choroid seen through the normal thin macular area ("cherry red macula") and the attenuated and segmented arteries.

Figure 47.2   Branch Retinal Artery Occlusion. This 75-year-old man presented with sudden blurring in one eye. Note the segmented blood column in the superior temporal retinal artery and pallor of the superior retina indicating early infarction.

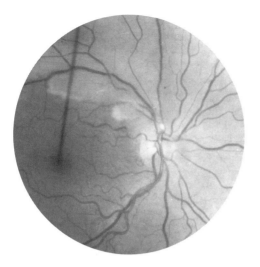

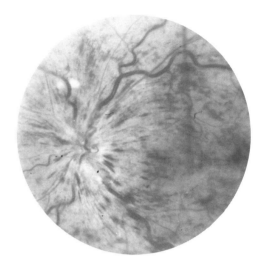

Figure 47.3 Branch Retinal Artery Occlusion. This 45-year-old woman with rheumatic mitral valve disease complained of black spots in the vision of her right eye. Note the calcific embolus at the disc margin, the attenuated and irregular caliber of the superior temporal retinal artery, and the associated pale infarcted retina.

Figure 47.4 Central Retinal Vein Occlusion. This 66-year-old man presented with sudden loss of vision in the left eye: VA 20/100. Note engorged tortuous veins, disc edema, and widespread, mostly flame-shaped hemorrhages.

F Common Fundoscopic Changes

Familiarity with the common expected pathologies and fundoscopic appearance will frequently allow even the nonexpert fundoscopist to make a secure diagnosis of the various conditions associated with both arterial and venous vascular insufficiency, which can cause sudden visual loss (see Table 47.1 and Figures 47.1 to 47.5). Central retinal artery and branch retinal artery occlusions are most frequently the result of hypertension and arteriolar sclerosis. Anterior or posterior ischemic optic neuropathy is especially important since this is frequently due to giant cell arteritis and demands rapid investigation, including ESR. If the ESR is elevated, temporal artery biopsy should be performed, and corticosteroid treatment should be initiated.[1] With severe visual loss seen in the first 24 hours high-dose intravenous corticosteroid treatment may be helpful in improving recovery.[2] Because retinal veins and arteries share a common adventitial sheath, and because the lamina cribrosa's sieve-like structure limits expansion and displacement of vessels within the optic nerve, the most frequent cause of retinal venous thrombosis is that of retinal arterial disease. Less frequently, hypercoagulable states and hyperviscosity states, including macroglobulinemia, are causative. In acute central retinal artery occlusions, maneuvers that are reported to be helpful include ocular massage and nitroglycerin.[3] Thrombolysis, although helpful in some cases, has been associated with significant risk of intraocular hemorrhage.

Formal ophthalmological consultation is recommended in patients suspected of having retinal vascular insufficiency. Such evaluation often includes fluorescein angiography, which has become indispensable in the diagnosis and evaluation of many retinal conditions. An ophthalmologist is also vital to the recognition and treatment of complications such as glaucoma and neovascularization.

G   Amaurosis Fugax

Amaurosis fugax can be defined as transient monocular visual loss attributed to ischemia or vascular insufficiency. Typically, patients describe diminished or absent vision in one eye, which develops over a few seconds and lasts for seconds to a few minutes. The impairment may involve the entire visual field or may selectively affect a sector of vision. Attacks are often described as being like a "curtain drawn downward," or less often sideways. A rare but unique symptom correlating strongly with high-grade ipsilateral carotid stenosis is loss of vision in conditions of bright light, such as going out of doors on a bright day. This is analogous to claudication of the retina where the metabolic demands cannot be met due to impaired arterial supply. Although systemic hypotension is a rare cause of monocular visual loss, when it is responsible, it generally causes a circumferential or iris-like loss of vision.

H   Biochemical Tests for Systemic Disease

The initial recommended blood work to detect systemic illness includes a complete blood count (looking for evidence of polycythemia or leukemia), platelet count (for evidence of thrombocytosis), a sedimentation rate (for evidence of giant cell arteritis), and blood sugar (for evidence of diabetes). The value of a routine search for a prothrombotic state has not been established, but such tests might be warranted

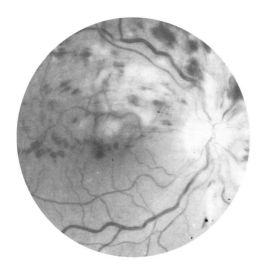

Figure 47.5   Branch Retinal Artery Occlusion. This 55-year-old woman presented with sudden painless loss of vision in her right eye. Note venous dilatation, hemorrhages, and cotton wool spots in the superior and nasal retina. Fluorescein angiography revealed capillary nonfilling in this area.

Acute Visual Failure

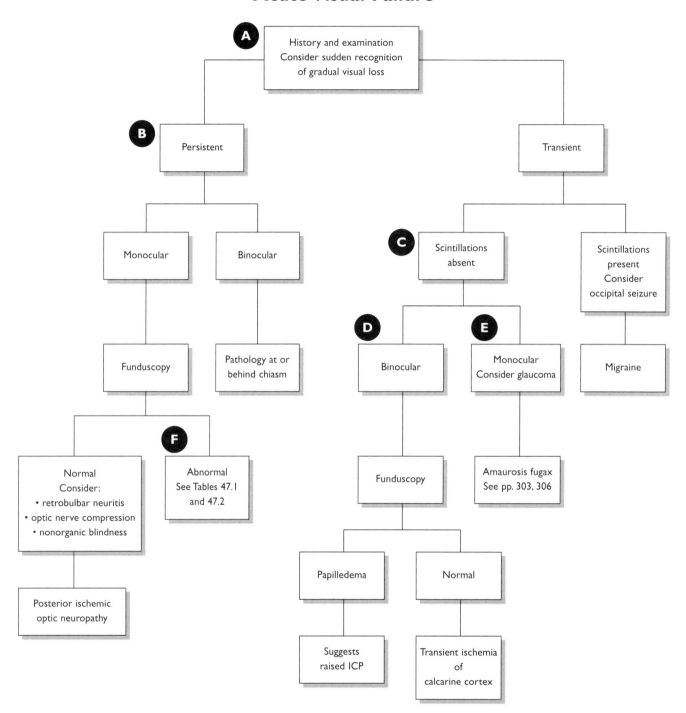

Amaurosis Fugax

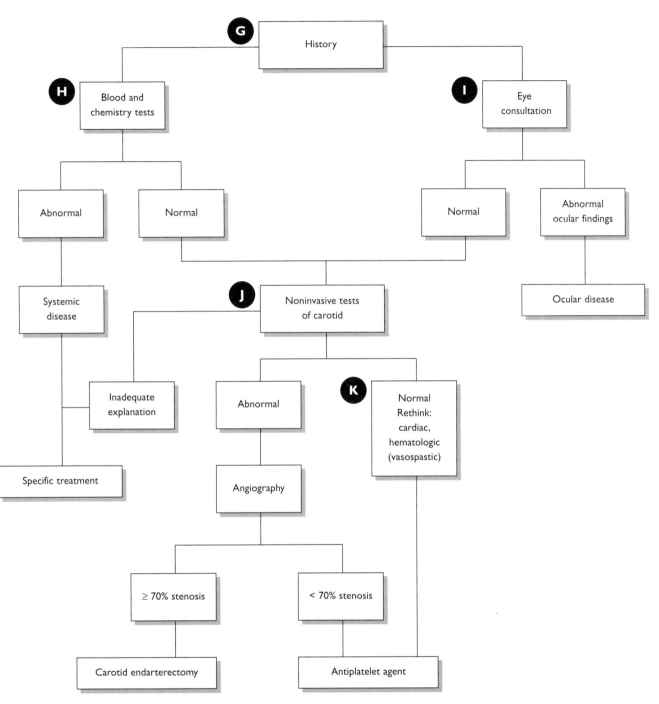

in younger patients or those with systemic symptoms, known malignancy, or other systemic diseases.[4]

I Ophthalmological Examination

An eye consultation is especially helpful in patients with atypical symptoms, or if one's own funduscopic skills are deficient. Rarely, glaucoma can produce episodes indistinguishable from amaurosis fugax.

J Investigation in Retinal Ischemic Syndromes

Patients with amaurosis fugax or other retinal ischemic syndromes, including asymptomatic retinal cholesterol emboli, are at significant risk of both stroke and coronary events.[5,6,7] Noninvasive investigations are useful in screening for significant atherosclerosis at the carotid bifurcation but in most instances, arteriography is advised before a final decision concerning endarterectomy is made (see Chapter 39).

K Treatment after Negative Workup

After extensive investigation, some patients with amaurosis fugax are found to have no definable abnormalities. Most such patients can be managed satisfactorily with antiplatelet medication but a small number who have had frequent and prolonged attacks and some of whom have had migraine appear to respond successfully to calcium channel blockers.[8]

Bibliography

1. Diamond JP. Treatable blindness in temporal arteritis. Br J Ophthalmol 1991;75:432.
2. Matzkin DC, Slamovits TL, Sachs R, Burde RM. Visual recovery in two patients after IV methylprednisolone treatment of central retinal artery occlusion secondary to giant cell arteritis. Ophthalmology 1992;99:68–71.
3. Charness ME, Liu GT. Central retinal artery occlusion in giant cell arteritis: treatment with nitroglycerin. Neurology 1991;41:1698.
4. The Amaurosis Fugax Study Group. Current management of amaurosis fugax. Stroke 1990; 21:201–8.
5. Bruno A, Jones WL, Austin JK, Carter S, Qualls C. Vascular outcome in men with asymptomatic retinal cholesterol emboli: a cohort study. Ann Intern Med 1995;122:249–53.
6. Chawluk JB, Kushner MJ, Bank WJ, et al. Atherosclerotic carotid artery disease in patients with retinal ischemic syndromes. Neurology 1988;38:858–63.
7. Hankey GJ, Slattery JM, Warlow CP. Prognosis and prognostic factors of retinal infarction: a prospective cohort study. BMJ 1991;302:499–504.
8. Gautier J-C. Amaurosis fugax. N Engl J Med 1993;329:426–7.

Additional Reading

Sandborn GE, Magargal LE. Arterial obstruction disease of the eye. In: Duane's clinical ophthalmology. Vol. 3. Lippincott-Raven, 1996.

Sandborn GE, Magargal LE, Jaeger EA. Venous occlusive disease of the retina. In: Duane's clinical ophthalmology. Vol. 3. Lippincott-Raven, 1996.

Wray SH. The management of acute visual failure. JNNP 1993;56:234–40.

Section 3

HEMOSTASIS

Chapter 48

Clinical Assessment
of Excessive Bleeding

Irwin Walker

The aim of the clinical assessment of excessive bleeding is to determine the likelihood, and the severity, of a bleeding disorder. The results of an accurate and detailed clinical assessment will indicate either that a bleeding disorder is unlikely, and thereby help avoid unnecessary investigation, or will guide the extent, type, and interpretation of subsequent laboratory tests. Also, the clinical assessment is critical, in conjunction with test results, in determining the severity of the bleeding disorder.

Bleeding disorders are characterized by (1) spontaneous bleeding into skin, mucous membranes, or internal organs, (2) excessive or prolonged bleeding following trauma or minor surgery, and/or (3) bleeding from more than one site.

Bleeding disorders are relatively uncommon, and most episodes of excessive bleeding result from trauma or local causes. Therefore, the occurrence of excessive bleeding should not automatically prompt an investigation for a bleeding disorder. Bleeding disorders may be suspected when episodes are spontaneous but certain types of bleeding, such as menorrhagia, epistaxis, and skin bruising, occur most commonly in the absence of a bleeding disorder. Bleeding that occurs immediately or soon after trauma or surgery is also most commonly due to a local cause; however, it may be the first manifestation of a bleeding disorder. In general, when the episode is unexpected, when the bleeding is repetitive, when the manifestations are suggestive, and/or when the background medical or family histories raise its likelihood, a bleeding disorder can be suspected.

Clinical assessment conventionally involves history followed by physical examination. However, when bleeding occurs, this sequence is often reversed or merged, and sometimes it is an abnormal laboratory test result that first prompts the assessment. Hence, this guide does not prescribe a rigid sequence to data gathering. The approach helps to identify critical questions and indicates the information needed to answer them. Though laboratory results may ultimately contribute valuable data to the answering of these questions, this guide concentrates on the clinical assessment.

A *Is a Bleeding Disorder Likely?*

Some situations are highly suggestive of a bleeding disorder and require immediate action and investigation. These include bleeding that is both spontaneous and occurring at multiple sites, is accompanied by petechiae or large or multiple ecchymoses, and is occurring in unusual sites, such as the stump of the umbilicus or the joints.

Bleeding that occurs at only one site, even if spontaneous, has a low likelihood of being due to a bleeding disorder. This is true for most sites of bleeding including the gastrointestinal, urinary, respiratory, and genital tracts. When bleeding occurs at a single site, additional evidence is required.

Evidence that increases the likelihood of a bleeding disorder includes a previous history of abnormal bleeding, a predisposing medical background, and a positive family history. Anticoagulant therapy or other medications, renal failure, liver failure, and diseases that predispose to thrombocytopenia, such as a hematological malignancy or systemic lupus erythematosus, may also increase the likelihood of a bleeding disorder. Evidence of lesser weight is repeated or prolonged bleeding in the face of negative investigations for a local cause or failure to control bleeding by local measures.

Spontaneous skin bleeding is frequent and readily attracts attention but it is not usually due to a bleeding disorder. Skin bruising occurs very commonly in women and children. In women, it is usually a manifestation of the benign "simple easy bruising" syndrome; in children, bruises are mostly due to trauma caused by the rough and tumble of play. In either case, bruises larger than 2 to 3 cm, more than two to three at once, bruises which are raised or bruises away from usual sites of trauma should lead to a consideration of either a bleeding disorder, or physical abuse. Physical abuse may also be suspected because of psychosocial circumstances. Bruising is uncommon in men, and its occurrence merits more detailed attention. Two types of skin bleeding that should be readily recognized as not being due to a bleeding disorder are bruises due to atrophy of subcutaneous tissue, occurring on the forearms of older individuals, and petechiae on the face following vomiting, particularly in children.

Abnormal bleeding following surgery or trauma may be the only manifestation of a bleeding disorder but is most often due to local causes. A single episode of bleeding, by itself, does not usually raise suspicion; however, suspicion should be higher if bleeding follows a first surgery, if bleeding continues despite corrective surgical measures, or if excessive bleeding has followed previous surgeries. Additional evidence is the presence of a predisposing medical condition or positive family history.

Certain operations are particularly prone to result in bleeding, both intra- and postoperatively; in these situations, bleeding, as a single event, does not constitute strong evidence of a bleeding disorder. Examples include wisdom tooth extraction, tonsillectomy, sinus surgery, major abdominal surgery, particularly hepatectomy and abdominoperineal resection, and major orthopedic procedures such as hip replacement. Conversely, absence of bleeding following these surgeries constitutes strong evidence against a bleeding disorder, and this is discussed further below.

The absence of supporting evidence, as outlined above, usually excludes major bleeding disorders. However, mild disorders may be missed because suitable hemostatic challenges may not have been encountered. Thus, a negative bleeding history can have different meanings, depending on whether the subject has been challenged. It is particularly important to obtain a history of hemostatic challenges because a bleeding disorder can often be excluded by a lack of bleeding following multiple or highly significant challenges. A lack of bleeding after one or more such challenges may exclude a congenital bleeding disorder or pinpoint the earliest time of onset of an acquired disorder.

B *What Type of Disorder is Present?*

The type of disorder—coagulation factor deficiency, platelet disorder, or vascular disorder—can best be ascertained when bleeding is spontaneous rather than when induced by surgery or trauma. Knowing that bleeding occurs only when induced is valuable because it suggests the type of disorder and also indicates that the disorder is likely mild in degree. An exception is delayed bleeding, which is much more suggestive of a coagulation disorder. The scope of surgery or trauma needed to induce the episodes helps to decide the severity of the disorder.

The type of disorder can often be ascertained when bleeding is spontaneous. Hemarthroses, large ecchymoses, deep hematomas, or major bleeding into multiple sites suggest the presence of a coagulation defect. Umbilical cord bleeding is highly suggestive of factor XIII deficiency, and bleeding into mucous membranes is typical of von Willebrand disease. Petechiae, which are not seen in coagulation disorders, indicate the presence of either a platelet or vascular disorder. Bleeding from vascular disorders usually take on specific appearances that are often sufficient for an accurate diagnosis. Examples are petechiae on the back of the legs and buttocks in Henoch-Schönlein purpura, perifollicular petechiae in scurvy, subdermal extravasations induced by steroids or occurring in aging skin, ecchymoses around the eyes (raccoon distribution) or in the skin folds in amyloidosis, small bruises, usually on the thighs or upper arms of women in "simple easy bruising," the typical angiomatous lesions of hereditary hemorrhagic telangiectasia (Rendu-Osler-Weber), and palpable petechiae of a vasculitis.

Finally, the family history may add information. For example, a history of dominant inheritance supports a diagnosis of von Willebrand disease, of sex-linked inheritance of hemophilia, while a recessive inheritance is more typical of a platelet function defect.

C Is the Disorder Congenital or Acquired?

The age at onset of bleeding and family history are the most important pieces of information when deciding whether the disorder is congenital or acquired. However, the information is often incomplete or ambiguous, and one should be aware of its limitations. With regard to family history, small families and recessive or sex-linked inheritances may result in a "false-negative" history. A complete history of surgeries and other challenges should be taken, as the absence of bleeding after one or more significant challenges earlier in life may effectively rule out a congenital disorder. When the bleeding defect is mild and there have been no significant hemostatic challenges, the first clinical manifestation may by delayed until adulthood, or even old age.

D Is the Bleeding Disorder Likely to Be Serious?

An assessment of the severity of the disorder is necessary to guide the speed with which investigation should proceed and to allow suitable counseling to the patient. In some instances, laboratory tests will provide an accurate measure of severity, for example, factor levels in the case of hemophilia. In other cases laboratory results need to be correlated with clinical history; for example, in factor XI deficiency, the severity of bleeding does not closely parallel the factor levels. If bleeding seems to be serious, rapid action is needed. Serious bleeding is suggested by spontaneous onset, involvement of multiple sites, major extent, occurrence in critical anatomic sites such as the mouth, neck, and internal organs, and by repetitive bleeding in response to multiple hemostatic challenges. The most serious and dramatic situation is the sudden onset of generalized bleeding in individuals who have no previous history of bleeding, and these cases demand immediate assessment and investigation. Most cases are due to one of three causes: disseminated intravascular coagulation, acquired factor VIII inhibitor, or severe thrombocytopenia.

Additional Reading

White II GC, Marder VJ, Colman RW, Hirsh J, Salzman EW. Approach to the bleeding patient. In: Colman RW, Hirsh J, Marder VJ, Salzman EW, eds. Hemostasis and thrombosis: basic principles and clinical practice. 3rd edn. Philadelphia: J.B. Lippincott Co., 1994.

Clinical Assessment of Excessive Bleeding

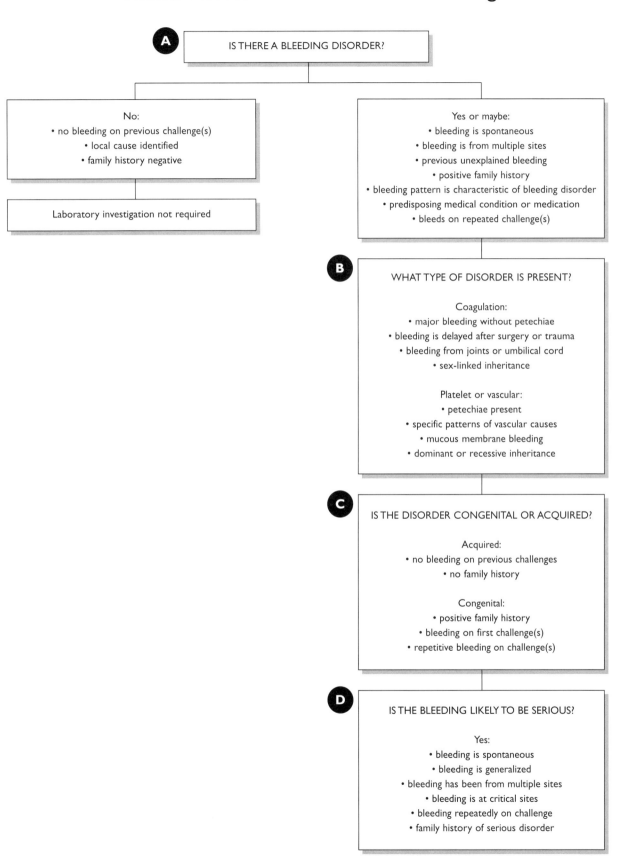

A IS THERE A BLEEDING DISORDER?

No:
- no bleeding on previous challenge(s)
- local cause identified
- family history negative

Laboratory investigation not required

Yes or maybe:
- bleeding is spontaneous
- bleeding is from multiple sites
- previous unexplained bleeding
- positive family history
- bleeding pattern is characteristic of bleeding disorder
- predisposing medical condition or medication
- bleeds on repeated challenge(s)

B WHAT TYPE OF DISORDER IS PRESENT?

Coagulation:
- major bleeding without petechiae
- bleeding is delayed after surgery or trauma
- bleeding from joints or umbilical cord
- sex-linked inheritance

Platelet or vascular:
- petechiae present
- specific patterns of vascular causes
- mucous membrane bleeding
- dominant or recessive inheritance

C IS THE DISORDER CONGENITAL OR ACQUIRED?

Acquired:
- no bleeding on previous challenges
- no family history

Congenital:
- positive family history
- bleeding on first challenge(s)
- repetitive bleeding on challenge(s)

D IS THE BLEEDING LIKELY TO BE SERIOUS?

Yes:
- bleeding is spontaneous
- bleeding is generalized
- bleeding has been from multiple sites
- bleeding is at critical sites
- bleeding repeatedly on challenge
- family history of serious disorder

Chapter 49

Investigation
of Abnormal Bleeding

Irwin Walker

A Pretest Stage

A thorough clinical evaluation, as outlined in Chapter 48, must precede the laboratory investigation. There is no single laboratory test which will establish, or exclude,
the presence of all bleeding disorders; that is, there is no universal screening test.
Neither is there a single test which will determine the type of disorder. The clinical
evaluation determines the likelihood that a bleeding disorder is present, its type,
and whether it is likely to be congenital or acquired. From this, the type and extent
of laboratory testing required is detemined. The routine use of preoperative global
tests, that is, testing in the absence of a clinical assessment of hemostasis, is discouraged. The performance of a platelet count is an exception.

B Hemostasis Screen

Hemostasis is a complex process involving vessel walls, platelets, and coagulation; it
is described in Chapter 51. Laboratory testing of hemostasis involves the performance of global function tests, usually called screening tests, followed by specific
testing of individual components, either qualitatively or quantitatively, and finally,
observing platelet morphology. Tests may be classified as those pertaining to the
coagulation system and those pertaining to platelets. Testing is mostly in vitro. A
number of in vivo tests, in previous use, have been discontinued, and only the
bleeding time and measurement of platelet life span continue to be performed.
Lately, the sensitivity and specificity of the bleeding time have been challenged, and
its use has decreased.

It is important to consider the sensitivity, specificity, and appropriateness of
screening tests. Screening tests of coagulation lack sensitivity to mild single factor
deficiencies, and specific factor assays should be performed if such defects are suspected. For some disorders, there are no satisfactory screening tests, and specific
tests need to be performed at the outset, for example, in factor XIII deficiency,

α_2-antiplasmin deficiency, and von Willebrand disease. On the other hand, screening tests are generally satisfactory to exclude acquired coagulation disorders, such as occur with liver failure, disseminated intravascular coagulation, and acquired factor VIII antibodies.

Before testing is performed, the clinical probability of a bleeding disorder and the nature of the disorder, either coagulation or platelet/vascular and either congenital or acquired, should be determined.

Three screening tests of coagulation are commonly performed: activated partial thromboplastin time (aPTT) tests the intrinsic pathway; prothrombin time (PT) tests the extrinsic pathway; and thrombin clotting time (TCT) tests the conversion of fibrinogen to fibrin, the final step in coagulation. For each screening test, coagulation is stimulated in a specific way and the time to clot formation is observed.

In aPTT, coagulation is initiated by the addition of a contact acting surface, such as kaolin or silica, calcium is added to reverse the action of the citrate anticoagulant, and phospholipid is added as a platelet substitute. In PT, tissue factor and phospholipid, usually obtained as an animal brain extract, are added to plasma along with calcium. Prothrombin time is reported as the International Normalized Ratio (INR). The final step of coagulation, the conversion of fibrinogen to fibrin, is tested by thrombin clotting time (TCT). In this test, coagulation is initiated by the addition of thrombin. A simple scheme of coagulation and the basic tests employed are summarized in Figure 49.1.

Some common coagulation defects and their pattern of tests results are as follows: liver disease affects the production of all factors except factor VIII; hence aPTT, PT, and TCT may all be prolonged (TCT is prolonged only in the late stages of liver disease as the fibrinogen level falls late). Vitamin K deficiency, including that induced by coumarin therapy, affects factors in both the intrinsic and extrinsic pathways (see Figure 49.1); thus, both aPTT and PT are prolonged but TCT is unaffected. Factor VIII or IX deficiency (as in hemophilia A and B), as well as the presence of factor VIII inhibitors, results in prolongation only of aPTT. Disseminated intravascular coagulation (DIC) causes multiple factor deficiencies; hence all tests may be prolonged, but classically it is the fibrinogen level, and hence TCT, which is most affected. Heparin inhibits thrombin and factor Xa; however, only aPTT and TCT are commonly prolonged, PT being prolonged only when heparin levels are high.

The tests, aPTT, PT, TCT, platelet count, and bleeding time (BT), are often combined and ordered together as a "hemostasis screen." However, this screen is not uniformly reliable. Negative results generally exclude thrombocytopenia and acquired coagulation disorders but the screen lacks sensitivity for mild hereditary bleeding disorders, von Willebrand disease in particular, and is inappropriate for the testing of factor XIII and α_2-antiplasmin deficiencies, for which specific assays must be performed.

The platelet count is a reliable test for thrombocytopenia. However, since the test, as performed by electronic counters, relies on the size difference between platelets and other cells, abnormally large or clumped platelets can give spuriously low counts (pseudothrombocytopenia). Conversely, fragmentary hemolysis can result in spuriously high counts. Examination of a blood smear should be carried out in every case of thrombocytopenia to identify these artifacts.

Bleeding time (BT) is the traditional global screening test of platelet function but, when evaluated by objective methods in a variety of clinical settings, it has been shown to lack both sensitivity and specificity. Therefore, BT should not be relied upon to exclude platelet function defects. A variety of in vitro alternatives are currently being tested but none have yet been validated for routine use.

The diagnosis of vascular causes of bleeding is usually established on the clinical features. The role of the hemostasis laboratory is limited to excluding disorders of coagulation and platelets. Many vascular causes of bleeding are acquired and are secondary to primary medical diseases. Therefore, much of the laboratory investigation is related to the underlying clinical disorder. Sometimes a biopsy will confirm a specific diagnosis, for example in amyloidosis or septic vasculitis.

C and D *Interpretation of the Hemostasis Screen*

The decision path to be followed after the performance of the hemostasis screen is outlined in the algorithm. An abnormal hemostasis screen should be interpreted in

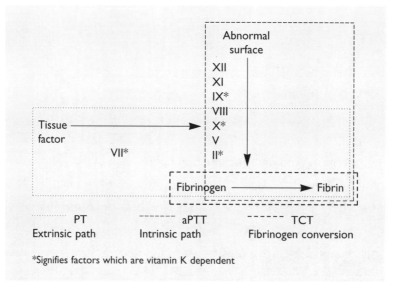

Figure 49.1   A basic outline of coagulation and screening tests.

conjunction with a review of the pretest diagnosis, which may then be modified. Extra testing is often required to confirm the diagnosis. A normal hemostasis screen should also be interpreted in light of the pretest diagnosis. The value of a normal screen is in excluding acquired coagulation abnormalities and thrombocytopenia; other abnormalities are not excluded, and the need for extra testing will depend on the level of clinical suspicion. In some cases, particularly when a congenital abnormality is suspected, special tests should be performed at the outset and not be dependent on the results of the screen.

E *Specific and Special Tests*

A summary of specific and special tests is provided in Table 49.1. These tests are more specific than the screening tests but can similarly be classified according to coagulation, platelet, or vascular functions. Therefore, the tests and their application to diagnosis will be described in that order.

Once fibrin is formed, it is stabilized by the formation of covalent cross-links and the incorporation of the fibrinolytic inhibitor α_2-antiplasmin, through the action of factor XIII, and becomes resistant to enzymatic degradation by the fibri-

Table 49.1   Tests of Hemostasis

Global Tests	Specific Tests	Special Tests
Hemostasis "screen"	Vascular	
Partial thromboplastin time (aPTT)	Biopsy	
Prothrombin time (PT)	Coagulation	Coagulation
Thrombin clotting time (TCT)	Fibrinogen level	Clot lysis time
Platelet count	Fibrin degradation products	Fibrin stability (factor XIII)
Bleeding time	Inhibitor assay	
Blood count and smear	Heparin assay or neutralization	
	Factor assays	
	Thrombocytopenia	
	Blood count, smear, reticulocytes	
	Marrow biopsy incl. karyotyping	
	Platelet survival test	
	Drug antibodies	
	Trial of steroids/immunoglobulin	
	Platelet function	Platelet function
	von Willebrand factor assays	Platelet aggregation
	Blood smear for platelet morphology	Platelet electron microscopy
		Platelet biochemical analysis
		Membrane glycoprotein analysis

nolytic system. Lack of factor XIII and of α_2-antiplasmin can be assessed by measuring clot lysis by urea, and α_2-antiplasmin can be measured more specifically either by immunoassay or chromogenic assay.

Disseminated intravascular coagulation is diagnosed by measuring the degradation of fibrin, the products of which are detected as fibrin degradation products.

Coagulation factors are assayed by determining the ability of the patient's plasma to correct the coagulation defect in a plasma which is deficient in the factor being assayed. The plasmas are mixed, a clotting test is performed, usually aPTT or PT, and the results are compared with those of a control test in which a normal plasma replaces the patient's plasma.

Suspected Bleeding Disorder

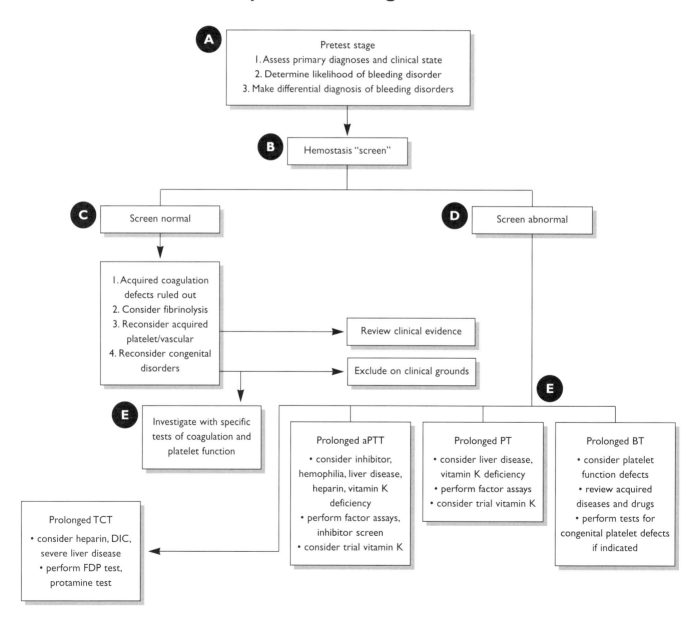

Circulating inhibitors of coagulation are detected by mixing the patient's plasma with normal plasma in equal volumes. Inhibitors in the patient's plasma affect the normal plasma; hence, the prolonged aPTT of the patient's plasma is not corrected. The control plasma, deficient in factors, is by contrast corrected by the normal plasma.

The commonest hereditary disorder affecting platelet function is von Willebrand disease. Deficiency of von Willebrand factor may cause a prolonged bleeding time. Von Willebrand disease is commonly associated with a mild deficiency of factor VIII; however, aPTT lacks sensitivity to mild depressions of single factor deficiency. Thus, when von Willebrand disease is considered, von Willebrand factor analysis must be performed. Such analysis includes quantitative measurement of von Willebrand antigen, functional assay by the ristocetin test or collagen binding assay, and von Willebrand multimer analysis by gel filtration. Coagulation assay of factor VIII completes the basic investigation. The mean and range of normal values of von Willebrand factor is lower in those with blood group O. Also, levels may fluctuate with time; therefore normal tests should be repeated if clinical suspicion remains.

Most other platelet function abnormalities result from defective platelet aggregation. While the causes are multiple, all can be screened for by the platelet aggregometer. In this test, platelets suspended in plasma are stimulated to aggregate by a variety of agonists of which the most important are adenosine diphosphate, adrenaline, and collagen. Further testing, to define specific defects, involves platelet biochemistry, assessment of platelet morphology by examination of blood smear and electron microscopy, and membrane glycoprotein analysis.

Finally, there are some very rare hereditary platelet function disorders, not detected by the above tests, such as Bernard-Soulier syndrome and Scott's syndrome. These should be considered if clinical suspicion remains, and tests for von Willebrand disease and platelet aggregation tests are normal.

Acquired platelet function disorders are associated with various disease states and drug therapy. Defects of function are common in these situations but a reliable test of bleeding tendency is lacking. Most testing is directed at the underlying disease and therapy is usually empiric.

Additional Reading

Broze GJ Jr. Tissue factor pathway inhibitor and the revised theory of coagulation. Ann Rev Med 1995;46:103–12.

Lind SE. The bleeding time does not predict surgical bleeding. Blood 1991;77:2547–51.

Rogers RPC, Levin J. A critical reappraisal of the bleeding time. Semin Thromb Hemost 1990;16:1.

Suchman AL, Mushlin AI. How well does the activated partial thromboplastin time predict postoperative hemorrhage? JAMA 1986;256:750.

Chapter 50

DIAGNOSIS AND TREATMENT OF DISSEMINATED INTRAVASCULAR COAGULATION

Theodore E Warkentin

Disseminated intravascular coagulation, or DIC, is a group of clinicopathologic syndromes characterized by dysregulated intravascular generation of thrombin, leading to intravascular fibrin formation and a reactive fibrinolytic response (plasmin generation). Clinical consequences include hemorrhage and multisystem organ dysfunction, the latter possibly related to microvascular thrombosis. Most commonly, clinicians face "acute DIC" related to abrupt-onset illness (e.g., septicemia, trauma). Less commonly, clinicians encounter "chronic DIC," which is often associated with adenocarcinoma and typically presents with macrovascular venous or arterial thrombosis.

A *History and Physical Examination*

Disseminated intravascular coagulation should be considered in patients with symptoms and signs of bleeding, thrombosis, or vital organ dysfunction. For example, generalized bleeding is suggestive of acute DIC, typically accompanied by thrombocytopenia, multiple coagulation factor deficiencies, and hyperfibrinolysis. Multiple organ failure in critically ill patients is often associated with thrombocytopenia and laboratory evidence of activation of the hemostatic system. Trousseau's syndrome (migratory thrombophlebitis in association with cancer) is strongly associated with chronic DIC.[1]

B *Screening Laboratory Studies*

The investigation of DIC should include the following screening tests: (1) complete blood count (CBC) and examination of the blood film; (2) prothrombin time (PT)—often expressed as the International Normalized Ratio (INR)—and activated partial thromboplastin time (aPTT); (3) thrombin clotting time (TCT) and/or fibrinogen; and, (4) a measure of fibrin(ogen) degradation products (FDPs). Three types of FDP assays are the most widely used to diagnose DIC.[2] A serum FDP assay uses polyclonal antibodies to detect fibrin(ogen) products D and E; this assay is sensitive for DIC but can give false-positive results under some circumstances (e.g., in vitro fibrinolysis if the sample is not drawn into a fibrinolytic inhibitor; residual fibrinogen caused by incomplete clotting of the sample due to heparin). Increasingly, laboratories perform an assay of plasma using a monoclonal antibody to detect the covalently linked D regions of FDPs (D-dimer). Finally, the addition of either protamine sulfate or ethanol can cause precipitation in plasma of fibrin monomers and other fibrin-containing complexes. Although these "para-coagulation" assays are less sensitive than both the plasma D-dimer and serum FDP assays to detect DIC, they usually provide clinically useful information because they are usually positive in patients with clinically significant DIC that is complicated by bleeding or thrombosis.

C *Clinical Disorders Associated with DIC*

Disseminated intravascular coagulation occurs in many clinical settings, which include trauma (especially brain injury, burns, heatstroke), shock/hypoxia caused by any etiology, obstetrical complications (particularly placental abruption, amniotic fluid embolism, retained dead fetus syndrome; eclampsia; saline abortion), malignancy, infection, acute hemolysis (ABO incompatible transfusions, thrombotic thrombocytopenic purpura [TTP]), heparin-induced thrombocytopenia [HIT], liver disease, vascular abnormalities (giant hemangiomas, abdominal aortic aneurysms), prothrombin complex concentrates, purpura fulminans (congenital and acquired) (Figure 50.1), and snake and spider envenomation, among others. The clinical spectrum of DIC caused by malignant disease can range from venous and arterial thrombosis (e.g., mucin-producing adenocarcinomas) to life-threatening hemorrhagic syndromes (especially, acute promyelocytic leukemia and prostatic adenocarcinoma). Some of the disorders listed are more often *not* associated with significant laboratory evidence for DIC even though they can have significant thrombocytopenia (e.g., TTP, HIT) or coagulation disturbances (e.g., liver disease).

D *Laboratory Abnormalities Consistent with DIC*

Although the platelet count, PT/INR, aPTT, TCT, and/or fibrinogen are routinely measured in the laboratory assessment of DIC, abnormalities in these parameters are neither sensitive nor specific for DIC. However, patients with clinically significant DIC that results in bleeding or thrombosis will usually have abnormalities in these measurements. The presence of FDPs is usually considered a sine qua non for the diagnosis of DIC. One suggested strategy—based on the greater sensitivity of the serum FDP assay and the greater specificity of the D-dimer assay for DIC—is to screen for DIC with the former and to confirm the diagnosis with the latter assay.[3]

Complete blood count and blood film examination. Thrombocytopenia occurs in many patients with DIC. The blood film sometimes shows red cell fragments in DIC, and may also reveal potential explanations for DIC (e.g., leukocytosis and "toxic" white cell abnormalities suggesting infection; primitive leukocytes signifying acute leukemia).

Global coagulation tests (e.g., PT/INR, aPTT) are variably prolonged among different patient populations with DIC but are useful in guiding plasma replacement therapy for bleeding patients.

Hypofibrinogenemia is found in a minority of patients with DIC although increased fibrinogen turnover is believed to occur in most patients.

Fibrin(ogen) degradation products should be elevated in almost all patients with DIC. In one study that used D-dimer detected by immunoblotting as the "gold standard" for defining DIC, a positive latex bead agglutination assay for D-dimer was strongly associated with DIC (odds ratio = 176).[3]

E *Combined Clinical and Laboratory Data Supportive of the Diagnosis of DIC*

Disseminated intravascular coagulation is a clinicopathologic syndrome, i.e., it can be diagnosed only when supportive laboratory abnormalities occur in the appropriate

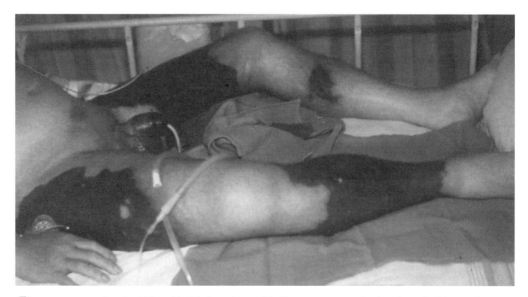

Figure 50.1   Acquired idiopathic fulminans in an adult. Postmortem examination showed widespread microvascular thrombosis and organ infarction involving skin, renal cortices, gastrointestinal tract, and prostate. Small bilateral pulmonary thromboemboli were also found.

clinical context. For example, a patient who is recovering normally from major surgery would not be considered to have DIC on clinical grounds; however, laboratory studies might well show thrombocytopenia and coagulopathy (secondary to hemodilution) and also elevated D-dimer levels (normal hemostasis of wound healing). Similarly, a patient who presents with symptomatic deep vein thrombosis is likely to have elevated D-dimer levels caused by the thrombosis. Indeed, elevated whole blood D-dimer levels have been used in diagnostic algorithms to help determine whether patients with leg swelling and dyspnea are likely to have deep vein thrombosis and pulmonary embolism, respectively.[4] Disseminated intravascular coagulation is an unlikely diagnosis, unless the patient had coexisting thrombocytopenia and coagulopathy to suggest chronic DIC of malignancy presenting as DVT.[1]

F *Specialized Laboratory Testing*

A large number of laboratory markers of activation of coagulation and fibrinolysis will be elevated in DIC. Used primarily for research purposes, these markers include byproducts of zymogen activation such as prothrombin fragment 1+2 and factor X activation peptide, enzyme-inhibitor complexes such as thrombin-antithrombin complexes and plasmin-antiplasmin complexes, and byproducts of the action of thrombin on fibrinogen such as soluble fibrin monomer, fibrinopeptide A, and Bβ15-42 peptide. (The Bβ15-42 peptide indicates the sequential action of thrombin and plasmin on fibrinogen; in contrast, the Bβ1-42 peptide indicates that plasmin alone has acted on the fibrinogen.) There has been recent interest in the possible diagnostic value of quantitative assays for soluble fibrin monomer to diagnose DIC.[5] Because soluble fibrin is generated by thrombin without the requirement for plasmin action, it could be a more sensitive marker for DIC in situations with impaired fibrinolysis (e.g., septicemia with elevated plasminogen activator inhibitor levels).

Perhaps more relevant to the clinician are assays of coagulation factor activity that can be reduced markedly in DIC. These include both procoagulant (e.g., factor V, factor VIII, prothrombin) and anticoagulant (antithrombin, protein C) activities. Depletion of plasminogen and α_2-antiplasmin can also occur in DIC. These assays are sometimes clinically useful. For example, some patients with overwhelming bacterial septicemia develop acral necrosis in the setting of shock and DIC; there is evidence that severe acquired protein C and protein S deficiency might contribute to such necrosis.[6] It has also been noted that α_2-antiplasmin levels are markedly reduced in some patients with predominant hyperfibrinolysis seen in prostate cancer or liver disease.[7] It may be useful to measure α_2-antiplasmin levels to monitor the effect of antifibrinolytic agents, such as ϵ-aminocaproic acid.

G *Treat the Underlying Disease*

Disseminated intravascular coagulation is caused by pathologic activation of the hemostatic mechanism. Accordingly, the cornerstone of treatment is the management of the underlying cause of DIC. Sometimes, specific therapy can have dramatic results. Examples include removal of retained placental products in missed abortion and retinoids to treat acute promyelocytic leukemia with DIC.

H *General Supportive Measures*

It is important to maintain adequate oxygenation (transfusion for anemia; ventilatory support) and tissue perfusion (adequate volume replacement; vasopressors) in patients with DIC, because persisting hypoxemia can lead to additional tissue damage, further promoting DIC.

I *Bleeding or Invasive Procedures*

Whenever possible, laboratory studies should guide blood product administration to patients with DIC who are bleeding or who require surgery or other invasive procedures. It is important to monitor closely the clinical and laboratory responses to blood transfusions as the abnormalities associated with DIC can worsen quickly.

J *Thrombocytopenia*

Patients with diffuse microvascular bleeding should receive platelets if the platelet count is below 50×10^9/L. A higher platelet count threshold ($75–100 \times 10^9$/L) should be considered for patients at risk for life-threatening bleeding (closed head injury; pericardial injury). Patients without bleeding should receive prophylactic platelet transfusions if severe thrombocytopenia occurs (platelet count less than 20×10^9/L).

K *Global Coagulopathy*

Prolonged INR/PT and aPTT values usually indicate deficiencies of numerous procoagulant and anticoagulant hemostatic factors. Accordingly, transfusion of fresh frozen plasma to DIC patients with bleeding is appropriate.

L *Hypofibrinogenemia*

The fibrinogen level should be assessed in patients with suspected DIC. This is because some DIC syndromes are associated with severe hypofibrinogenemia and bleeding (placental abruption; acute head injury; prostatic adenocarcinoma with hyperfibrinolysis). The goal of treatment is to raise the fibrinogen at least to above 0.75 g/L. Cryoprecipitate provides a more concentrated source of fibrinogen than fresh frozen plasma: 10 units of cryoprecipitate (150 ml blood product) contains approximately 2.5 grams of fibrinogen, the same as 4 units of frozen plasma (1000 ml blood product).

M *Pharmacologic Adjuncts*

Under special circumstances, pharmacologic adjuncts to control DIC should be considered. For example, some patients with bleeding and DIC have excessive fibrinolysis (e.g., promyelocytic leukemia; vascular malformations; prostatic adenocarcinoma); antifibrinolytic agents such as ε-aminocaproic acid (EACA) or tranexamic acid can benefit these patients.[8,9] Antifibrinolytic therapy is not recommended as a general treatment in DIC because of the potential risk for causing thrombosis.

N *Vitamin K and Folic Acid*

Vitamin K deficiency is not uncommon in critically ill patients.[10] Administration of vitamin K (10 mg SQ once daily for 2 to 3 days) to patients at risk for DIC will minimize the risk of exacerbating hemorrhagic or thrombotic sequelae due to acquired deficiencies of the vitamin-K-dependent procoagulant and anticoagulant factors. Routine folic acid administration to critically ill patients will prevent thrombocytopenia caused by folate deficiency.

O *Thrombosis*

Otherwise unexplained thrombocytopenia or coagulopathy should always suggest the possibility of chronic DIC and underlying malignancy in a patient who presents with venous and/or arterial thrombosis. A clue to this possibility is a dramatic increase in the platelet count that occurs when heparin is initially used to treat the thrombosis. Typically, the thrombocytopenia recurs after heparin is stopped. Many of these patients develop new or progressive thrombosis on warfarin anticoagulation. Sometimes, these unfortunate patients develop venous limb gangrene, possibly because of warfarin-induced protein C deficiency. Subcutaneous, low-molecular-weight heparin is often useful to treat these patients.

P *Purpura Fulminans*

Purpura fulminans is a rare syndrome characterized by necrosis of the skin in multiple sites associated with DIC. When this syndrome begins within hours or days of birth, homozygous protein C deficiency is the likeliest diagnosis; this illness can be controlled with lifelong protein C replacement. Postinfectious purpura fulminans occurs in older children, typically 1 week after varicella infection. It could

Patient with Bleeding, Thrombosis, or Organ Failure

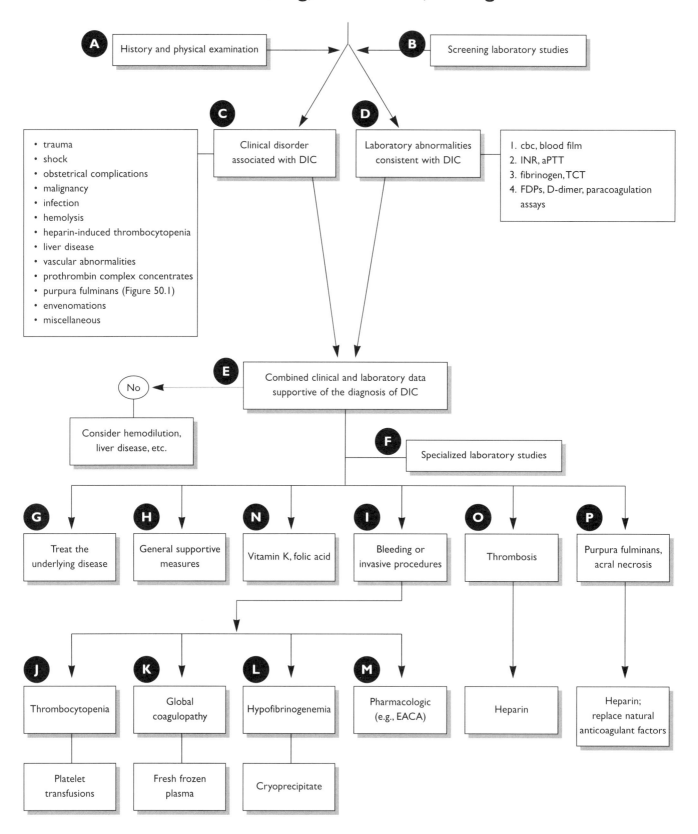

A History and physical examination

B Screening laboratory studies

C Clinical disorder associated with DIC

- trauma
- shock
- obstetrical complications
- malignancy
- infection
- hemolysis
- heparin-induced thrombocytopenia
- liver disease
- vascular abnormalities
- prothrombin complex concentrates
- purpura fulminans (Figure 50.1)
- envenomations
- miscellaneous

D Laboratory abnormalities consistent with DIC

1. cbc, blood film
2. INR, aPTT
3. fibrinogen, TCT
4. FDPs, D-dimer, paracoagulation assays

E Combined clinical and laboratory data supportive of the diagnosis of DIC

No → Consider hemodilution, liver disease, etc.

F Specialized laboratory studies

G Treat the underlying disease

H General supportive measures

N Vitamin K, folic acid

I Bleeding or invasive procedures

O Thrombosis

P Purpura fulminans, acral necrosis

J Thrombocytopenia → Platelet transfusions

K Global coagulopathy → Fresh frozen plasma

L Hypofibrinogenemia → Cryoprecipitate

M Pharmacologic (e.g., EACA)

Heparin

Heparin; replace natural anticoagulant factors

represent an immune-mediated disturbance in the protein C anticoagulant pathway. Acral necrosis resembling purpura fulminans can also occur in the setting of overwhelming septicemia, where limb gangrene can occur, likely as a result of the combination of poor tissue perfusion (hypotension) and of microvascular thrombosis resulting from acquired natural anticoagulant deficiency.[6] It is possible that protein C or antithrombin III concentrates will be effective in some patients with purpura fulminans.

Bibliography

1. Sack GH, Levin J, Bell W. Trousseau's syndrome and other manifestations of chronic disseminated coagulopathy in patients with neoplasma: clinical, pathophysiologic, and therapeutic features. Medicine 1977;56:1–37.

2. Hathaway WE, Goodnight SH Jr. Disorders of hemostasis and thrombosis. A clinical guide. New York: McGraw-Hill, 1993:219–29.

3. Carr JM, McKinney M, McDonagh J. Diagnosis of disseminated intravascular coagulation. Role of D-dimer. Am J Clin Pathol 1989;91:280–7.

4. Wells PS, Brill-Edwards P, Stevens P, et al. A novel and rapid whole blood assay for D-dimer in patients with clinically suspected deep vein thrombosis. Circulation 1995;91:2184–7.

5. Okajima K, Uchiba M, Murakami K, Okabe H, Takatsuki K. Determination of plasma soluble fibrin using a new ELISA method in patients with disseminated intravascular coagulation. Am J Hematol 1996;51:186–91.

6. LeClerc F, Hazelzet J, Jude B, Hofhuis W, Hue V, Martinot A, van der Voort E. Protein C and S deficiency in severe infectious purpura of children: a collaborative study of 40 cases. Intensive Care Med 1992;18:202–5.

7. Williams E. Plasma α_2-antiplasmin activity: role in the evaluation and management of fibrinolytic states and other bleeding disorders. Arch Intern Med 1989;149:1769–72.

8. Schwartz BS, Williams EC, Conlan MG, Mosher DF. Epsilon-aminocaproic acid in the treatment of patients with acute promyelocytic leukemia and acquired alpha-2-plasmin inhibitor deficiency. Ann Intern Med 1986;105:873–7.

9. Avvisati G, Ten Cate JW, Buller HR, Mandelli F. Tranexamic acid for control of haemorrhage in acute promyelocytic leukaemia. Lancet 1989;2:122–4.

10. Alperin J. Coagulopathy caused by vitamin K deficiency in critically ill, hospitalized patients. JAMA 1987;258:1916–9.

Additional Reading

Baglin T. Disseminated intravascular coagulation: diagnosis and treatment. BMJ 1996;312: 683–7.

Staudinger T, Locker GJ, Frass M. Management of acquired coagulation disorders in emergency and intensive-care medicine. Semin Thromb Hemost 1996;22:93–104.

Bauer KA. Laboratory markers of coagulation activation. Arch Pathol Lab Med 1993;117:71–7.

Chapter 51

CLASSIFICATION
OF BLEEDING DISORDERS

Irwin Walker

Bleeding disorders are classified according to the normal hemostatic mechanisms they affect, i.e., platelets, vessels, or coagulation factors. The following simplified description of the normal mechanisms of hemostasis provides sufficient background to understand most bleeding disorders.

Hemostasis is normally maintained by the supportive connective tissue surrounding blood vessels, by the vascular endothelium and, within vessels, by platelets and the clotting factors of the coagulation system. When the endothelium is intact, inhibitory substances, such as prostacyclin, thrombomodulin, and protein C, prevent intravascular coagulation and platelet aggregation. When the endothelium is breached or damaged, activators overcome these inhibitory mechanisms.

The first response to bleeding is contraction of blood vessels. This restricts the flow of blood to the damaged vessel, tightens gaps in the endothelium, and alters flow so as to favor activation of coagulation and platelets.

Breaches of the endothelium expose subendothelial tissues and intracellular substances. These interact with platelets and coagulation factors leading to the formation of a thrombus. In this process, platelets first adhere to the subendothelium through molecular bridges. These bridges, composed mainly of von Willebrand factor, span between subendothelial tissues and platelet glycoprotein Ib receptors. Platelet adhesion results in the deposition of a monolayer of platelets across the site of the breach; various agonists from the vessel wall activate additional platelets, and these bind to the existing monolayer and to each other. During this latter process, referred to as platelet aggregation, molecular bridges, composed mainly of fibrinogen, are formed between glycoprotein IIb-IIIa receptors on adjacent platelets. The result is a platelet plug.

The processes which occur during platelet aggregation are complex. The platelet agonists, which include collagen, thrombin, and adenosine diphosphate, bind to membrane receptors, which transmit signals internally to biochemical pathways. These trigger various effectors, principally thromboxane A_2, which is produced by the phospholipase A_2 pathway. The effectors cause the release of platelet aggregating and procoagulant substances from the platelet granules and expose glycoprotein IIb-IIIa membrane receptors. The result is twofold: first, the platelet membrane is altered to facilitate binding and interaction of coagulation factors, thereby promoting fibrin formation; and second, platelets become bound to each other by bridges of fibrinogen between glycoprotein IIb-IIIa surface receptors on adjacent platelets.

Once a platelet plug is formed, coagulation may be activated by substances from the vessel wall, such as tissue factor. Activated platelets attract the activated clotting factors, promote their adhesion and interaction, and this in turn leads to cleavage of fibrinogen, and thus fibrin formation. Fibrin strengthens the platelet plug and the extending thrombus. Fibrin is then either stabilized by the formation of covalent crosslinks between its chains, through the action of factor XIII, or lysed through the action of the fibrinolytic system, which is initiated by plasminogen activator from the endothelium.

The classification of bleeding disorders is based on alterations in the normal mechanisms of either the vessel wall, platelets, or coagulation. Within these general categories, single specific biochemical defects have been identified that explain many congenital disorders. However, acquired disorders, which occur in association with many medical diseases, often cause multiple abnormalities. In these cases, the primary disease, rather than a biochemical defect, is listed under the appropriate general category. Some diseases may cause multiple defects and are listed more than once. For example, liver disease may cause multiple coagulation defects and both qualitative and quantitative platelet defects.

A description of vascular, platelet, and coagulation disorders as well as von Willebrand disease, follows.

A *Vascular Disorders*

Vessel walls include a layer of endothelium, surrounded by connective tissue, and, to a variable extent, smooth muscle. Bleeding results either from stress fractures of unsupported, inflamed, or infiltrated vessels, or from abnormal permeability of the vessel wall.

B *Platelet Disorders*

Platelet disorders are either quantitative, involving a decrease in the number of circulating platelets (thrombocytopenia), or qualitative, involving an impairment in function.

Thrombocytopenia is due either to increased peripheral destruction or to decreased production and may be congenital or acquired. Increased platelet destruction is associated with a decreased platelet lifespan, measurable by an isotope-labeled platelet survival test. Decreased production of platelets is associated with a normal platelet lifespan and, in most cases, with a decrease in production of leukocytes and/or red cells. A mild thrombocytopenia may also accompany some types of congenital qualitative platelet disorders and some cases of congenital deficiency of platelet adhesive protein (von Willebrand disease).

Platelet function disorders may also be congenital or acquired.[1] Congenital disorders can often be subclassified by a specific biochemical or structural defect. Acquired platelet function disorders, on the other hand, cannot be conveniently classified in this way, either because the main defect has not been delineated, or because multiple mechanisms exist. Acquired disorders are listed according to the disease under which they arise.

Vascular Disorders

CONGENITAL
Hereditary hemorrhagic telangiectasia
• Rendu-Osler-Weber syndrome
Ehlers-Danlos syndrome
Other rare tissue disorders

ACQUIRED
Cushing's syndrome
Amyloidosis
Anaphylactoid purpura
Simple easy bruising
Senile purpura
Scurvy
Mechanical purpura
Schamberg's disease
Infections
Allergic purpura
• Henoch-Schönlein
• drugs
Factitious purpura
Dysproteinemias
Psychogenic purpura

C *Abnormalities in Platelet Adhesive Protein (von Willebrand Disease)*

Von Willebrand disease is a group of genetic disorders resulting from abnormalities in the gene for von Willebrand factor, found on chromosome 12. It is the commonest congenital disorder affecting platelet function. Rare cases are acquired rather than congenital, resulting from premature removal or neutralization of circulating von Willebrand factor. Von Willebrand factor is a protein responsible for the binding of platelets to the subendothelium, i.e., platelet adhesion. It circulates as multimers of various sizes, the largest of which are most effective in causing platelet adhesion. Von Willebrand factor also binds and stabilizes coagulation factor VIII, and deficiency of von Willebrand factor often results in a secondary decrease of circulating factor VIII. Abnormalities of von Willebrand factor, either congenital or acquired,

Platelet Disorders

THROMBOCYTOPENIA	DEFICIENT PLATELET FUNCTION
Decreased production Diseases causing pancytopenia Amegakaryocytic thrombocytopenia Myelodysplastic syndrome	**CONGENITAL** **Decreased adhesion** Bernard-Soulier syndrome
Shortened lifespan Immune thrombocytopenia • idiopathic • drugs, including heparin • infections, including HIV • autoimmune diseases • post transfusion • passive neonatal	**Decreased aggregation** Glanzmann's thrombasthenia **Release defects** Prostaglandin pathway defect Gray platelet syndrome Storage pool deficiency
Nonimmune thrombocytopenia • massive hemorrhage • pre-eclampsia ("HELLP") • congenital platelet disorders • von Willebrand disease • infections • microangiopathy (TTP, HUS) • DIC • drugs, alcohol	**Decreased procoagulant activity** Scott's syndrome **ACQUIRED** Hyperglobulinemia Renal failure Liver failure Myeloproliferative disorders Acquired von Willebrand disease Leukemias and myelodysplasias Cardiopulmonary bypass Drugs Antiplatelet antibodies
Abnormal distribution Hypersplenism **Hemodilution**	

are responsible for the majority of known defects of platelet adhesion. Other instances of defective adhesion have been described, usually in conjunction with other defects in platelet function but their importance has not been established.

Congenital von Willebrand disease has a variable phenotype, reflecting a wide variety of molecular alterations which are classified into a few broad groups.[2] The most common clinical phenotype is Type 1, which occurs in about 70% of cases and manifests as a mild or moderate deficiency of the von Willebrand factor. It is inherited in an autosomal dominant pattern. Type 3 is a severe, or even complete, absence of the protein and is inherited in a recessive pattern.

While Types 1 and 3 represent quantitative deficiencies in von Willebrand factor, Type 2 represents a qualitative abnormality of the protein, leading to a corresponding loss of function. In type 2A there is a deficiency of high-molecular-weight multimers, due either to defective multimer formation or their premature proteolysis.

von Willebrand Disease

CONGENITAL

Quantitative defects

Type 1: Mild defect; decrease of all multimers
Type 3: Severe defect

Qualitative defects

Type 2A: Decrease in high-molecular-weight multimers
due to defective production or premature proteolysis

Type 2B: Decrease in high-molecular-weight multimers
due to promiscuous platelet binding and clearance

Type 2N: Abnormal factor VIII: C binding and clearance
with resultant low levels of factor VIII: C;
mimics hemophilia but with autosomal inheritance

Type 2M: Abnormal function but normal multimer pattern
Probably due to mutation(s) at platelet binding site

ACQUIRED

Either idiopathic, or secondary to various disease,
commonly lymphoproliferative disorders

Type 2B also represents a loss of high molecular multimers but the mechanism is different. The characteristic finding is an increased affinity of von Willebrand factor to platelets. There is probably an alteration in the normal sequence by which von Willebrand factor binds first to the vessel wall and then to platelets. Instead, von Willebrand factor, mainly comprising high molecular multimers, binds directly to circulating platelets. Both platelets and high molecular multimers are prematurely cleared from the circulation leading to low levels of high-molecular-weight von Willebrand factor and often of platelets also. In Type 2N there is defective binding of factor VIII, which is prematurely cleared. The phenotype is similar to mild hemophilia, and specific tests of von Willebrand factor quantitation and function are normal but the inheritance pattern is autosomal rather than sex-linked. In Type 2M there is a qualitative abnormality with loss of function but the multimeric pattern is normal. The mechanism may be alteration of the binding site for platelet glycoprotein Ib.

Deficiency of von Willebrand factor may occur as an acquired abnormality. It is often associated with primary diseases, particularly lymphoproliferative disorders and is due to premature clearance of von Willebrand factor, either by antibodies or through binding to abnormal sites.

Bernard-Soulier syndrome is a rare bleeding disorder, characterized by large platelets, and defective binding to von Willebrand factor due to abnormality of glycoprotein Ib. The pathogenesis of bleeding thus mimics that associated with lack of von Willebrand factor; hence it is usually classified with these disorders although it could also be classified with disorders of platelet function.

D *Coagulation Disorders*

In almost all cases, bleeding is a result of lack of coagulation factors. In a small minority of instances, a fibrin clot forms but rapid lysis follows, due either to a lack of cross-links from deficiency of factor XIII, or to increased activity of the fibrinolytic system. Lack of coagulation factors may be congenital, in which case only single factors are usually involved, or acquired, in which case multiple deficiencies often occur. Lack of factors may be the result of subnormal production, or reduced life span. Reduction in life span may be due either to neutralization with antibodies or to increased utilization.

The most common congenital coagulation factor deficiencies are of factor VIII, leading to the disorder of hemophilia A, and of factor IX, leading to hemophilia B or Christmas disease.[3] As well as being the most common disorders, they are also the most serious and life threatening. Both are inherited in sex-linked patterns and are graded by the degree of factor deficiency: severe, with levels < 1%; moderate, with levels of between 1 and 5%; and mild, with levels of > 5%. In 10 to 15% of cases of severe hemophilia A, and 2% of hemophilia B, antibodies to these factors develop, making the replacement by infused factors ineffective.

Acquired deficiency of coagulation factors is commonly a result of liver failure, the sole site of production of all factors except factor VIII. Vitamin K deficiency, due either to dietary deficiency, or inhibition of production by oral anticoagulants, results in lack of production of factors II, VII, IX, and X. Excessive consumption of factors is mostly the result of disseminated intravascular coagulation,[4] which may be induced by a variety of clinical situations. The commonest cause of bleeding due to neutralization of coagulation factors is heparin therapy; rarely, it is due to neutralization by antibodies to coagulation factors, usually factor VIII. Even rarer is the abnormal absorption of factors, as has been described for factor X, in amyloidosis.

Not included in this discussion are abnormalities that result in impaired coagulation in vitro but do not result in bleeding, such as the presence of lupus-like inhibitors or factor XII deficiency.

Coagulation Disorders

CONGENITAL
Factor production deficiency
Hemophilia A and B
Other factor deficiencies

Coagulation inhibitors
Secondary to hemophilia A or B

Increased fibrinolysis
Deficiency of inhibitors

ACQUIRED
Factor production deficiency
Liver failure

Increased consumption
Disseminated intravascular coagulation
Massive hemorrhage

Increased fibrinolysis
Increased activators—various causes

Coagulation inhibitors
"Lupus-like" inhibitors
Factor VIII inhibitor
Other inhibitors

Bibliography

1. Rao AK, Holmsen H. Congenital disorders of platelet function. Semin Hematol 1986;23:102.

2. Sadler JE. A revised classification of von Willebrand disease. Thromb Haemost 1994; 71:520–525.

3. Hoyer LW. Hemophilia A. N Engl J Med 1994;330:38–47.

4. Bick RL. Disseminated intravascular coagulation: objective clinical and laboratory diagnosis, treatment, and assessment of clinical response. Semin Thromb Hemost 1996;22:69–88.

Chapter 52

Approach to the Patient with Thrombocytopenia

Margaret Warner

John G Kelton

I. DECISION TREE FOR THROMBOCYTOPENIC PATIENTS

Physicians managing patients with thrombocytopenia must simultaneously resolve two issues: first, the risk posed by the thrombocytopenia and, second, the cause of the thrombocytopenia itself. Like all cytopenias, thrombocytopenia is *always* caused by some disease or disorder. Often, the underlying cause poses a greater risk to the patient than the thrombocytopenia itself.

A *Exclude Pseudothrombocytopenia*

The first step when faced with a patient with thrombocytopenia is to exclude pseudothrombocytopenia. When blood is collected into the anticoagulant EDTA, the platelets sometimes form clumps, leading to a false low platelet count when enumerated by an automated cell counter. Platelet clumping is caused by an antibody in the serum of some patients, which binds to sites on platelet glycoproteins IIb/IIIa. These sites are unmasked by conformational changes induced by the EDTA. This antibody is only active in vitro and is of no clinical significance to the patient. Platelet clumping can be overcome by drawing blood samples from affected patients into different anticoagulants such as citrate or heparin.

B *Urgency of Intervention*

Thrombocytopenic bleeding is associated with a hierarchy of signs that approximately parallel the degrees of thrombocytopenia. For example, moderate thrombocytopenia (platelet count $50-80 \times 10^9/L$) is usually asymptomatic. More severe thrombocytopenia (platelet count of $10-20 \times 10^9/L$) usually is associated with petechiae, which are tiny collections of blood caused by capillary leaks and usually found on the most dependent regions of the body. These patients also have scattered bruises that tend to be on the lower limbs. Severely thrombocytopenic patients have platelet counts less than $10 \times 10^9/L$ and can have mucous membrane bleeding in addition to petechiae and purpura. Often, these patients have blood blisters along the bite margins in their mouths. These patients are at high risk of severe and potentially life-threatening bleeding and require urgent intervention to raise the platelet count.

Causes of thrombocytopenia can be divided into four categories: (1) increased platelet destruction, (2) decreased platelet production, (3) platelet sequestrations, or (4) hemodilution. In assessing thrombocytopenic patients, it is useful to distinguish between *inpatients* and *outpatients* because the common causes of thrombocytopenia differ between the two groups. It is our opinion that in the vast majority of outpatients, the thrombocytopenia is caused by increased platelet destruction. Thrombocytopenia in inpatients is usually more complex and can be caused by many different factors.

A functional approach to thrombocytopenias. The physician managing a patient with thrombocytopenia must first determine if the patient has true as opposed to pseudothrombocytopenia. Each thrombocytopenic patient must be categorized into underproduction, sequestration (typically with an enlarged spleen), and increased destruction. However, another useful approach is to distin-

I. Decision Tree for Thrombocytopenic Patients

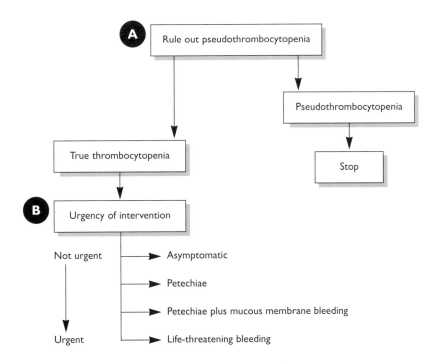

guish thrombocytopenic patients according to their mode of presentation. For example, those patients who seek medical attention as outpatients most frequently will have thrombocytopenia that was discovered because of a bleeding or bruising tendency. In contrast, thrombocytopenia which occurs in hospitalized inpatients more commonly is identified through a routine laboratory test. In this chapter, we will divide the mechanisms responsible for thrombocytopenia into inpatient or outpatient thrombocytopenic patients.

II. THROMBOCYTOPENIA IN NONHOSPITALIZED OUTPATIENTS

For most patients, the thrombocytopenia is identified because it has become symptomatic. Typically, the patient has evidence of hemostatic impairment. Less commonly, the patient will have evidence of a thrombotic platelet disorder such as thrombotic thrombocytopenic purpura or hemolytic uremic syndrome. The vast majority of these patients will have immune thrombocytopenia, which is typically idiopathic but can be secondary to drugs, other immunological disorders, or infections such as HIV.

A *Drug-Induced Thrombocytopenia*
For isolated and unexpected thrombocytopenia, immune mechanisms are almost always causative. Drug-induced thrombocytopenia, most frequently caused by quinine and quinidine, and gold-induced thrombocytopenia are encountered in outpatients. By far the most common inpatient drug-induced immune thrombocytopenia is caused by heparin; this will be discussed subsequently. The diagnosis of drug-induced thrombocytopenia is based on a history of drug exposure (which can include the ingestion of quinine in tonic water) plus the resolution of thrombocytopenia after discontinuing the drug. The diagnosis can be confirmed in specialized laboratories by demonstrating drug-dependent binding of antibodies to platelets. The patients with drug-induced thrombocytopenia (excluding heparin) should be managed by discontinuing the drug and induction of reticuloendothelial cell blockade through high-dose intravenous IgG or anti-D (in an Rh-positive individual). Corticosteriods have not been shown to be effective. Rarely, for those patients with persisting and potentially life-threatening drug-induced thrombocytopenia, removal of the offending drug–antibody complex can be accomplished by plasma exchange. Gold-induced thrombocytopenia can induce chronic autoimmune thrombocytopenia, which behaves similarly to idiopathic thrombocytopenic purpura (ITP).

Most patients with gold-induced thrombocytopenia have a genetic predisposition to the disorder and carry the HLA-B8, Dr3 haplotype.

Isolated thrombocytopenia which is caused by marrow underproduction can rarely be caused by excessive and acute alcohol intake.

B Infection-Induced Thrombocytopenia

Infection-induced thrombocytopenia can be associated with chronic infections such as HIV or transient infections such as infectious mononucleosis. Young people at risk for infectious mononucleosis should be investigated serologically for the disorder if they present with isolated and severe thrombocytopenia. The thrombocytopenia associated with infectious mononucleosis typically resolves spontaneously but resolution may not occur for several months. These patients have other typical features of infectious mononucleosis.

Thrombocytopenia associated with HIV is common but, fortunately, very severe thrombocytopenia is uncommon. In these patients, the platelet count often rises with antiviral therapy but sometimes more definitive intervention such as RE blockade or splenectomy is required. We have tried to avoid corticosteriods in these patients.

C Hypersplenism

Patients with thrombocytopenia caused by hypersplenism typically have mild to moderate thrombocytopenia, and very severe thrombocytopenia makes the diagnosis unlikely. A proportion of these patients will also have mild leukopenia and sometimes anemia. The diagnosis is made by documenting an enlarged spleen and can be confirmed with a radiolabelled platelet survival study. These patients virtually never require intervention to correct the thrombocytopenia itself, and the thrombocytopenia is not progressive.

D Thrombocytopenia Associated with Microangiopathic Hemolytic Anemia

The presence of schistocytes, also known as red cell fragments, on the peripheral blood film in conjunction with thrombocytopenia is diagnostic of a microangiopathic or macroangiopathic process such as disseminated intervascular coagulation, thrombotic thrombocytopenic purpura (TTP), hemolytic uremic syndrome (HUS), pre-eclampsia, or malignant hypertension. Almost always, the history and physical examination as well as routine laboratory screening will clarify the diagnosis. Very occasionally, patients with TTP can also have disseminated intravascular coagulation (DIC). Thrombotic thrombocytopenic purpura is characterized by thrombocytopenia, schistocytic hemolytic anemia, and less commonly neurological or renal impairment and fever; TTP is managed by plasma exchange and possibly corticosteroids. The treatment of DIC is by managing the underlying disorder; HUS is treated supportively, with consideration of dialysis or plasma exchange, if appropriate.

II. Thrombocytopenia in Nonhospitalized Outpatients

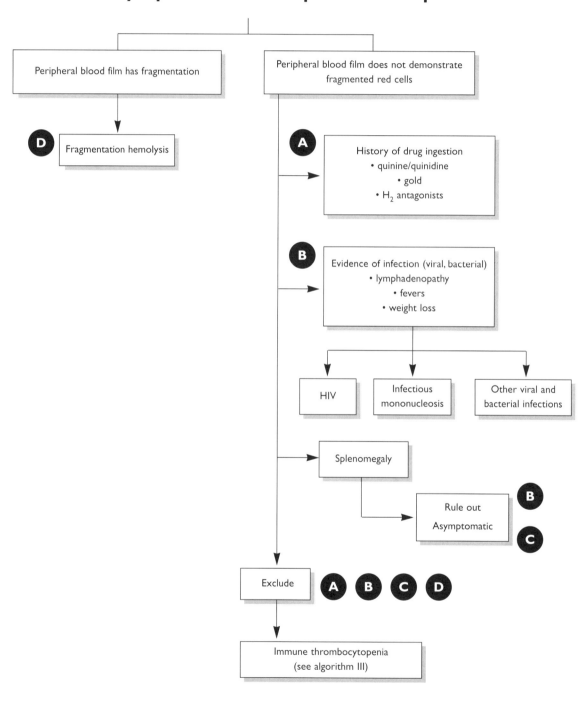

III. IMMUNE THROMBOCYTOPENIA

Immune thrombocytopenia is defined as a thrombocytopenic disorder caused by an increased rate of platelet destruction, which is mediated through immune mechanisms. The destruction usually is caused by antibodies which target platelet proteins. The diagnosis is made by demonstrating isolated thrombocytopenia, which is associated with normal or increased numbers of megakaryocytes in the bone marrow. Recent advances in serological testing have made it possible for the diagnosis to be confirmed serologically by detecting antibodies bound to certain platelet-specific glycoproteins such as IIb/IIIa.

Immune thrombocytopenia can be separated into primary and secondary thrombocytopenia. Primary immune thrombocytopenia is also known as idiopathic thrombocytopenic purpura (ITP). Secondary immune thrombocytopenia represents those disorders associated with an underlying condition such as lymphoproliferative disorders, systemic lupus erythematosus, and a variety of bacterial and viral infections, notably the human immunodeficiency virus (HIV).

A *Idiopathic Thrombocytopenic Purpura*

Idiopathic thrombocytopenic purpura (ITP) is a common disorder of children and adults. More frequently (80%) acute ITP in children is triggered by vaccination or viral infection and typically resolves within 1 to 3 months. In contrast, about 80 to 90% of adults who present with ITP will be found to have a chronic illness that may require more definitive therapy.

Patients with ITP present in one of three ways: first, they may have a long history of easy bruising; second, they may have acute bleeding, which not infrequently is triggered by the ingestion of an antiplatelet agent such as aspirin or alcohol; and third, they may have mild thrombocytopenia discovered on routine blood testing. In our experience, at least half the patients with ITP do not require specific therapy.

The diagnosis of ITP is one of exclusion. These patients have a normal physical examination, with the exception of a hemostatic defect. The majority of these patients will have autoantibodies against glycoprotein IIb/IIIa, which is relatively a specific test for ITP. Platelet-associated IgG measurements are not helpful. Bone marrow examination is usually not required unless there are abnormalities of the blood film, or the patient has an atypical course. For those patients in whom a bone marrow examination is performed, we have found cytogenetic analysis helpful to exclude myelodysplasia.

The first and most important step in determining intervention for a suspected ITP patient is to decide whether any therapy is required. Those patients with low platelet counts, but who are asymptomatic (typically their platelets are about $30-40 \times 10^9$/L), can be monitored. Sometimes, the platelet count must be raised if the patient has to undergo a dental or surgical procedure. For those patients with severe thrombocytopenia (platelets less than 10×10^9/L) or less severe thrombocytopenia but with clinical signs of hemostatic impairment, the platelet count can be raised by corticosteriods (Prednisone, 1mg/kg/day or equivalent dose), or by RE blockade (high-dose intravenous IgG or anti-D in an Rh-positive patient). After the platelet count has been raised by either maneuver, the patient is monitored. About 80 to 90% of ITP patients will have a relapse of their thrombocytopenia when therapy is discontinued and the corticosteroids tapered. For these patients, particularly if very severe thrombocytopenia recurs, we move more quickly to splenectomy rather than continue with multiple courses of immunosuppression or RE blockade. Splenectomy should be preceded by vaccination against encapsulated bacteria. Laparoscopic splenectomy is an effective and low-morbidity maneuver.

III. Immune Thrombocytopenia

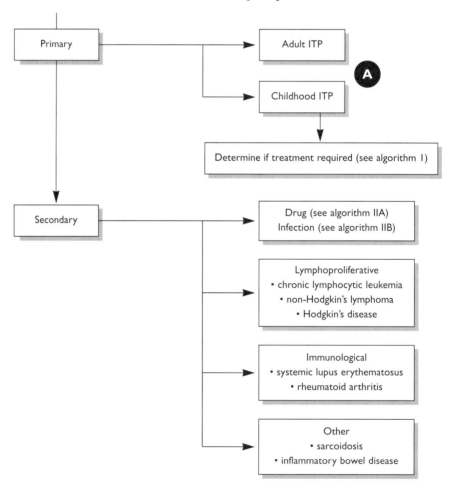

IV. THROMBOCYTOPENIA IN HOSPITALIZED PATIENTS

There are several other steps that should be taken as soon as thrombocytopenia is identified in a hospitalized patient. First, the platelet count should be evaluated longitudinally. For example, if the patient had thrombocytopenia at the time of admission, then the mechanism responsible is likely to be one of those discussed under the thrombocytopenia in an outpatient section, such as ITP. The review of the clinical situation will almost always define the mechanism responsible for the thrombocytopenia; for example, recent surgery suggests dilutional thrombocytopenia. The temporal association with a drug can identify the drug responsible; the administration of a previous blood product, particularly in women with previous childbirths, is consistent with post-transfusion purpura. In the next section, we will describe the more common causes of thrombocytopenia in hospitalized patients.

A Infection-Induced Thrombocytopenia

A bacterial infection is one of the most common causes of isolated thrombocytopenia in a hospitalized patient. These patients typically have isolated thrombocytopenia that usually is moderately severe but can be very severe. Almost always, there is evidence for a systemic bacterial infection but, occasionally, the first signs of a bacteremia is the thrombocytopenia. Treatment of these patients requires the successful treatment of the underlying infection. Infected patients with very severe thrombocytopenia should also be investigated for evidence of disseminated intervascular coagulation, which itself may require specific therapy.

B Dilutional Thrombocytopenia

Dilutional thrombocytopenia is typically seen in a postoperative patient, and the onset is at the time of surgery or shortly after surgery. Virtually every patient who has a major surgical procedure will have a fall in platelet count. For some patients, the administration of large amounts of crystalloids or blood products has contributed to the thrombocytopenia through a dilutional mechanism. This thrombocytopenia is not severe, and the patient's platelet count will progressively rise over the next few days. No treatment is required.

C Drug-Induced Thrombocytopenia

Drug-induced thrombocytopenia is a common and important cause of thrombocytopenia in hospitalized patients. The "classic" immune thrombocytopenia can be seen with many agents including H_2 antagonists and certain antibiotics such as sulfonamides. However, virtually any drug can cause immune thrombocytopenia.

These patients present and are managed similar to immune thrombocytopenia in the outpatients population.

D *Heparin-Induced Thrombocytopenia*

Heparin-induced thrombocytopenia (HIT) is a special type of drug-induced thrombocytopenia. The onset of HIT is typically 5 or more days after heparin exposure. These patients have mild to moderate thrombocytopenia with typical platelet counts of $60–80 \times 10^9$/L. Bleeding is not a problem for these patients; rather, it is the thrombotic complications which cause major morbidity. The thrombi are clinical situation dependent and can include venous thromboembolic events, particularly in orthopedic patients, and arterial thromboembolic events, especially in patients who have had surgical procedures in the arterial circulation. The intensely prothrombotic nature of heparin-induced thrombocytopenia has led to a reappraisal in management. First, patients with HIT should never be started on warfarin during the acute thrombocytopenic episode. Warfarin can be slowly introduced after the HIT has resolved and the platelet count has returned to normal levels. Heparin should be stopped as soon as possible after the diagnosis is made. Platelet transfusions should be avoided unless the patient has life-threatening hemorrhage. Low-molecular-weight heparin should not be used. There are three treatment options, each of which carries advantages and disadvantages and none of which has been compared in a head-to-head therapeutic trial. Danaparoid, a heparinoid, has been used in patients with HIT but carries approximately 10% cross-reactivity. A defibrinogenating agent, ancrod, has also been used but has the disadvantage of not inhibiting thrombin generation and should not be used if the patient has DIC. Recent studies have described the successful use of thrombin-specific inhibitors such as argatroban and hirudin.

E *Thrombocytopenia in Pregnancy*

Thrombocytopenia occurs in about 5% of otherwise well pregnant women. The most common cause is incidental thrombocytopenia of pregnancy, which is defined as mild thrombocytopenia (platelets greater than 70,000 to 80,000/mL). These patients require no further investigation or treatment for their fetus or themselves.

The next most common cause of thrombocytopenia in pregnancy is thrombocytopenia associated with hypertensive disorders including pre-eclampsia. These patients have thrombocytopenia complicating the hypertension and are managed by the standard approach to patients with hypertension in pregnancy, which includes a prompt and early delivery and control of the hypertension.

IV. Thrombocytopenia in Hospitalized Patients

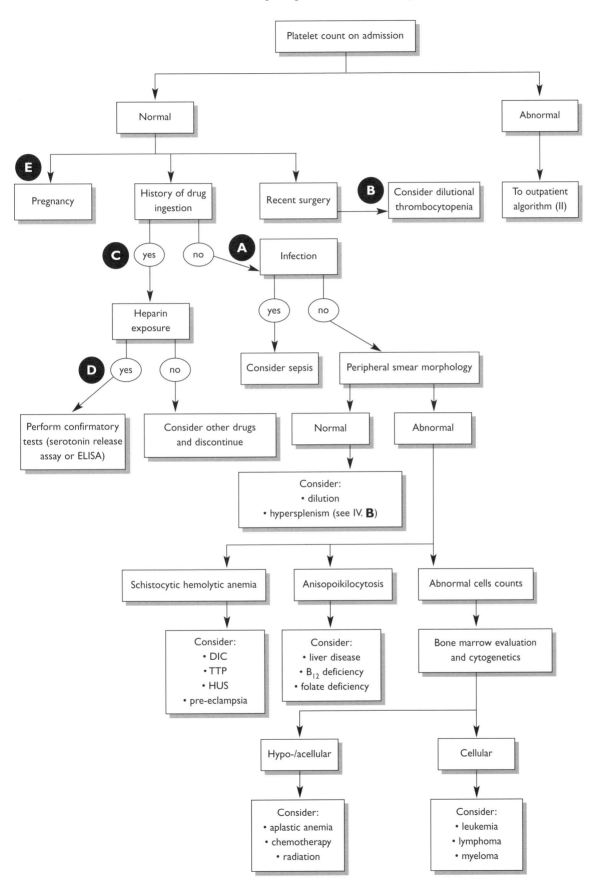

The third most common cause of thrombocytopenia in pregnancy is immune thrombocytopenia; in these patients, the thrombocytopenia is treated directly in the mother as in the management of ITP except that preference is given to the use of high-dose intravenous IgG over corticosteriods. Thrombocytopenia occurs in a small proportion of the infants of these women but very severe thrombocytopenia is distinctly uncommon and requires no special mode of delivery or fetal monitoring.

Additional Reading

Blanchette VS, et al. A prospective randomised trial of high-dose intravenous immunoglobulin G (IV-IgG), oral prednisone and no therapy in childhood acute immune thrombocytopenic purpura. J Pediatr 1993;123:989.

George JN, et al. Idiopathic thrombocytopenic purpura: a practice guideline developed by explicit methods for the American Society of Hematology. Blood 1996;88:3.

Kelton JG, Warkentin TE. Diagnosis of heparin-induced thrombocytopenia: still a journey, not yet a destination. Am J Clin Pathol 1995;104:611.

Mueller-Eckhardt C, et al. Recent trends in platelet antigen/antibody detection. Blut 1989;59:35.

Index